HEALING WHAT HURTS

Fast Ways to Get Safe Relief from Aches and Pains and Other Everyday Ailments

David Y. Wong, M.D., and Deborah Mitchell

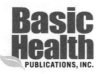

Basic Health
PUBLICATIONS, INC.

The information contained in this book is based upon the research and personal and professional experiences of the authors. It is not intended as a substitute for consulting with your physician or other healthcare provider. Any attempt to diagnose and treat an illness should be done under the direction of a healthcare professional.

The publisher does not advocate the use of any particular healthcare protocol but believes the information in this book should be available to the public. The publisher and authors are not responsible for any adverse effects or consequences resulting from the use of the suggestions, preparations, or procedures discussed in this book. Should the reader have any questions concerning the appropriateness of any procedures or preparation mentioned, the authors and the publisher strongly suggest consulting a professional healthcare advisor.

Basic Health Publications, Inc.
28812 Top of the World Drive
Laguna Beach, CA 92651
949-715-7327 • www.basichealthpub.com

Library of Congress Cataloging-in-Publication Data
Wong, David Y.
   Healing what hurts : fast ways to get safe relief from aches and pains
and other everyday ailments / David Y. Wong and Deborah Mitchell.
      p. cm.
   Includes bibliographical references and index.
   ISBN 978-1-59120-192-2 (alk. paper)
   1. Medicine, Popular. 2. Self-care, Health. 3. Alternative medicine.
4. Naturopathy. I. Mitchell, Deborah R. II. Title.

   RC81.W85   2006
   616--dc22
                                        2006036138

Editor: Tara Durkin
Typesetting and Book design: Gary A. Rosenberg
Cover Design: Mike Stromberg

Printed in the United States of America

10   9   8   7   6   5   4   3   2   1

Contents

Foreword, vii

PART I

The Foundations of Health

1. **The Four Pillars of Health, 3**

   Eating for Maximum Health, 4

   Living a Healthy Lifestyle, 7

   Stress and Stress Management, 14

   Attitude and Spiritual Health, 17

2. **How to Treat Yourself Using Natural and Conventional Medicine, 21**

   Taking Care of Yourself, 22

   Herbal Medicine, 22

   Homeopathy, 24

   Essential Oils and Aromatherapy, 25

   Nutritional Supplementation, 26

   Acupressure, 28

   Other Self-Help Therapies, 28

   Over-the-Counter Medications, 33

   Preparing a Self-Care Remedy Kit, 35

PART II
How to Heal Naturally, Head to Toes

---

3. From the Neck Up, 39

Bad Breath, 39

Bleeding Gums, 41

Canker Sores, 43

Cataracts, 45

Cold Sores, 47

Conjunctivitis, 49

Dandruff, 51

Dry Eyes, 52

Dry Mouth, 54

Ear Infections, 56

Glaucoma, 58

Hair Loss, 60

Laryngitis, 64

Lice (Head), 65

Macular Degeneration, 66

Nosebleed, 69

Tinnitus, 70

Yellow Teeth, 72

---

4. Aches and Pains, 76

Back Pain, 76

Headache, 79

Migraine, 81

Osteoarthritis, 84

Repetitive Strain Injury, 87

Restless Legs Syndrome, 89

Rheumatoid Arthritis, 90

Shingles, 94

Sore Nipples, 96

Temporomandibular
Disorder, 98

Tendinitis and Bursitis, 100

---

5. The Nether Regions, 103

Erectile Dysfunction, 103

Genital Herpes, 106

Hemorrhoids, 109

Jock Itch, 110

Menopause, 112

Premenstrual Syndrome, 114

Prostate Problems, 116

Stress Incontinence, 119

Urinary Tract Infections, 121

Vaginitis, 124

6. Tummy Troubles, 127

Belching, 127

Constipation, 129

Diarrhea, 132

Flatulence, 136

Food Poisoning, 139

Heartburn, 143

Hiccups, 145

Inflammatory Bowel Disease, 147

Irritable Bowel Syndrome, 149

Nausea, Vomiting, and Morning Sickness, 151

Ulcers, 153

7. Itchy, Bumpy, Flaky All Over, 157

Abscesses, 157

Athlete's Foot, 159

Boils, 161

Bunions, 163

Calluses and Corns, 165

Eczema, 168

Hives, 171

Insect Bites and Stings, 173

Poison Ivy, Oak, and Sumac, 176

Psoriasis, 178

Warts, 180

8. Feeling Down and Out, 183

Anemia, 183

Caffeine Withdrawal, 186

Chronic Fatigue Syndrome, 188

Common Cold, 192

Depression, 196

Hangover, 200

Insomnia, 202

Jet Lag, 205

Lactose Intolerance, 208

Nicotine Withdrawal, 211

9. Look, Smell, and Feel Good, 213

Acne, 213

Body Odor, 216

Burns, 219

Hangnail, 221

Ingrown Nail, 222

Liver Spots, 224

Nails (Chipped, Soft, Brittle), 225

Obesity, 227

Skin Tags, 232

Smelly Feet, 233

Varicose Veins, 235

10. Take a Deep Breath, 239

Asthma, 239   Hay Fever, 246

Bronchitis, 244   Sinusitis, 249

Snoring, 251

11. The Body Internal, 255

Cold Hands, 255   High Blood Pressure, 270

Diabetes (Type II), 257   High Cholesterol, 273

Fibrocystic Breasts, 260   Hypoglycemia, 276

Gallstones, 263   Hypothyroidism, 279

Hepatitis C, 266   Kidney Stones, 282

Osteoporosis, 284

Resources and Further Reading, 289

Index, 293

About the Authors, 309

Foreword

ne of my greatest joys in life is helping people realize and utilize their own potential for wellness. I have been fortunate to be able to live this joy every day for more than three decades. As a board-certified family practice physician and cofounder and director of the Health Integration Center in Torrance and Santa Monica, California, I use a variety of healing practices, including acupuncture, natural hormones, herbal and homeopathic remedies, nutrition, and stress management, to help men and women realize their greatest gift in life—health.

Each and every person has great abilities to become an active participant in his or her own health and well-being—to nurture and take control of one's own physical, emotional, and spiritual natures—yet many people fail to do so. Too often, people rush to doctors when they experience minor symptoms because they are fearful of what may be "wrong." Symptoms—be they fever, aches and pains, depression, or a rash—indicate that something may be off balance in people's bodies or lives. When symptoms come knocking, it's a good opportunity for individuals to listen to their bodies and learn how they can work on regaining balance and harmony in all three realms of their being.

One way to achieve that balance, or homeostasis, is to tap into the body's ability to heal itself. Everyone has that ability, and in this book, we present natural ways for you to help your body heal from many different ailments. Rather than run to the doctor every time you get a cold, we show you ways to banish your symptoms and strengthen your immune system. If you're fretting about back pain, we'll help you harness your discomfort. Instead of dosing yourself with antibiotics for an ear infection, we offer alternatives that are friendly to the body and that don't compromise your immune system.

Speaking of antibiotics, I am reminded of the age-old adage familiar to physicians: "The symptoms will abate in a week with antibiotics and in seven days without." Unfortunately, many doctors seem to forget this truism, and they prescribe antibiotics liberally to patients, even when they are completely inappropriate, such as in the case of the common cold or flu. Why are they inappropriate in these cases? Because antibiotics kill bacteria only, and cold and flu are caused by viruses. Yet many patients will insist their doctors give them antibiotics for these ailments.

In today's healthcare environment, it's becoming more and more feasible and practical for men and women to take charge of their own health whenever possible. Why?

♦ *Time.* Most people are very busy, and finding the time to go to the doctor can be a problem.

♦ *The healthcare system itself.* Often people must wait days and more commonly weeks to get an appointment with a doctor.

♦ *Cost.* Natural therapies are very often more inexpensive than over-the-counter or prescription medications.

♦ *Side effects.* When you take over-the-counter and prescription drugs, you run the risk of experiencing side effects. Natural remedies are associated with a much lower risk, and in many cases there are none.

♦ *Empowerment.* You can achieve a great sense of satisfaction from taking charge of your own health. It's your body, and no one knows it better than you do.

Naturally, there are times when you have symptoms that require professional care. For each ailment in this book, we help you determine which symptoms are urgent and when you should seek advice from a knowledgeable healthcare practitioner.

While the majority of this book—Chapters 3 through 11 (Part II)—discusses how to use natural methods to heal what hurts, it is prefaced by two important chapters. Chapter 1 lays a solid foundation for overall health. It explains how to stay physically, emotionally, and spiritually balanced through good nutrition, healthy lifestyle choices, stress management, and positive attitude. This holistic approach is the only one that can truly bring about health and well-being, because our physical, emotional, and spiritual components work together to make up who we are.

It is all well and good to practice natural medicine and help your body heal naturally. Yet if your body—your foundation—is weak or compromised, because of poor nutrition, bad sleeping habits, lack of exercise, or ill-chosen lifestyle choices, then your efforts to heal naturally, or even conventionally, will not be successful. It's like an individual with bronchitis who takes slippery elm to stop his hacking cough. The herb can be very effective, but if the individual continues with a poor lifestyle choice—like smoking—he isn't going to get the relief he's looking for.

In Chapter 2, we introduce you to the natural treatments that are mentioned throughout Part II. You'll learn about herbal and homeopathic remedies and essential oils and how to use them, what to look for when purchasing nutritional supplements, how to do acupressure and reflexology on yourself, and the basics of other self-help therapies. You'll also learn about the benefits and side effects of some common over-the-counter medications, and how to assemble your own self-care remedy kit with natural items.

Once you've finished Chapters 1 and 2 (Part I), you'll be ready to explore Part II, which covers the ailments that may concern you or your loved ones. Included are conditions that affect everywhere from the top of your head—like hair loss and dandruff—to the tips of your toes—like athlete's foot and smelly feet—and everything in between. And should you want more information about any of the ailments or treatments we've discussed, you can turn to Resources and Further Reading on page 289.

It is our hope that you will not only find relief when using the techniques discussed in this book, but that you will also better appreciate the wonder of your body, mind, and spirit as one in health.

PART I

The Foundations of Health

CHAPTER 1

The Four Pillars
of Health

What is health? For many years, in Western society the definition of health has been something like "the absence of illness or disease," and that seemed to satisfy most people. This way of thinking is the essence of mainstream, or allopathic, medicine, the approach that is the basis of health care in the United States today. Mainstream medicine focuses on the physical body: doctors evaluate a patient's symptoms, run medical tests to help identify the problem, and prescribe drugs, surgery, or other medical treatments to relieve the symptoms. This approach addresses only one aspect of people's essence—their physical being—and ignores and neglects the emotional and spiritual natures of the individual. Yet all three elements play a critical role in a person's overall health and well-being.

Any approach to health that considers the physical, emotional, and spiritual aspects of a person's essence is generally considered to be *holistic,* meaning that it deals with a person as a whole, not just as fragmented symptoms that need to be "fixed." It recognizes that the body has a natural tendency toward balance or "homeostasis." To attain and maintain homeostasis, we need to strengthen the pillars of health—diet, lifestyle, stress management, and attitude/spirituality. These pillars are the foundation upon which health and well-being rest. The bottom line is, health is a matter of balance.

In this chapter we look at the four pillars of health and explain guidelines in each area that can help you restore and keep your body in balance. When you have a strong foundation—when your physical, emotional, and spiritual natures are in harmony—you are better able to fight off potential health problems. These problems can range from invading viruses and bacteria to broken bones, stomach disorders, and muscle pain. Attention to your diet, lifestyle, stress levels, and spiritual health also makes you better equipped to bounce back from disease—when the body is out of harmony—if and when it strikes.

EATING FOR MAXIMUM HEALTH

Every day of our lives, each of us has a unique opportunity to nourish and nurture the body with nutritious, life-sustaining foods. Yet most Americans choose a less healthy path, consuming high-fat, low-fiber foods, lots of sugar, and highly processed foods, all of which contribute to a variety of illnesses, including heart disease, stroke, cancer, diabetes, gallstones, osteoporosis, high blood pressure, various intestinal problems, and obesity.

In particular, Americans consume too much fat, most of which is found in meats, dairy products, fried foods, and desserts. The American Cancer Society, the American Heart Association, and the Center for Science in the Public Interest noted in a joint report that if Americans consumed about 20 percent of their calories from fat, the healthcare costs in the United States would fall by $17 billion per year. Yet most Americans are regularly consuming nearly twice that amount of fat calories, and it shows in the increasing waistlines in both adults and children, and in the consistently high rates of food-related diseases.

A Balanced Diet

The recipe for a healthy, balanced eating plan is simple: 60 percent of calories from carbohydrates, 20 percent from fats, and 20 percent from protein, plus plenty of pure water. The food choices you make in each of these categories is important, because you want to select foods that are good sources of vitamins, minerals, fiber, and other essential elements. First, let's look at each of these categories, starting with carbohydrates.

Carbohydrates

Carbohydrates are our most abundant source of energy. When you ingest carbohydrates, your body converts them into glucose (which the body uses as immediate fuel) and glycogen (which the body stores and transforms into glucose when needed). Carbohydrates come in two forms—simple and complex—and are found in a wide variety of foods. Simple carbohydrates are basic sugars, which have no nutritional value by themselves. They include cane sugar (common white table sugar), beet sugar, and honey, and are also found in fruits and to a lesser degree in vegetables and milk. Simple sugars are found in many processed foods: simply look on the label for the telltale words "sucrose," "fructose," "glucose," "dextrose," as well as "sugar." Simple carbohydrates provide a quick source of energy because they are rapidly absorbed by the body. However, the energy surge is short-lived, and soon after consuming foods high in simple carbohydrates (for example, a candy bar or can of orange soda) your energy level can drop dramatically.

Complex carbohydrates are processed much more slowly by the body, which means they provide a steady source of longer-term energy. These carbohydrates are found in starchy foods such as brown rice, whole-grain breads and pasta, legumes, root vegetables, and potatoes. Unlike simple carbohydrate foods, those containing complex carbohydrates provide essential fiber, vitamins, minerals, and other important nutrients.

Protein

Protein, which consists of elements called amino acids, is necessary for the growth, maintenance, and repair of the body's cells. The average American needs about 0.38 grams of protein per pounds of body weight. Therefore, a 150-pound individual requires 57 grams of protein per day. Yet most Americans eat excessive amounts of protein, and the extra is either burned as energy or stored as fat. Protein foods include meat, poultry, fish, soybeans, cereal grains, legumes, nuts, eggs, and cheese.

Fats

Fats are a necessary part of our diet, yet the amount and type of fat you consume is important if you are concerned about your health. Saturated fat, found in meat, cheeses, and butter, contribute to high cholesterol, heart disease, stroke, and obesity. Trans fats, found in margarine and processed foods, are produced when unsaturated vegetable oils are converted into saturated fats. Unsaturated fats, which consist of monounsaturated and polyunsaturated fats, are considered to be the healthy fats. Monounsaturated fat is found in avocados, nuts, seeds, and olives. Polyunsaturated fat contains essential fatty acids, which are critical for health. They can be found in oily fish (for example, sardines, tuna, salmon) and most vegetable oils.

A Healthy Eating Plan

Countless studies of different dietary habits from around the world have shown that the best nutritional advice can be boiled down to three easy-to-implement and practical concepts. First, eat simple, unprocessed foods, preferably organic. Processed foods contain additives, such as artificial flavorings, preservatives, and colorings, as well as added salt, sugar, and other unhealthy ingredients.

Choosing organic foods, when available, reduces your exposure to pesticides, herbicides, fungicides, and other toxins. If you eat meat or dairy products, they also should be organically produced (that is, without hormones, steroids, pesticides, and antibiotics). Second, eat in moderation. Overeating causes obesity and contributes to various diseases. Third, enjoy your food. Eat slowly, in pleasant, stress-free surroundings, to aid the digestive process.

Now let's look in more detail at the types of foods you should choose to promote health and well-being.

◆ Choose the majority of your foods from plant sources. These include fruits, vegetables, rice, soy-based foods, whole grains, legumes, seeds and nuts, and foods that have been made from whole grains (for example, whole-grain cereals, pastas, and breads). Whenever possible, all of these sources should be organic. Plant foods are an excellent source of fiber, which helps pass food through the intestinal tract and may help prevent the accumulation of cancer-causing substances in the colon. Fiber also lowers cholesterol levels and helps maintain sugar levels in the bloodstream, which is especially important for people who have diabetes.

◆ Eat five to seven servings daily of fruits and vegetables. These are an excellent source of nutrients, especially antioxidants, which help fight free-radical damage. Free radicals are molecules that damage the cells and contribute to heart disease, cancer, and many other health problems, as well as aging. Fruits and vegetables are also a good source of fiber.

◆ Protein sources should include beans, split peas, lentils, soybeans and soy-based foods (including tempeh, soymilk, and tofu), wheat gluten, nuts and seeds, and fish (oily, cold-water fish). If you eat meat, choose organically raised poultry; avoid red meat.

◆ Limit dairy consumption. If you eat dairy foods, choose no- or low-fat varieties. Healthy alternatives to dairy are soy, rice, and nut milks; soy cheeses, soy yogurt, rice and soy milk frozen desserts, and soy margarine.

◆ Use extra-virgin olive oil or other monounsaturated oils for salads and vegetables.

◆ Steam, quick stir-fry, or broil your food; do not fry. Also, do not boil vegetables, as they lose much of their nutritional value.

◆ Limit consumption of sugar, salt, and caffeine.

◆ Limit alcohol consumption to no more than one drink daily.

As a final suggestion, if at all possible, grow some of your own vegetables and herbs. You don't need a lot of space; even apartment dwellers can have a few window boxes or large pots with pepper, cherry tomato, basil, and oregano plants. Growing some of your own food not only provides you with fresh produce and herbs, it can give you a sense of accomplishment and pride. Working with plants is a connection with Nature, a connection that many people find helps reduce stress and brings joy into their lives.

LIVING A HEALTHY LIFESTYLE

If you think of your diet as the fuel you put into your car, then your lifestyle is how you treat your car. Do you run it regularly? Do you put a lot of stress on the engine by not changing the fluids when recommended? Do you keep it in a garage out of the elements? How you answer these and other questions determines how long your car will stay in optimal condition.

Likewise, your lifestyle choices have a major impact on your health and well-being. A proper balance of rest and activity, stress and relaxation, and exposure and avoidance to certain lifestyle choices can determine the strength of this second pillar of health. Let's look at some of those choices.

Exercise

The overall health benefits of regular exercise are hard to ignore. Here are just a few of them:

- Improves the function of the lungs and heart

- Strengthens muscles, which improves stamina

- Enhances blood circulation, which helps prevent heart disease and several types of cancer, plus gives your skin a healthy glow

- Lowers high blood pressure

- Reduces cholesterol levels

- Reduces the risk of diabetes

- Reduces weight and helps prevent obesity

- Strengthens bones and helps prevent osteoporosis

- Improves flexibility and balance

- Helps alleviate menstrual cramps and other menstrual symptoms

◆ Reduces depression and improves mood

◆ Relieves tension and anxiety

◆ Improves self-esteem

◆ Helps maintain mental alertness by improving the flow of blood and oxygen to the brain

Naturally, these benefits aren't possible if the most exercise you get is walking from your house to the car. In order to be of benefit, exercise should meet several criteria.

Exercise should be *regular.* Jogging once a week is okay, but it shouldn't be the only exercise you get during a seven-day period. Plan to exercise at least three, and preferably five or six times per week for at least thirty minutes each time.

Exercise should be *varied.* Your body needs aerobic, strength-building, and flexibility exercises. Aerobic exercise (for example, walking, jogging, swimming, cycling, dancing) improves your heart and lungs, blood circulation, muscle endurance, flexibility, and strength. Aerobic exercise should be practiced regularly, but there are also strength-building exercises (for example, working with weights) and flexibility exercises (for example, yoga, stretching) to be considered. When you combine all three—perhaps aerobic exercise for twenty to thirty minutes three times a week along with stretching exercises; and then strength-building exercises two to three times a week, with some stretching— you give your body a complete workout.

Exercise should be *enjoyable.* Exercise should be a part of your life, so you should choose activities that are as pleasurable as possible. Varying your activities is one way to keep yourself motivated; exercising with a friend is another way. If you enjoy exercising with others, you might consider joining a community softball, tennis, or basketball team, or finding a running or cycling club. If you enjoy exercise equipment, you may want to join a gym or health club.

Exercise should be *sufficiently intense.* When doing aerobic exercises you should raise your heart rate for at least twelve minutes to a level that allows you to carry on a conversation without puffing or gasping for breath. When doing strength-building exercises, you want to work your muscles hard but not so hard that you injure yourself. Consulting with an exercise trainer can be helpful for many people.

Most important of all, talk to your healthcare practitioner before you start any type of exercise program, especially if you've been sedentary.

Sleep

America is a nation of sleep-deprived and overstressed individuals. If you have trouble sleeping, you probably worry about your lack of sleep, and being sleep-deprived likely affects your work, energy level, and other aspects of your life. If you are overstressed, you probably have trouble falling asleep or staying asleep. So regardless of which comes first—the stress or the lack of adequate sleep—your health and well-being are in jeopardy.

Sleep has the power to rejuvenate the body. Research shows that during dreamless sleep (also known as non-rapid-eye-movement sleep, or NREM), the body builds bone and muscle, repairs tissue, and may also enhance the immune system. That's because the immune system has a variety of cells that follow a daily rhythm. When you get too little sleep, the levels of certain cells get out of synch and can weaken the immune system. For example, the levels of catechol-amines (chemicals involved in nerve transmission) can rise, which causes the immune system to be suppressed and thus increases your risk of succumbing to infection. The levels of other cells responsible for fighting disease also are disrupted, again increasing your chances of becoming ill.

During dreaming, or REM sleep, experts are less clear about what occurs. Some say that dreaming helps people work through psychological troubles and thus acts as an emotional release mechanism, even if we don't remember the dreams. Another theory is that nerve cells in the brain are stimulated in order to remain healthy.

Regardless of what does or does not occur in the brain and the rest of the body during sleep, researchers believe that most people need an average of seven to eight hours of sleep per twenty-four-hour cycle for optimal health. There are exceptions, however. Some people may need up to ten hours while others seem to operate very well on six.

Alcohol

When we talk about drinking alcohol, moderation is the key word. Various studies have demonstrated that moderate consumption of beer, wine, or spirits may be beneficial to the heart because it raises the levels of good cholesterol (high-density lipoproteins). Moderate consumption is two drinks daily for men, one for women; a drink is defined as 5 ounces of wine, 12 ounces of beer, or 1.5 ounces of 80-proof liquor. However, alcohol also has some very real downsides:

◆ Drinking and driving, or operating other potentially dangerous equipment, is a major cause of automobile accidents, deaths, and other injuries.

♦ Drinking alcohol during pregnancy can have severe negative effects on the unborn child. Fetal alcohol syndrome is the primary known cause of mental retardation. When a pregnant woman drinks alcohol, the alcohol enters her bloodstream, which supplies her growing fetus through the placenta. Thus, when the mother drinks, so does her baby. Forty-four percent of women who drink heavily during pregnancy give birth to babies with fetal alcohol syndrome. The remaining 56 percent will have children with learning disabilities, attention and behavioral problems, or other abnormalities.

♦ Alcohol can cause sleep disturbances, resulting in lack of adequate sleep and various related problems. It may cause problems with concentrating and sleepiness during the day, especially while driving.

♦ Excessive consumption of alcohol can lead to addiction and the problems associated with it, including malnutrition, liver damage, gastrointestinal problems, high blood pressure, and social problems (including crime and violence).

♦ Drinking to excess results in a hangover and can cause you problems with your job, relationships, and family.

♦ Moderate to heavy alcohol consumption also appears to increase a woman's risk of breast cancer.

Women and men are not equal when it comes to how the body treats and reacts to alcohol. Women absorb and metabolize alcohol differently than men and there are several reasons for this difference. One is that, generally, women have less body water than men of similar weight, thus they achieve higher concentrations of blood alcohol. Women also seem to eliminate alcohol from their blood faster than men.

If you believe you have a problem with alcohol and you want help, contact Alcoholics Anonymous (most cities have local chapters; check your phone book) or the National Clearinghouse for Alcohol and Drug Information (800-729-6686).

Home, Safe Home?

According to the National Safety Council, every year in the United States, there is a fatal injury every eighteen minutes and a disabling injury every four seconds. Topping the list of deadly events is poisoning, followed by falls, burns and fires, and suffocation by ingesting an object. In 2002, a total of 13,900 people lost their lives to poisoning when they ingested drugs, medicines, foods (such as shellfish or mushrooms), or chemicals. Falls claimed the lives of 16,200 people, most of whom were older than sixty-five years. Smoke inhalation is the cause of most deaths associated with fires at home, while young children are the ones most likely to choke on objects, such as small pieces of toys or food.

You can make your home a safer place for you and your family and help eliminate injuries by following these tips.

◆ If you have throw rugs, only use those with no-skid backs. If there are individuals in your home who use a walker or cane, throw rugs should be eliminated because it is easy to trip over them.

◆ Use a bath mat or place no-slip stickers on the bottom of the bathtub.

◆ Install handrails for all stairs.

◆ Make sure all stairways are well lit and free of items that people can trip over, such as toys and clothes.

◆ Make sure all electrical wires are out of walkways. Use cord shorteners on cords that children can reach, and tape down cords when necessary.

◆ Check electrical wires regularly for damage and plugs to make sure they are secure.

◆ Install smoke detectors in your home: a minimum of one per level of the house, and adjacent to bedrooms.

◆ If there are young children at home, place childproof latches on all cabinets and drawers, the main circuit breaker box, and windows.

◆ Keep all plastic bags locked away from children.

◆ Keep a fire extinguisher in your kitchen.

◆ Lock up all sharp objects if there are young children in the home.

◆ Put safety locks on all toilets if you have toddlers at home.

◆ If there are young children at home, keep your blind cords out of reach.

◆ Ideally, do not keep guns in the house. If you do have guns in the house, they should be emptied of ammunition and locked away with a safety lock.

The Air You Breathe

According to the Environmental Protection Agency (EPA), the level of air pollutants indoors can be two to five times, and sometimes as high as a hundred times worse than that outdoors. How is that possible?

Consider the items in your home or office. Carpets, upholstery, tile, paint, varnishes, cleaning products, furniture, copy machine chemicals, plastics, and dozens of other items emit toxins into the air. These chemicals include benzene, hexanes, formaldehyde, toluene, and xylene, among many others, that can cause and contribute to various symptoms and ailments. There is strong evidence, in fact, that environmental toxins are involved in cancer and many of the autoimmune diseases (for example, lupus, rheumatoid arthritis, multiple sclerosis, Graves' disease, chronic fatigue and immunodeficiency syndrome, type II diabetes, and others). If you or your neighbors spray pesticides and herbicides around or near your home, you are exposed to those poisons as well.

To improve the quality of air in your home or office and reduce your exposure to environmental toxins, apply the following suggestions:

- ◆ Do not smoke, and do not allow others to smoke in your home. Cigarette smoke generates the production of free radicals, which damage your cells.

- ◆ Use natural cleaning supplies, such as vinegar, lemon, baking soda, and Borax. Most cleaning supplies contain ingredients that are not only harmful to you and the environment, but they also cost much more than natural, environmentally friendly items.

- ◆ Use natural products for personal cleaning and health needs as well, such as natural soaps, deodorants, toothpaste, and shampoo. Many conventional products contain aluminum, mercury, and other chemicals.

- ◆ Use only nontoxic paints, varnishes, and stains in your home.

- ◆ Do not use detergents or fabric softeners that contain formaldehyde.

- ◆ Vacuum your home often. Vacuums that have a dust sensor can detect when all the particles have been extracted from the carpet.

- ◆ Install HEPA (high-efficiency particulate arresting) filters in your home. These filters remove virtually all the pollutants in the air within an enclosed space. Portable units can be placed in individual rooms or brought to your office.

- ◆ Certain plants, such as English ivy, corn plants, bamboo palm, spider plants, and wandering Jew, help remove chemicals such as formaldehyde and benzene from the air. Place them in your home or office.

- ◆ If pest control is needed, use natural methods, such as heat or boric acid. Some exterminators specialize in natural approaches.

◆ Check for radon. The EPA reports that radon exposure is the second leading cause of lung cancer in the United States: about 15,000 lung cancer deaths are attributed to radon exposure annually. Radon is an extremely toxic, odorless and colorless gas that is found in well water and is emitted from the earth and rock. The gas can enter your house, and because buildings are enclosed, the gas is more highly concentrated than it is in the outdoors. You can check for possible radon toxicity in your home by purchasing a radon testing kit from a hardware store, or contacting your state radon office for names of radon contractors.

Smoking

One of the first things that come to mind when people talk about smoking is lung cancer. Eighty-five percent of lung cancer cases are associated with smoking. Yet smoking has also been linked with many other health problems, some of which we mention here:

◆ Smoking damages blood vessels and makes them constrict (become narrow), which restricts blood flow and can cause stroke.

◆ Ninety percent of people who undergo heart bypass surgery are smokers or ex-smokers.

◆ Nearly 95 percent of people who smoke one pack of cigarettes or more per day have emphysema, even though not all of them display the symptoms of the disease.

◆ People with diabetes who smoke are three times more likely to die of heart disease than people who don't have diabetes. Smokers with diabetes are also more likely to have kidney disease and to suffer nerve damage.

◆ Low-birth-weight and premature infants are twice as likely to be born to women who smoke. These children are at high risk of jaundice, low blood sugar, respiratory conditions, and other medical problems.

◆ Sudden infant death syndrome occurs twice as often among children who have parents who smoke.

◆ Smokers are more susceptible to colds and respiratory infections, and they tend to have them longer.

◆ Smoking has been linked to cervical cancer. Cancer-causing substances found in tobacco have been found in the cervix of women who smoke.

◆ Smoking increases the risk of getting mouth and throat cancer. Both of these cancers rarely affect nonsmokers.

Sun Exposure

Exposure to the sun's natural light can be both beneficial and detrimental. On the positive side, sun exposure helps the body manufacture vitamin D, which is why this vitamin is called the sunshine vitamin. On the downside, the sun's ultraviolet rays accelerate aging of the skin and promote skin cancer. Thus, the key to worshipping the sun is moderation and protection.

To get both, follow a few simple rules. Ten to fifteen minutes of daily unprotected sun exposure (before 10 A.M. or after 4 P.M.) to the face and hands is all your body needs to manufacture vitamin D. After that, you want to apply sunscreen with a sun protective factor (SPF) of at least 15, even if it's cloudy, because ultraviolet rays can penetrate the clouds. Other protectants against skin cancer include clothing that covers the arms and legs and a wide-brimmed hat. Because sun exposure can contribute to cataracts and other vision problems, sunglasses are also recommended.

STRESS AND STRESS MANAGEMENT

Stress is an important and natural part of life, and a certain amount is healthy and positive. It can keep us motivated, lift our spirits, and bring us joy. The stress associated with being in love, learning how to drive, or playing in a big tennis match are typically thought of as positive stress.

But in today's fast-paced society, we are surrounded by many stressors, from having to clean out the cat's litter box every day, to sitting in rush-hour traffic five days a week or having a fight with family members. There are also environmental stressors, such as air pollution, noise pollution, and odors; chemical stressors such as alcohol, caffeine, sugar, and nicotine; as well as internal stressors, including feelings of guilt, fear, and sorrow. All of these can accumulate and leave us feeling highly stressed, anxious, and depressed unless we learn how to manage our stress.

The human body was designed to react to stress with a simple response called "fight-or-flight." This is a chemical reaction in the body that sends the message to run. This reaction worked very well when our ancestors were fleeing from dangerous animals, but in today's world, most stress is emotional and spiritual, and so we internalize our stress. When we "stuff" our stress, we impact various parts of the body, including the immune, nervous, and endocrine systems, all of which work together and communicate via neurotransmitters—special chemical messengers.

How Stress Works

The body is equipped with a system of checks and balances to deal with stress. During a stressful situation, the sympathetic nervous system, which is part of the central nervous system, sends the hormones adrenaline and noradrenaline into the bloodstream. This raises heart rate, breathing rate, and blood pressure, and causes people to feel tense. In an effort to relieve that feeling, the parasympathetic nervous system secretes a hormone called acetylcholine, which can reduce heart rate and improve digestion.

However, if you continue to feel stressed, the parasympathetic nervous system can't do its job well, and your body tries to adapt to your higher level of stress. Although the body can usually adapt well to occasional stress, chronic stress, which many people experience today, drains the body and throws it out of balance. Nutritional deficiencies are common among people who do not adequately manage their stress, because stress can increase the need for certain nutrients, especially B vitamins and vitamin C. Other signs of imbalance caused by stress are depression, fatigue, physical pain (for example, headache, migraine, muscle spasms), loss of appetite, and a greater susceptibility to illness, such as the common cold and flu.

Stress also affects the endocrine system, which is composed, in part, of the pituitary, thyroid, and adrenal glands. Each of these glands secretes different hormones, and stress can affect the levels of each of them. When one hormone level is disrupted, it affects others, and the body can get out of balance.

When you're under stress, your adrenal glands secrete many hormones, including adrenaline, noradrenaline, and cortisol. Cortisol plays a critical role in the function of the immune system. If you experience severe or chronic stress, your body can produce too much cortisol (as well as other hormones), which can interfere with the function of immune system cells that are responsible for warding off infection. Adrenaline, which in low amounts helps the body during stressful situations, can suppress the immune system when levels rise due to chronic stress.

Managing Stress

What makes one person feel stressed and anxious when a phone rings every few minutes while another person takes it in her stride? The answer lies in our perception of and attitude toward the stressor and life in general, and how we choose to manage the stress in our lives. Stress itself does not make us sick; rather, it's our reaction to it that can cause the body to become unbalanced.

To avoid negative reactions to stress, we can learn to respond positively to it and to manage it. Meditation, deep breathing, yoga, tai chi, visualization, dance, massage, progressive relaxation, and biofeedback are a few effective ways to manage stress. Regular practice of one or more methods can restore balance to your physical, emotional, and spiritual essence. We explain two of these methods—meditation and deep breathing—below. We encourage you to explore any of the other options mentioned by reading, watching videos, attending workshops, or joining groups that participate in these activities.

Meditation

Research shows that regular meditation reduces blood pressure, lowers the levels of stress hormones, slows the heart rate, and increases alpha brain waves, all of which are associated with relaxation. There are many ways to meditate; for example, you can focus on your breathing, repeat a word or phrase, gaze at a candle flame or other object, chant, meditate while walking, or practice tai chi. Regardless of your approach, the concept of meditation is to focus the mind and enter a state of relaxed awareness and increased mental clarity. There are many books and other instructional materials on how to meditate, as well as community and private classes in meditation. Here is one simple example:

1. Choose a place where you will not be distracted for at least fifteen or twenty minutes. That means get away from the phone, kids, and other intrusions.

2. Sit in a comfortable position in a chair or on the floor or on a pillow. If you lie down, you may fall asleep. Allow your hands to rest on your lap or on your legs.

3. Close your eyes.

4. Breathe slowly and deeply (see the next section, "Deep Breathing") and allow yourself to relax.

5. As you continue to breathe slowly and deeply, focus on a word or phrase every time you exhale. "Om" is the word used by many Hindus during meditation, but you can choose anything that is calming for you.

6. If your mind begins to wander, simply refocus on your breathing and the word or phrase you've chosen. It is very common for the mind to wander, especially when meditation is new to you.

7. When you reach the time you've allotted to meditation, sit quietly for a few minutes before you get up.

Meditate for at least fifteen to twenty minutes, twice a day if possible. Many people find that meditating early in the morning before work and breakfast, and when they get home before dinner are good times.

Deep Breathing

Although everyone does it all the time and without thinking about it, the majority of people don't breathe very efficiently. Most people breathe from the chest, which supplies the body with much less oxygen than abdominal breathing and also requires more effort. When you practice deep breathing, especially deep abdominal breathing, you send more oxygen to your brain, reduce stress, and help stimulate the flow of lymphatic fluid, which promotes the elimination of waste products from the lymph nodes. Deep breathing is easy to do and can be done just about anywhere: sitting in traffic, at your desk, in the kitchen waiting for your toast to pop up, or in bed to help you drift off to sleep at night. Here's how easy it is to do:

1. After a normal inhalation of breath, exhale through your nose and mouth and get rid of all the air in your lungs.

2. Place one hand over your abdomen and the other on your chest. Take several deep breaths from your abdomen. Take each breath slowly, breathing in through your nose and allowing your abdomen to expand with each inhalation and fall with each exhalation. You'll know if you're breathing correctly if the hand on your abdomen moves out while the one on your chest doesn't. Practice several times.

3. Repeat ten to fifteen times, and you should feel more relaxed and alert.

4. Do deep-breathing exercises several times a day. Deep breathing can be used as an introduction to or during meditation.

ATTITUDE AND SPIRITUAL HEALTH

One of the most powerful tools you have to attain and maintain health is literally in your head—your brain. Specifically, your attitude toward yourself, your life, and the world, as well as having supportive and loving relationships, have a significant impact on your physical, emotional, and spiritual health and your body's ability to heal.

Attitude Is Everything

Your attitude toward yourself and everything around you is shaped by your experiences, education, and environment. A positive attitude can help you cope with the curves life throws you, be they relationship or work challenges, or health problems. If you are continually negative or pessimistic about life—or if you feel anxious much of the time—your physical, emotional, and spiritual health will suffer.

It's been shown that attitude and emotional state affect the immune system—the more stress you experience and the longer it lasts, the more you beat up your body (see "How Stress Works" on page 15). But if you can improve your attitude toward yourself and how you approach your life, you can enhance your health. Study after study indicates that an overall positive outlook is linked with a longer life in general. A study published in the *Journal of the American Heart Association* reported that attitude improves your chances of longer-term survival after a stroke. Several studies have shown that women with breast cancer who maintained a positive outlook survived longer than women who had a pessimistic and negative perspective on their situation.

To nurture a positive attitude, try the following:

- ◆ Live in the present; don't dwell on the past or worry about the future.

- ◆ Set reasonable goals for yourself. Assess your lifestyle, thoughts, and emotions (writing them down can help) and then make plans that are logical for you.

- ◆ Exercise daily: it raises your endorphin levels (natural painkillers), improves your self-esteem and self-confidence, and increases alpha waves in the brain, which is a sign of relaxation.

- ◆ Help others; giving of yourself lifts your spirits. Studies show that people who volunteer their time to help others feel better about themselves.

- ◆ Practice stress-reduction techniques. Choose one or more techniques and practice them daily.

- ◆ Spend time with Nature and take time to learn about how all living things are interconnected. Having a spiritual connection with Nature can provide inner peace and satisfaction.

- ◆ Laugh. It's been shown that laughter stimulates the immune system by lowering cortisol levels and increasing the number of certain cells that help the body fight infection.

◆ Tackle creative projects, such as painting landscapes, planting a garden, sewing, sculpting, or writing poetry. These can stir your imagination and boost your self-esteem.

Emotional and Spiritual Guidance

Having faith in God, Nature, your personal concept of a higher power, or having a spiritual foundation can promote healing and sustain physical and emotional health. People who embrace faith or spirituality have a sense of purpose in life and a feeling that they belong to the world. Those positive feelings translate into better health as well.

At Duke University Medical School, a study showed that people with rheumatoid arthritis could control and reduce their pain using spiritual coping strategies, such as feeling close to God and enjoying the beauty of Nature. Other studies show that people who attend church suffer less depression, have lower blood pressure, and half the risk of dying from coronary artery disease than people who rarely go to church. According to psychiatrist David Larson, president of the National Institute for Healthcare Research, "a solid majority of studies that examine the effects of religious commitment on life satisfaction have found the two positively linked."

Connecting and forming meaningful relationships with others is a critical part of balanced well-being. Each of us needs the emotional and spiritual support we get from our family, friends, neighbors, coworkers, and members of any groups to which we belong. If we isolate ourselves, especially in times of stress, we make ourselves more vulnerable to illness. People who have intimate friends are happier overall and less likely to die prematurely. Studies also show that married people are happier than people who are divorced or who never married.

CHAPTER 2

How to Treat Yourself Using Natural and Conventional Medicine

or thousands of years, the art of healing and medicine has had its roots in Nature. Herbal medicine has been around as long as humans have inhabited the Earth. Traditional Chinese medicine has been practiced for more than four thousand years and embraces herbal and nutritional remedies, as well as acupuncture. Massage has been practiced since the days of the ancient Romans and Greeks and is an integral part of Ayurveda, the traditional Indian system of medicine that also makes extensive use of herbs and nutrition. Ayurveda has been practiced since about 2500 B.C.

Naturopathy, which is based on the ancient belief that the body has the ability to heal itself, was developed in the late nineteenth century and brought to the United States from Europe in the 1890s. In some ways it is similar to traditional Chinese medicine and to Ayurveda. In naturopathy, treatments focus on diet, herbal remedies, hydrotherapy (use of water as therapy), yoga, and various physical therapies such as chiropractic, acupressure, massage, and reflexology.

Yet, especially in the United States, we look upon any medical or healing practice that is not allopathic (conventional) as the new kid on the block. In one sense, this is appropriate because we have grown up in a society in which allopathic medicine has been our primary healthcare option. But as scientific studies on natural healing approaches prove that herbal remedies and other healing methods have validity, conventional physicians are adopting some of the natural ways into their practices. And the public is demanding it. Results from a 2002 survey released by the National Center for Complementary and Alternative Medicine shows that 62 percent of Americans had used some form of alternative or natural treatment for a medical problem.

Both allopathic and alternative medicine have a place in our lives. Herbs or massage certainly can't set a fractured bone, so we must seek help from allopathic physicians, but both herbal remedies and massage do offer something that can complement the healing process. Likewise, when an individual has a heart attack, mainstream medicine steps in to monitor heartbeat and prescribe medication to correct heart rhythm problems. However, natural approaches, such as nutritional therapy, dietary changes, stress-reduction techniques (for example, yoga and breathing exercises), and herbal remedies can play a significant role in an individual's recovery process and in preventing recurrence.

TAKING CARE OF YOURSELF

Many of the common ailments that afflict people can be managed effectively, safely, and efficiently at home, using various natural therapeutic approaches. In most cases, you can get significant relief, and even eliminate, health problems as diverse as acne, bloating, diarrhea, headache, osteoporosis, sunburn, tendonitis, and warts without drugs or going to your doctor. Use of natural approaches can save you time and money, and best of all, allows you to take control of your health. (Conditions and treatment methods are discussed in Part II of this book.)

While self-care is highly desirable, it may not be the healthiest or safest way when complications or certain symptoms arise, or when your efforts at self-care aren't working. For example, you may use an herbal remedy to treat a boil, but despite your best efforts the boil doesn't go away and you develop a fever and night sweats. These symptoms are signals that you should seek a doctor's help. Advice on what to look for and when to consult a healthcare professional is a key part of each entry in Part II and is appropriately labeled "When to See a Doctor." You should always seek your doctor's help for serious symptoms or when your efforts at self-care aren't working.

But for the many times that self-care is possible, you need to have a good understanding of the basic techniques of the natural therapies you may use. If you've typically treated common ailments with over-the-counter drugs and you now want to try a natural approach, you should learn how to use herbal, homeopathic, or nutritional remedies, or understand how acupressure or massage works. The sections below explain the general principles of various natural therapies and offer guidelines on how you can use them if the need arises.

HERBAL MEDICINE

There's no doubt about it: herbal medicine is strong medicine. This is a fact our ancestors knew well. People around the world have been using herbal remedies for thousands of years to treat ailments from the common cold to heart disease. Today, more than 80 percent of the world's population uses herbs for health, although in the United States the figure is closer to 20 percent.

Because herbal remedies are derived from plants, many people have the misconception that they are 100 percent safe and free of side effects. However, even though herbal remedies are associated with far fewer problems than conventional medications, they can cause problems if they are taken incorrectly (i.e., overdose or allergic reaction). Therefore, it's always best to consult a knowledgeable professional about herbal remedies before you take them.

When using herbal medicine, keep the following precautions in mind:

◆ Avoid taking herbal remedies along with over-the-counter or prescription medications without first consulting your doctor. Some herbs and conventional medications can interact with negative results (see "Herb-Drug Interactions" on page 34).

◆ If you are pregnant or breast-feeding, consult with your doctor before taking herbal remedies.

◆ More is not better. Always follow the package directions or the instructions from your physician.

◆ Many herbal remedies can be given to children; however, check with your doctor for the proper dosing instructions.

Forms of Herbal Remedies

When you shop for herbal remedies, you'll find that they are available either processed or raw. Processed remedies include tablets, capsules, liquids (tinctures and extracts), powders, teas, and creams. Raw, unprocessed remedies include dried roots, flowers, leaves, and stems. Many herbs are available in more than one form, so in Part II we note the most popular and effective forms of each remedy. You should take herbal remedies as directed by your doctor or according to the package instructions.

Buying Herbal Remedies

When buying herbal remedies, you may come across some terms that are unfamiliar to you. Here are explanations of some of those terms.

Tinctures—This herbal form is prepared by soaking an herb in alcohol, water and alcohol, or glycerin. On the label, you should see a ratio, such as 1:3 or 4:1. The first number refers to the amount of herb in the formula; the second is the amount of alcohol, water, or glycerin. Thus, a 4:1 ratio means there are 4 parts herb to 1 part alcohol in the tincture. If you want to avoid alcohol, look for glycerin products.

Tablets and *capsules*—These two forms contain powdered herbs.

Standardized—Herbal remedies that are standardized have been guaranteed by the manufacturer to contain a specified potency, which means you are more likely to get results. However, because herbal remedies are not regulated by the Food and Drug Administration (FDA), you cannot be certain you are getting the potency stated on the label. Additionally, not all herbal remedies are available in standardized form.

Using Herbal Remedies

If you choose to prepare unprocessed herbs, there are two different kinds of "teas" you can make: infusions or decoctions. An infusion is made by pouring boiling water over the soft parts of an herb, typically the flowers or leaves. A decoction uses the hard parts of an herb, such as the bark, seeds, or roots, and involves simmering these parts in water.

Here are a few simple steps for making an infusion or decoction from an unprocessed herb. The directions given here are general; some herbs require a different amount of steeping or simmering time. Use a glass or ceramic pot.

◆ For an infusion, pour 16 ounces of boiling water over 1 ounce of dried herb, or 2 ounces of fresh herb, that you have placed in a glass or ceramic pot. Cover and allow the herbs to steep for five to ten minutes. Pour the infusion through a fine strainer to remove the herb parts.

◆ For a decoction, place 1 ounce of the herb in 16 ounces of simmering water and continue to simmer for at least fifteen minutes. Pour the decoction through a fine strainer to remove the herb parts.

HOMEOPATHY

The concept that "like cures like" is the basis of homeopathy, a system of medicine that was developed in Germany in the eighteenth century and soon thereafter spread to the United States. Basically, this concept says that a substance that causes symptoms of an illness or disease in a healthy person can also be used to treat the same symptoms in a person who is sick. This idea is similar to that used in mainstream medicine when it comes to vaccinations. To prevent people from becoming afflicted with, say, the measles, they are given a vaccine that contains a tiny amount of the measles virus. Similarly, in homeopathy, a remedy contains a minute amount of the substance that, in much higher amounts, would cause the symptoms or illness it is treating.

Buying and Using Homeopathic Remedies

Ideally, before taking a homeopathic remedy, you would go to a homeopath who would conduct an in-depth consultation to determine your overall condition. Such a consultation would take into account your diet, emotional state, social activities, exercise, stress levels, and other lifestyle factors. Then, the homeopath would choose a remedy that best suits your profile.

However, there are some basic homeopathic remedies that have proven to be effective for many common ailments. They can be purchased at health food stores and pharmacies, and from homeopaths and naturopaths. They are available as tablets, powder, granules, and liquid. A few are available as ointment or cream.

When shopping for a homeopathic remedy, the label will say something like "6c" or "12c." This refers to how much the remedy has been diluted. A remedy that is 1c contains 1 part of the substance and 99 parts of water, alcohol, or both. Taking 1 part of that solution and mixing with 99 parts diluting agent results in a 2c potency. According to homeopathic theory, the higher the dilution rate, the greater the potency. Thus a 30c remedy is more potent than a 12c.

Taking and Caring for Homeopathic Remedies

When taking and storing homeopathic remedies, there are some specific guidelines you need to follow.

◆ Homeopathic remedies should be taken at least fifteen minutes either before or after you have any food, beverages, or other substances in your mouth. Substances such as toothpaste, gum, tobacco, and mouthwash may counteract the effect of the remedy.

◆ Take the remedy on a clean, dry spoon or use a dropper if it is a liquid. Do not touch the remedy with your hands or fingers.

◆ Allow the remedy to dissolve in your mouth. Do not chew tablets or granules.

◆ Some healthcare practitioners advise patients to avoid use of caffeine products if they are taking homeopathic remedies, because they believe it reduces the effectiveness of the remedy.

◆ Store remedies in a dark, cool place.

ESSENTIAL OILS AND AROMATHERAPY

Essential oils—the oils that are extracted from the roots, stems, leaves, seeds, and flowers of plants—have been used for medicinal purposes since 4500 B.C.

They can help heal by affecting hormones and other chemical messengers throughout the body once they enter through the skin (either through massage or while bathing) or the lungs (via inhalation).

Buying Essential Oils

Essential oils are potent, yet fragile substances. Therefore, when purchasing essential oils, look for those that are sold in dark glass bottles. The label should say "pure" or "true" essential oil, and preferably indicate that the oil was derived from organic plants. Store the bottles in a cool, dark place.

Using Essential Oils

When using essential oils for respiratory ailments, you can use them one of two ways: The first option is to place a few drops of the oil on a tissue or piece of cloth and inhale the aroma from the tissue or cloth. Alternatively, add a few drops of essential oil to a bowl of hot water, place a towel over your head and the bowl, and inhale the vapors for five minutes.

When adding essential oils to bath water, always mix the oils with a carrier oil (for example, almond, sunflower, extra-virgin olive oil, jojoba oils) before adding them to the bath water. The carrier oil helps disperse the essential oils more evenly in the water. A typical mix for bathing is 7 tablespoons carrier oil plus 30 drops essential oil.

When using essential oils for massage, mix 8 to 12 drops of essential oil with 6 to 8 teaspoons of carrier oil.

NUTRITIONAL SUPPLEMENTATION

Nutritional supplements, be they vitamins, minerals, amino acids, enzymes, phytochemicals (chemicals derived from plants), or other substances, can be instrumental when it comes to healing. But when you walk into your neighborhood health food store, pharmacy, or grocery store and see the tremendous number of different types of supplements on the shelves, it's easy to feel overwhelmed. Equally confusing can be the meaning of the different terms used on the labels. What does "chelated" mean? What does "USP" stand for and is it important? What does "DV" stand for? Here we answer these and other questions about nutritional supplements so you can feel confident when it's time for you to make a purchase.

What does % Daily Value (DV) mean? Supplement containers have a boxed area entitled "Supplement Facts," and in this box is a list of the supplements and their corresponding % daily value. The % daily value reflects how much one serving (for example, one tablet or capsule) contributes to a 2,000 calorie diet. If you need more or less than 2,000 calories daily to maintain your weight, then you will also require more or less of the supplement.

What is a high-potency supplement? According to government regulations, a high-potency supplement contains at least 100 percent of the daily value (see above) for the nutrients in a given product. In supplements that contain many nutrients (for example, a multivitamin and mineral supplement), at least two-thirds of the nutrients must meet or exceed 100 percent of the DVs for the product to be identified as "high potency."

What are chelated minerals? "Chelated" means that the mineral is bound to a protein molecule. Theoretically, this allows the mineral to be absorbed better by the body, although some experts say this is not true.

What does "USP" mean? This acronym on a supplement label stands for United States Pharmacopeia, an independent nonprofit corporation that was established in 1820. Its members, which number more than 100 from various medical institutions, national associations, and federal government departments, determine the quality, purity, packaging, potency, and labeling standards for drugs and nutritional supplements. A product that has "USP" on its packaging has met the standards of this institution.

How safe are the fillers that are in some supplements? Supplements can contain a variety of fillers and other added ingredients, most of which do not cause problems for the vast majority of people. If you have a food allergy or food sensitivity, however, read the label carefully for allergenic substances such as yeast, milk, wheat, salt, soy, starch, sugar, or soy. Other ingredients such as talc or artificial colors should be avoided if possible. Tablets usually contain ingredients that are part of the production process and considered to be safe; these include cellulose and magnesium stearate.

If nutritional supplements aren't regulated by the Food and Drug Administration, how can I know they are safe and effective? In 1994, the United States government passed the Dietary Supplement Health and Education Act (DSHEA). This act provides some protection to consumers by requiring manufacturers to provide specific information, such as serving size, dosing information, ingredients, storage instructions, additives, and the manufacturer's name. The information also should be in a certain format (that is, a box titled "Supplement Facts" lists the amount of each ingredient and its % DV). But the DSHEA does not address questions of potency or purity of a product. That means consumers must trust the manufacturers of the products they buy. Therefore, purchase your supplements from well-established companies. If you have any questions about a supplement, contact the customer service division of the company (contact information should be on the packaging or can be accessed through the Internet). You can also get unbiased information about nutritional supplements from Consumer Lab, an independent testing organization that can be accessed at www.consumerlab.com.

ACUPRESSURE

The healing art of acupressure is a part of traditional Chinese medicine and has been practiced for thousands of years. It is often described as acupuncture without needles, because the points, or sites, where pressure is applied are the same as those used to insert the needles used in acupuncture. Both acupressure and acupuncture are based on the concept of *chi,* or life energy, which flows throughout the body along channels known as meridians. When pressure is applied to specific points along the different meridians, people can influence the flow of chi and thus restore or help maintain balance in the body.

Ailments such as muscle pain, fatigue, headache, depression, high blood pressure, nausea, and menstrual problems, among others, are indications that the body is out of balance. Acupressure can be used to relieve the pain and discomfort associated with these conditions and to help restore balance to the body, mind, and spirit.

Acupressure can be done at home to help treat minor ailments. The advantage to being treated at least once or twice by a professional acupressure therapist is that you will then know how to apply pressure; however, many people learn from books or video tapes and refer to meridian and acupoint charts to find the proper points to treat. (See Figure 2.1 on page 29 for acupressure points referred to in Part II of this book.)

Although professional acupressure therapists may use their fingers, palms, knuckles, feet, and knees to treat their clients, you will use your index or middle finger or knuckles for self-treatment. The points to be stimulated vary according to the ailment, but the technique remains the same: apply steady, firm pressure that is uncomfortable but not painful. Press each point for about three minutes. You can also massage the point by moving your finger in a circle without moving it from the point; that is, massage in place.

OTHER SELF-HELP THERAPIES

Here's a brief look at a few additional natural self-help therapies you may come across in this book. We encourage you to read more about these and other ways to improve your health and well-being.

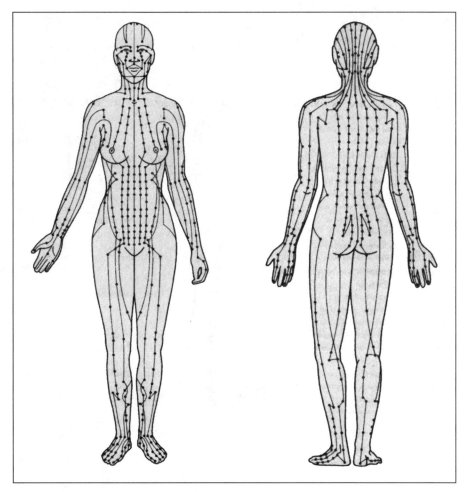

Figure 2.1. Acupressure Point Chart

Hydrotherapy

The use of water in its various forms (liquid, ice, steam) as therapy has been valued throughout history. The use of hot compresses, for example, can relieve pain and muscle tension. Ice packs are used to reduce swelling and pain. Saunas (hot, dry environment, with temperatures of 100°F or higher) promote sweating, which helps the body eliminate toxins. Sitz baths, in which two hip baths are placed side by side, one filled with hot water and the other with cold, are used to treat menstrual cramps, cystitis, hemorrhoids, and incontinence. To stimulate blood circulation, reduce swelling, relieve tension, and heal infected wounds, whirlpool baths can be used.

Reflexology

Drawings in the tombs of ancient Egyptians show that the practice of foot manipulation has a long history. Reflexology is based on the belief that the feet and hands have specific sites that correlate to certain areas of the body. When pressure is applied to these sites, the individual experiences relief from particular symptoms. Certain points on the bottom of the big toe, for example, correspond to the pituitary gland, nose, sinuses, and throat. (See Figure 2.2 below and right.) To do reflexology on yourself, apply pressure with your thumb to each point, pressing until it "hurts good" and then releasing. Repeat several times for each point.

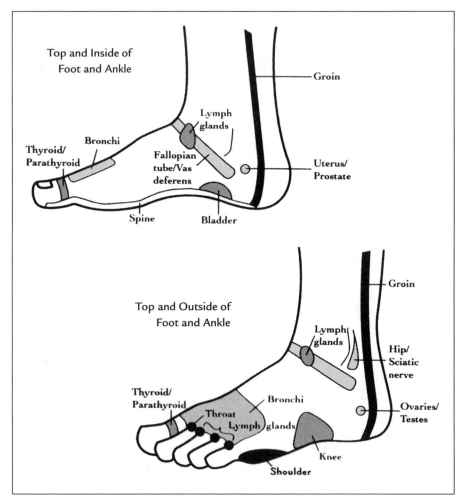

Figure 2.2. Reflexology Chart

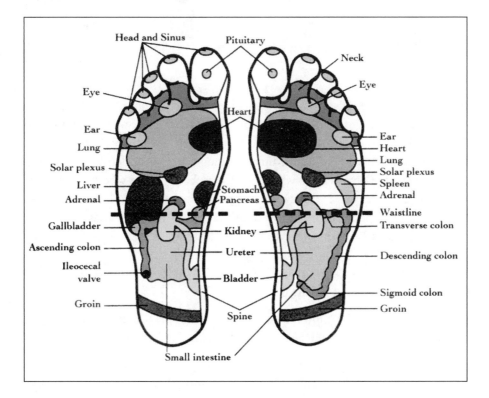

Tai Chi

Tai chi is an ancient Chinese movement therapy that relaxes the muscles and nervous system, improves posture, balance, breathing, and joint flexibility, and reduces stress. According to traditional Chinese medicine, tai chi promotes the flow of *qi* (chi), or life energy, and thus helps the body regain and maintain homeostasis. Tai chi can be learned from classes, videos, or books.

Visualization

In this technique, you use your imagination to help you cope with tension, stress, pain, and other symptoms. Visualization requires no special tools, just a comfortable, quiet place to go on your internal journey. Once you are relaxed, you will close your eyes, breathe slowly, and focus on a mental image that will help you achieve your goal. If you want to relieve stress, you can envision a beautiful, calm scene, such as a mountain retreat or a deserted beach. If you are trying to relieve pain or heal an ailment, you may imagine that you are packing up your illness in a suitcase and sending it away, or shooting it up into space on a rocket. Visualization can be learned from audiotapes, books, or with the help of a practitioner.

Yoga

Yoga is another ancient system that has many overall mental, physical, and spiritual benefits. It originated in India about 4,000 years ago, and was brought to the United States in the nineteenth century. There are many types of yoga, including some that integrate meditation along with controlled breathing and specific postures. Research shows that yoga can help people who have asthma, back pain, rheumatoid arthritis, depression, and heart disease. It also improves posture, flexibility, and energy level. Yoga can be learned from classes, videos, and books. For maximum benefit, you should practice yoga daily for at least thirty minutes.

Progressive Muscle Relaxation

Progressive muscle relaxation is a very simple technique to release tension from your body, which in turn relieves pain and fatigue. Here are the steps:

1. Lie on your back on a comfortable surface with a small pillow under your head if desired. Your arms should be comfortably at your sides, and your feet should be bare.

2. Close your eyes and be aware of the weight of your body. Focus on your breathing as your abdomen rises and falls with each breath.

3. Tense the muscles in your left foot. Hold for a few seconds, then release. Then tense the muscles in your calf, hold, then release. Do the same with your thigh muscles. Repeat the sequence with your right foot, calf, and thigh.

4. Tense, hold, then release each buttock.

5. Tense, hold, then release your stomach muscles.

6. Clench your left fist, hold, then release. Repeat for the muscles in your left arm. Then repeat the entire sequence with your right fist and arm.

7. Scrunch up your shoulders toward your ears. Hold for several seconds, then release. Repeat this three times.

8. Gently roll your head to the left, hold, then roll it to the right, hold, then return to your original position.

9. Open your mouth as wide as you can, hold, then close it. Raise your eyebrows, hold, and release. Yawn as wide as you can, then relax.

10. Take several slow, deep breaths, letting the air out slowly each time. Focus on your breathing.

11. When you are ready, gently wiggle your toes and fingers, roll onto your side, and get up slowly.

OVER-THE-COUNTER MEDICATIONS

Americans use a lot of over-the-counter (OTC) medications. According to the American Pharmaceutical Association, people in the United States spend more than $30 billion per year on OTC drugs. Overall, OTC medications are convenient, usually less expensive than prescription drugs, and can be used without having to see your doctor. To help ensure these drugs are safe, the Food and Drug Administration requires that OTCs meet specific standards.

Despite their advantages, OTC drugs can cause serious harm if not taken correctly. Therefore, if you choose to take an OTC medication, take it as directed on the package or by your doctor. Always check with your doctor or pharmacist before combining any prescription drugs or herbal remedies with OTCs, as many drugs and herbs have interactions.

Even when taken as directed, OTC medications can cause side effects. Below is a list of common OTC drugs, what they are designed to do, and the side effects associated with them.

◆ *Acetaminophen* (for relief of mild to moderate pain and reduction of fever). Side effects are rare and can include fatigue, rash, itching, hives, sore throat, fever, bruising, painful urination, jaundice, and blood in urine.

◆ *Antacids* (for relief of heartburn and gassy stomach). Side effects are infrequent and can include mild constipation, unpleasant taste in the mouth, stomach cramps, increased thirst.

◆ *Antibacterials and antifungals, topical* (for skin infections). Side effects are infrequent and can include rash, itchy skin, and redness.

◆ *Antihistamines* (reduces symptoms of hay fever, hives, common cold, motion sickness, and nausea). Side effects can include drowsiness, dizziness, dry mouth, dry throat, vision changes, rash, and loss of appetite.

◆ *Laxatives* (for short-term relief of constipation). Side effects are infrequent and can include stomach cramps, belching, nausea, diarrhea, increased thirst, and throat irritation (if taking a liquid form of the drug).

♦ *Nonsteroidal anti-inflammatory drugs, or NSAIDs* (for relief of various types of pain such as joint, menstrual, headache, or muscle pain, as well as fever and inflammation). Side effects can include dizziness, nausea, stomach cramps, diarrhea, and rash. Infrequent side effects may include drowsiness, ringing in the ears, depression, constipation, diarrhea, vomiting, dry mouth, tremors, and insomnia.

Herb-Drug Interactions

Herbal remedies have been with us much longer than have conventional drugs, but experts know less about herb-drug interactions than they do about drug-drug interactions. Fortunately, research into herb-drug relationships is ongoing, and new information is being accumulated all the time. This is important, because about 20 percent of Americans use some type of herbal remedy at one time or another, and most take some kind of conventional medication—whether it be over-the-counter or prescription—at least occasionally.

Before you take any herbal remedy while also taking a conventional medication, you should consult with your physician or pharmacist about any possible herb-drug interactions. Some consumer drug books also list known herb-drug interactions, but you should still check with a knowledgeable healthcare practitioner for the latest information.

Here are a few general guidelines to consider if you plan to take herbal remedies and conventional medications together:

♦ *Antihypertensive drugs* (taken to lower blood pressure). Avoid herbs that are known to raise blood pressure, such as licorice, hawthorn, saw palmetto, ma huang, goldenseal, and ginseng.

♦ *Acetaminophen* (for pain relief). Avoid the herbs comfrey and chaparral, which may increase the risk of liver damage.

♦ *Antipsychotic drugs* (to treat schizophrenia and other types of psychosis). Avoid use of herbs that are often used to treat depression or low mood, such as kava, St. John's wort, valerian, passionflower, and hops. Risks include sedation, increased severity of psychotic symptoms, or development of a movement disorder called tardive dyskinesia (associated with use of kava).

♦ *Corticosteroids* (anti-inflammatory, immunosuppressive). Use of licorice with corticosteroids can increase the risk of serious drug side effects.

◆ *Nonsteroidal anti-inflammatory drugs* (for relief of pain, inflammation, and fever). Do not use feverfew, garlic, or ginkgo because of an increased risk of stomach bleeding.

◆ *Protease inhibitors* (to manage HIV [human immunodeficiency virus] infection). Do not use St. John's wort, as it can significantly reduce the effectiveness of these drugs.

PREPARING A SELF-CARE REMEDY KIT

Every home should have a basic first aid kit, stocked with items such as cotton, bandages, and scissors for minor injuries such as cuts, scrapes, and splinters (see "First Aid Kit" below). However, if you want to be prepared for many more ailments, you should prepare a self-care remedy cabinet or box equipped with some basic nutritional, herbal, homeopathic, essential oil, and everyday remedies and supplies.

Get a sturdy, lightweight container that has a secure lid. Plastic toolboxes and fishing tackle boxes fit the bill. You may want to combine your regular first aid

---

FIRST AID KIT

Every home should have a basic first aid kit consisting of the following:

◆ Adhesive tape
◆ Adhesive bandages (several sizes)
◆ Sterile gauze pads
◆ Sterile gauze rolls
◆ Sterile cotton balls
◆ Sterile eye patch
◆ Triangular bandage (for making a sling) and safety pins
◆ Tweezers
◆ Scissors
◆ Antibiotic cream
◆ Ibuprofen and acetaminophen
◆ Syrup of ipecac (for poisonings; use only with the advice of a poison control specialist or a doctor)

kit with your self-care remedies so they will all be in one place. Once your self-care kit is stocked, store it in a cool, dry place that is out of reach of small children and pets.

Here are some suggestions for your self-care remedy kit. You'll see these items mentioned throughout Part II of this book as remedies for specific ailments. You may want to add other items, depending on your personal and family needs.

◆ Vitamin C tablets (500 milligrams): to be taken at the first sign of a viral or bacterial infection, for inflammatory conditions, and many other uses

◆ Aloe vera gel: for burns or many types of irritated skin conditions

◆ Arnica cream: for bruises and sprains

◆ Chamomile (tea or dried leaves): for nausea, diarrhea, indigestion, and sleep difficulties

◆ Echinacea tincture: for allergic reactions and to help resist infections

◆ Lavender essential oil: for burns, insect bites, cold sores, sleep difficulties

◆ Tea tree essential oil: for bacterial and fungal skin infections

◆ Ginger (capsules or dried): for nausea and gas

◆ Nux vomica: homeopathic remedy for nausea; 12c potency

◆ Extra-virgin olive oil: for diluting essential oils

◆ Garlic (capsules): for bacterial and viral infections, and fungal skin infections

Also, in your kitchen, keep the following:

◆ Frozen peas: to be used as an ice pack, because the package easily molds around body parts

◆ Honey: for coughs and colds

◆ Lemons: for indigestion, sore throat

◆ Salt: for mouth and throat rinse

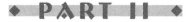

PART II

How to Heal Naturally, Head to Toes

CHAPTER 3

From the Neck Up

Have you ever asked someone, "How do you feel?" and you got the reply, "Okay from the neck down"? We've all had days when we would have gladly traded in our head for another model, when something was amiss with our ears, eyes, mouth, hair, throat, or nose. In this chapter we look at annoying ailments that can affect those areas. If you're looking for painful conditions that affect the area from the neck up, turn to Chapter 4.

BAD BREATH

Morning breath. Dragon breath. The "fog." Is your breath "foul?" If you believe the commercials and magazine advertisements, you might think everyone has bad breath. Apparently enough people do believe the ads: Americans spend $1 billion a year on items such as pleasant-smelling mouthwashes and other breath-freshening products.

True, most people wake up with a stale taste in their mouth, and with breath that doesn't smell sweet. But that staleness goes away quickly enough once you brush your teeth, have a cup of tea, or start harping on your kids to get ready for school. That's because morning breath is simply the result of bacteria that have gathered overnight while you slept. Once those bacteria are swept away—even through talking—the odor usually disappears.

But some people have persistent bad breath, or halitosis. If your breath could make an elephant faint, even after you've brushed your teeth and sucked on peppermint drops, it's probably time to look into the possible causes. Those could be:

◆ *Gum disease.* Food particles can become trapped in your gums and collect bacteria, which cause odor. Your dentist or a periodontist can examine your gums and treat them if necessary.

◆ *Sinus infection (sinusitis).* If you have sinus problems, notice if your bad breath occurs at the same time as your sinusitis episodes. This could indicate that a sinus infection is the culprit.

◆ *Tonsillitis.* A tonsil infection, or food particles getting caught in the tonsils, can cause bad breath.

◆ *Diabetes, kidney infection, and liver disease.* These are less common causes of halitosis.

◆ *Medication use.* Some drugs, such as tricyclic antidepressants, antihistamines, pain relievers, and decongestants, can interfere with saliva production and thus make your mouth dry.

◆ *Natural aging process.* Production of saliva, which helps ward off bacteria, declines as we age.

Remedies

You've already tried the obvious solutions—toothpaste, mouthwash, and breath mints—and they haven't worked. That's probably because they only mask the problem instead of attacking the cause. So what's next? Bring in the reinforcements!

Best Bets

◆ Take chlorophyll. It's the pigment that makes plants green, and it can make your breath springtime fresh, too. Chlorophyll is very effective at eliminating odors caused by garlic and infections. Contrary to popular belief, garlic odor comes from the lungs, not the mouth, so brushing your teeth will not get rid of it. You can either take chlorophyll capsules or tablets (three before every meal) or chew parsley. Parsley is one of Nature's richest sources of chlorophyll. Chew a few sprigs after eating or whenever you have halitosis.

◆ Use a tongue scraper. Don't laugh—the majority of people in the world scrape their tongues to eliminate bad breath. According to Ayurveda, the ancient natural healing system that originated in India, a silver or copper tongue scraper is best. A silver scraper is said to emit ions that kill bacteria that hide in tiny pockets in the tongue. A copper scraper is also effective and tones the taste buds. Both the top and sides of the tongue should be scraped after every meal. If you prefer, you can use a spoon or a toothbrush instead of a tongue scraper; just don't use these items for anything else.

♦ Take activated charcoal. No, not the charcoal briquettes you use in your barbecue, but the kind that comes in capsules. Take one capsule daily until your bad breath disappears. If you don't have any success after ten days, try another method or see your dentist.

Other Options

♦ Supplement with digestive enzymes. If your bad breath is caused by poor digestion, you may get relief by taking special enzymes that aid digestion. Look for a supplement that contains the following ingredients: amylase, cellulase, lipase, and protease. These substances are able to dissolve carbohydrates (amylase and cellulase), fat (lipase), and protein (protease). Dissolve the contents of one capsule in 4 ounces of water and drink before each meal. Continue taking the enzymes until your bad breath disappears.

♦ Wet your whistle. If your bad breath is caused by dry mouth, you need to stimulate the flow of saliva or keep your mouth moist. Chewing sugar-free gum can get the saliva flowing. You can also keep a bottle of water handy and take frequent sips (a good way to get your daily requirement of water as well) or suck on (don't chew!) ice chips. If you are taking medication that causes dry mouth, ask your doctor if you can take an alternative drug. Also, if you drink alcohol or use an alcohol-containing mouthwash, you may eliminate dry mouth if you stop using these items. Both are known to cause dry mouth and can worsen bad breath.

When to See a Doctor

If you've tried home remedies and nothing works, see a medical doctor or your dentist. If you have any of the diseases mentioned above, or if you have any dental problems, they may be causing your chronic bad breath. If a bacterial infection is the cause of your bad breath, your doctor can prescribe antibiotics, which may kill the infection, and with it, your halitosis.

BLEEDING GUMS

You take good care of your teeth: you brush after every meal and floss every day. Well, maybe you skip the floss once in a while. And brushing after every meal . . . well, it just isn't practical. So now your gums are red and puffy and they bleed when you brush. Are you in trouble? Do you have to go to the— don't make me say it—dentist?

Bleeding gums is a very common problem, especially among people age thirty-five years and older. In a way, it's a good sign, because your gums are letting you know that you are either in the beginning stages of gingivitis (gum disease), or eating a poor diet. In either case, there are several things you can do to bring your gums back to a healthy pink. But first things first.

Causes of Bleeding Gums

Gingivitis, or inflamed gums, develops when bacteria and food residue, known as plaque, accumulates on your teeth. If you fail to remove it regularly by brushing and flossing, plaque turns into tartar, which irritates your gums, making them swollen and red. Then when you brush or floss, your gums bleed.

But what if you really do brush and floss faithfully and your gums still bleed? Some dentists and physicians believe that the problem could be what you're putting in your mouth—besides your toothbrush, floss, and toothpaste. A diet that is high in sugar, fat, and processed foods and low in fiber creates digestive problems, which in turn produce toxic gases that can harm the gums. A poor diet also creates a welcome environment for gum-destroying bacteria in the mouth.

Remedies

Are your gums mildly tender and bleeding? Do you notice that your gums only bleed occasionally? The remedies listed here are recommended for mild bleeding or to help prevent gums from bleeding at all. If your gums are painful and bleed often, see "When to See a Doctor" below.

Best Bets

◆ Coenzyme Q_{10} has been used for gum problems throughout the world, although few studies have been done in the United States. The recommended dosage is 50 to 100 milligrams (mg) daily. This enzyme increases circulation, which brings more oxygen to the gums.

◆ Use an oral irrigator to clean deep inside the tiny spaces where bacteria hide in the gums.

◆ An herbal combination of echinacea, thyme, and cinnamon bark tinctures (2.5 ounces each) mixed with four to six drops each of lavender oil, peppermint oil, eucalyptus oil, and vegetable glycerin can reduce inflammation and swelling of the gums. Apply the solution using a perio-aid, a wooden toothpick that has a plastic handle. Hold the perio-aid at the crevice that surrounds each tooth and use it as if you were cleaning your cuticles. Work gently just below the gum line, being careful not to tear the gums. Use the perio-aid every night before going to bed.

Other Options

◆ Take a vitamin C supplement with bioflavonoids. Vitamin C helps produce collagen, which is the foundation of gum tissue, and bioflavonoids help with clotting and promote healthy tissue. Take 500 mg twice daily.

◆ Reduce your protein intake. Too much dietary protein creates saliva that is friendly to gum-destroying bacteria. Adults need an average of 0.38 grams of protein per pound of body weight. Therefore, a 150-pound individual needs 57 grams of protein daily.

When to See a Doctor

If you have chronic swollen, red, irritated gums that bleed, see your dentist. Left untreated, this condition can lead to periodontitis, in which the gums shrink and teeth can become loose and fall out. Research conducted at the University of Michigan School of Dentistry also suggests that older men whose gums bleed regularly are at high risk of coronary artery disease and stroke, although the reason for this association is not clear.

CANKER SORES

Your mouth speaks volumes . . . and not just with words. The next time you get tiny white painful eruptions on the inside of your lips or cheeks or on the loose part of your gums, you not only have canker sores, but your body is trying to tell you something is wrong. That's because the mouth is one of the first parts of the body that react strongly to excess emotional, physical, or mental stress in your life. Your mouth is telling you to "deal with it."

Emotional or mental stress is believed to be one of the main culprits of canker sores. Working too much overtime? Cramming for exams? Going through a divorce? These are times when canker sores have a tendency to appear in some people. Physical stress, such as a vitamin deficiency, digestive problems, or infection, are also thought to cause these annoying sores.

Don't confuse canker sores with cold sores, which are caused by the herpes virus and which appear on the outside of the lips and on the hard part of the gums. (See COLD SORES on page 47.)

Remedies

If you're hoping medical science has come up with some surefire ways to cure canker sores, we're sorry to disappoint you. Although doctors prescribe antibiotics, steroids, anti-inflammatory gels, silver nitrate, and other remedies, none of them seems to be the answer. In fact, many natural and homespun treatments appear to work just as well, if not better. If you think stress is causing your canker sores, then your number-one remedy is to relax! Okay, you say, but what else can I do to help speed up the healing process? And what can I do to prevent canker sores? Here are a few suggestions.

Best Bets

♦ Whenever you feel a canker sore coming on, place a tablet of activated charcoal on the spot and keep it there for fifteen to twenty minutes, or until the discomfort stops. If you need to repeat the process, do not use more than one tablet per hour. The only two minor—and temporary—side effects of activated charcoal are that the treated area turns black and your stools may turn black as well.

♦ Recurring canker sores may be caused by a deficiency of folic acid and vitamin B_{12}. Take 400 micrograms (mcg) of folic acid and 200 mcg of vitamin B_{12} daily.

♦ Dab some myrrh on the affected areas. Myrrh is an herb that is rich in tannin, a substance that dries the skin and repairs injuries. Take a dropperful of a tincture of myrrh and place it on a small piece of cotton gauze. Place the soaked gauze on the sore and leave it there for ten to fifteen minutes, if possible. Shorter treatments are also effective, but longer is preferred. Repeat four times daily. You can also apply witch hazel in the same way. Make sure you get herbal witch hazel (look for *Hamamelis virginiana* on the label) and not the alcohol-based product.

Other Options

♦ The amino acid lysine may help. Stress and fatigue can cause the body to lose much of its supply of lysine, and a deficiency of this amino acid causes canker sores. Consult your doctor before taking a lysine supplement. A typical dosage is 500 mg once or twice daily with food.

◆ Probiotics (good bacteria) are excellent natural antibiotics. Get a probiotic liquid or powder (mix with water according to package directions) and swish a tablespoon or two around in your mouth for about sixty seconds, then spit. Do this several times a day.

When to See a Doctor

Canker sores aren't serious, but they can be annoying and frustrating. If canker sores are chronic (which means they keep coming back), then you may have a food or medication sensitivity, which is a source of chronic stress to your body. Ask your doctor or dentist to conduct an allergy test that detects IgA antibodies in the immune system.

CATARACTS

Cataracts are an age-related clouding of the eye's lens that are most common in people older than sixty-five. Cataracts are responsible for blindness in about 20 million people around the world. It is believed that everyone who lives long enough will experience some degree of cloudy vision.

The lens is composed mainly of water and protein, and when the protein clumps together, it forms "clouds," or cataracts. These cataracts inhibit the lens' ability to focus light onto the retina in the back of the eye.

Symptoms of Cataracts

The first thing you may notice if you have cataracts is that you can't read as well as you used to because there is a haze or cloud across your vision. You may see haloes around the moon or around lights at night, especially when driving. During a bright day, you may find it difficult to see clearly because your pupils constrict, which limits the amount of light that enters your eyes.

Causes of Cataracts

Although cataracts are related to aging, other factors can increase your risk for their development. If you smoke, don't protect your eyes from the sun, have been taking corticosteroids for a long time, or have certain vitamin deficiencies (for example, deficiencies in vitamins C and E, beta-carotene, and zinc; see "Remedies" below), you should think about correcting these harmful habits.

One thing you can't do anything about is genetics. A British study conducted at St. Thomas' Hospital in London reports that genes are responsible for about 50 percent of the variation in severity of cataracts in women.

Remedies

Although many people believe that surgery is the only solution for cataracts, some healthcare practitioners don't agree. John D. Huff, M.D., an ophthalmologist and codirector of the Prather-Huff Wellness Center in Sugarland, Texas, believes that 90 percent of patients who have their cataracts diagnosed in the early stages can reverse the problem using natural treatments. Here are some suggestions from natural healthcare practitioners.

Best Bets

◆ Take antioxidant supplements. Because most cataracts are the result of oxidation—damage done to cells by molecules called free radicals—antioxidants can stop or reverse cataract formation. Take the following antioxidants daily: 1,500 mg vitamin C, 500 mg bioflavonoids, 12 mg beta-carotene, 400 IU (international units) vitamin E, 200 mcg selenium, 30 mg zinc, 2 mg copper, and 6 mg lutein.

◆ Take sulfur in the form of MSM (methylsulfonylmethane). It is one of the most important nutrients for vision. Use MSM powder dissolved in water: $\frac{1}{2}$ teaspoon per 100 pounds body weight per day. MSM is virtually tasteless.

Other Options

◆ Follow a vision-friendly lifestyle: if you smoke, stop; wear sunglasses that block out both ultraviolet A and B rays outdoors, and reduce or eliminate your consumption of fried foods and saturated fats.

◆ Include the antioxidant glutathione in your regimen. Many people with cataracts have low levels of this nutrient in their systems. Take 50 mg daily along with 500 mg n-acetylcysteine (NAC) and 100 mg alpha-lipoic acid (ALA), which are needed to metabolize glutathione.

When to See a Doctor

If you are experiencing hazy or blurred vision, impaired vision that is caused by bright lights, double or triple vision in one eye only, or you feel as if you are looking through a fog, see your eye doctor for an examination. If you are in the early stages of the condition, you most likely can avoid surgery and take a nutritional and lifestyle approach to treatment, under the guidance of a knowledge-able physician. If surgery is inevitable, you can be reassured by the fact that about 95 percent of people who undergo the surgery report an improvement in vision. Cataract surgery is a relatively simple procedure that can be done on an outpatient basis at a hospital or clinic.

COLD SORES

Many a date or social engagement has been marred by the sudden appearance of a cold sore, or fever blister, as they are also commonly called. Unlike canker sores, which erupt inside the mouth, cold sores announce themselves boldly and painfully on the outer lips, on the hard area of the gums, or on other parts of the face. So where do these nuisances come from?

Herpes Simplex Virus

Cold sores are infectious and are caused by the herpes simplex virus, which, once it invades your body, stays forever. That means there is no known cure for cold sores. Eighty percent of adults in the United States carry the herpes simplex virus, and 20 to 40 percent of those people—about 50 million Americans—develop cold sores occasionally. Most people get the virus during childhood, and then it can lie dormant for years before it causes symptoms. Stress, fever, sunburn, infection, menstruation, or anything that lowers your resistance can trigger an outbreak of cold sores. These sores are called "cold sores," because they often come out when the immune system is compromised with a cold or flu. Some people experience an outbreak once or twice a year; others get them as often as once or twice a month. A slight fever or a general sick feeling can accompany a cold sore.

Managing Cold Sores

While you're treating cold sores (see "Remedies" below), here are some things you can do to help prevent them from spreading:

◆ Do not touch the sores unless you are treating them. After you apply lotion or cream, or if you touch them accidentally, immediately wash your hands.

◆ Avoid skin contact, such as kissing.

◆ Do not share pillowcases, towels, eating utensils, or toothbrushes.

- Eat foods that are rich in the amino acid lysine, such as yogurt, fish, beans, and eggs. Avoid foods that are rich in the amino acid arginine (chocolate, peanuts, nuts, seeds).

- Eating lots of fruits and vegetables can supply the vitamins and antioxidants needed to boost your immune system. If you can't manage that, at least take a high-potency multivitamin and mineral supplement daily.

- Avoid eating spicy, sour, or acidic foods as they can irritate cold sores.

Remedies

Will you get a cold sore on the day of your big sales presentation? Will one pop out the day you're a bridesmaid for your best friend? The uncertainty of when a cold sore will emerge is something that people who harbor the type 1 herpes virus live with all the time. The good news is that cold sores usually clear up on their own within seven to ten days. The bad news: it can take seven to ten days. Here are some remedies that can significantly reduce the number of outbreaks and the pain and discomfort. For best results, always treat cold sores as soon as you notice that they're coming. Early treatment can reduce the length of time you have them.

Best Bets

- The first over-the-counter drug approved by the Food and Drug Administration (FDA) for cold sores is Abreva, a 10 percent docosanol cream. Studies show that the cream, when applied five times daily, reduces pain, burning, and tingling, and the length of time someone has a cold sore by one day.

- At the first sign of a sore, apply ice to the affected area. Wrap an ice cube or a small ice pack in a washcloth and hold it on the area for as long as you can stand it. Take a break and apply it again for a total of fifteen to thirty minutes. Because viruses don't respond well to cold, the ice can prevent blisters from developing.

- Apply a mixture containing equal amounts of lemon juice and water directly to the sores. This combination promotes healing.

Other Options

- Apply lotion containing the herb melissa (lemon balm). This is especially soothing to cold sores and can be used as needed.

◆ Take a supplement that contains 15 mg zinc daily (either a multiple or single supplement). This nutrient boosts the immune system, speeds up healing, and can help prevent cold sores.

When to See a Doctor

You should consider contacting your doctor about your cold sores if you experience frequent or severe sores, or if they develop near your eyes where they can be extremely painful if not treated quickly. The eye can become infected, in which case you may need antiviral drops.

CONJUNCTIVITIS

Conjunctivitis is the most common eye disease in the Western hemisphere, and it may also be one of the most annoying. Depending on which type of conjunctivitis you have, your eyes may itch, water, swell, or burn. Sometimes there is a discharge from the eye when you wake up in the morning, or pus may have formed a crust that sealed it shut. You may feel as if something is in your eye. Regardless of the type of disease, the whites of your eyes will turn red.

Types of Conjunctivitis

You can probably identify which type of conjunctivitis you have by the symptoms. Once you know the type, you can decide on your course of action, if any. *Bacterial conjunctivitis* is associated with a discharge of pus from the eye or a crust that forms on the eyelashes during sleep. Other symptoms include irritation or a gritty feeling in the eye, tearing, and swelling. It usually affects only one eye, but it can spread easily to the other one, as it is highly contagious. *Viral conjunctivitis* is accompanied by a watery discharge, usually from one eye only, and sometimes crusting. It typically begins in one eye but may spread easily to the other one, as it is highly contagious. A sore throat and a runny nose are common. *Allergic conjunctivitis* usually affects both eyes and causes itching, tearing, and swollen eyelids. It typically appears during allergy season.

How to Prevent Conjunctivitis

You can prevent conjunctivitis and reinfection if you practice a few precautions. If you have conjunctivitis or live with someone who does, for example, wash your hands often, as conjunctivitis spreads very easily and quickly. This means if one eye is infected, do not touch the uninfected eye. You should also stop using eye makeup while you have the infection and throw away the makeup you were using to avoid reinfecting yourself. You should also never share eye makeup or eye drops.

Remedies

The treatment approach depends on which type of conjunctivitis you have. Unfortunately, bacterial conjunctivitis usually responds best to prescription antibiotics.

Best Bets

- For viral conjunctivitis, there is no cure, but you can get relief by applying cool compresses to the affected eye(s) and using artificial tears. This form of conjunctivitis usually resolves within three weeks.

- For all three types of conjunctivitis, use one of the following herbal eye-washes several times a day. In each case, cool the solution and strain it through coffee filter paper before using it. One teaspoon dried eyebright steeped in 1 pint boiling water; or 2 to 3 teaspoons chamomile in 1 pint boiling water.

- For allergic conjunctivitis, cool compresses and artificial tears can provide relief.

Other Options

- Take one of the following homeopathic remedies four times a day for one or two days. If your eyes sting and your eyelids are red and puffy, take apis mellifica 30c. If your eyes are itchy and there is a sticky, yellow discharge, try pulsatilla 30c. For eyes that are bloodshot and have a gritty feeling, use argentum nitricum 30c.

- An over-the-counter boric acid eyewash can cleanse and soothe irritated eyes. Follow the directions on the package.

When to See a Doctor

Contact your ophthalmologist if your vision is affected or you experience eye pain, as you may have a staph or strep infection; or if the redness is accompanied by blurred vision and sensitivity to light, as you may have glaucoma.

DANDRUFF

Are you afraid to wear dark blouses, shirts, jackets, or dresses because your shoulders will look like they've been dusted with snow, even in the summer? Are your eyebrows flaky?

Although dandruff is a harmless health problem, it can be a source of embarrassment and frustration. But it doesn't have to be. One myth we want to dispel right away is the one that says dandruff is caused by a dirty comb or brush or by poor grooming habits. Dandruff is a skin problem, caused by excessive drying of the scalp and overactive oil glands, which produce a substance called sebum. Severe cases of dandruff, called seborrheic dermatitis, are caused by a fungus called *Pityrosporum ovale*. This fungus penetrates the scalp and causes itching, scaling, and inflammation. Some doctors say this fungal infection may be responsible for milder forms of dandruff as well.

Remedies

Eliminating dandruff is a two-step process: getting rid of the dry skin or excess oil, and then restoring moisture and body to your hair.

Best Bets

♦ For severe dandruff, try a shampoo that controls the fungal infection, such as Nizoral (contains ketoconazole) or products that contain zinc pyrithione (ZPT), such as Head and Shoulders and Zincon.

♦ Try a homemade shampoo, composed of 1 part propylene glycol (100%) and 4 parts baby shampoo. Both products are available in drugstores. Mix together and use as you would a dandruff shampoo.

♦ Use a shampoo that contains tea tree oil, or make it yourself by mixing 2–4 drops of tea tree oil in 1–2 ounces of baby shampoo. Tea tree oil kills fungus.

Other Options

♦ Tackle your dandruff from the inside out: take 400 IU vitamin E, 15–20 mg zinc, 200 micrograms (mcg) selenium, and 1–2 tablespoons of flaxseed oil daily. Vitamin E relieves dryness, zinc rebuilds skin, selenium relieves itching and flaking, and flaxseed oil is good for dryness and flaking.

♦ Massage your scalp with warm sesame oil twice a week before you go to bed.

Spend about ten minutes doing the massage, then wrap your head in a towel. Wash out the oil in the morning.

WASH THAT DANDRUFF OUT OF YOUR HAIR

- ◆ Wash your hair with an unmedicated shampoo to get rid of oils and dirt. Then use a dandruff shampoo. After lathering, leave the shampoo in your hair for three to five minutes, then rinse.

- ◆ Towel dry. Never use a blow-dryer, as it will dry out your hair and scalp.

- ◆ Rotate the type of dandruff shampoo you use. Some people develop a tolerance for certain ingredients after a few months. If you do, change your shampoo.

When to See a Doctor

If your dandruff has not responded to self-treatment after two to three months, see a dermatologist. You may have a fungal infection that requires a prescription. In some cases, persistent dandruff is caused by a hormone imbalance, which may need professional care.

DRY EYES

If you work at a computer monitor, chances are you experience dry eyes. That's because people who stare at a computer screen for hours on end tend not to blink often enough to allow tears to bathe their eyes. The result can be dry, red, gritty, burning eyes, a condition sometimes referred to as dry eye syndrome, or keratoconjunctivitis sicca.

Causes of Dry Eyes

Of course, we can't blame computers for every case of dry eyes. Dry eyes occur whenever the liquid supply to the eye is compromised. Thus, there can be either an insufficient amount of fluid being secreted by the lacrimal glands, or the fluid that is produced evaporates because of a problem with the meibomian (oil) glands. The American Optometric Association estimates that 59 million people in the United States suffer with dry eyes. Most cases are among people older than sixty-five, primarily because tear production decreases by about 60 percent between ages eighteen and sixty-five. But the rising use of computers is making dry eyes more common among young adults as well.

Often, dry eyes are part of another medical condition. For example, approximately 3 million Americans have dry eyes as a secondary symptom of Sjögren's syndrome. In this disease, the lacrimal gland is damaged. Some other medical problems and situations associated with dry eyes include:

◆ Rheumatoid arthritis, lupus, thyroid disease, allergies, asthma, which all have dry eyes as a symptom

◆ Wearing contact lenses

◆ Hormone fluctuations, especially during pregnancy, breast-feeding, and menstruation

◆ Use of medications such as antihistamines, oral contraceptives, antihypertensives, and antidepressants

◆ Exposure to smoke, air pollution, bright lights, and dry, dusty environments

◆ Eye diseases, such as meibomianitis, which interferes with tear evaporation; and blepharitis, a bacterial infection of the eyelid

ARE DRY EYEJ JERIOUJ?

Tears serve a critical purpose: they moisten the eyes and clear out irritants that can harm them. A mild, intermittent dry eyes condition is annoying, but chronic dry eyes can be damaging. Dry eyes should definitely be treated to avoid harming your eyes and vision.

Remedies

Most people think of eye drops when they want to soothe their dry eyes, but something that simply "gets the red out" isn't very effective. That's because such products constrict the blood vessels—which makes the red go away—but they don't moisten the eyes effectively. Here are some ways to keep your eyes moist.

Best Bets

◆ Use artificial tears. More than a dozen different products can be used to replace the tears your body isn't making. Be sure to get a brand that does not contain preservatives, such as EDTA or benzalkonium chloride, as they can irritate the eyes. Two examples of preservative-free artificial tears are Similasan and Viva-Drops.

◆ Promote tears from the inside out by taking daily supplements of evening primrose oil (1,500 mg), vitamin C (1,500 mg), and vitamin B$_6$ (500 mg). If you can't find evening primrose oil, you can substitute black currant seed oil or borage oil.

◆ A traditional Chinese medicine remedy called Lycii-Rehmannia can relieve dry eyes. Take according to package directions.

Other Options

◆ If the oil glands become clogged, as they often do, tears evaporate quickly. To prevent this from happening, place a very warm washcloth over your eyelids for three to four minutes twice a day. With your eyes closed, gently rub the washcloth over your eyelids and lashes from left to right several times.

◆ Foods to avoid because they can worsen dry eyes include dairy products, sugar, artificial sweeteners, fried foods, and hydrogenated oils in shortening and margarine. These foods interfere with the metabolism of fatty acids and can thus indirectly cause dry eyes.

When to See a Doctor

If artificial tears and other self-treatments don't offer relief and your eyes hurt, or if there is a discharge from the eye or if your vision changes, see your doctor.

DRY MOUTH

You feel as if the Mojave Desert moved into your mouth, and your tongue is dry and swollen. Your breath may smell like sweaty camels, and the corners of your mouth crack when you talk or smile. But you don't feel like smiling, because you have dry mouth, a common condition in which the salivary glands don't produce enough saliva. It can be caused by several different situations and remedied with several more.

Causes of Dry Mouth

The number-one nonmedical cause of dry mouth is stress and nervousness. Few things can dry out your mouth faster than having to give a speech in front of hundreds of people or going on an important job interview. Your adrenaline is flowing, but the saliva isn't, at least for the time you are under stress.

Most people who have chronic dry mouth also have a medical condition for which dry mouth is a symptom. For example, people who have rheumatoid arthritis, lupus, allergies, diabetes, asthma, or Sjögren's syndrome typically have dry mouth as part of their medical condition. Dry mouth is also a very common side effect of dozens of commonly used over-the-counter and prescription drugs. Drugs known to cause dry mouth include calcium channel blockers (for example, verapamil), high blood pressure medications like prazosin or pro-pranolol, diuretics like chlorothiazide or furosemide, antidepressants like amitriptyline, and over-the-counter antihistamines that contain chlorpheni-ramine, brompheniramine, or diphenhydramine. Check labels before you make a purchase.

Even everyday beverages can cause dry mouth in some people. The caffeine in coffee and tea, as well as the acid in soft drinks and other carbonated drinks can dry out your mouth. Alcohol, whether it's in a drink or in your mouthwash or medicines, can also cause dry mouth.

Chronic Dry Mouth

If you suffer with chronic dry mouth, you probably also experience other symp-toms caused by the excessively dry environment in your mouth. Bad breath, a burning tongue, cracks in the corners of the mouth, and gum disease are com-mon in people who do not treat chronic dry mouth. You don't have to be one of them.

Remedies

If your dry mouth is the result of nervousness and stress, then the first remedy listed below is for you. For all other reasons, try the other suggestions.

Best Bets

◆ *Breathe.* To relieve both dry mouth and the jitters, breathe deeply through your nose for about ten minutes. This is an Ayurvedic approach that works by filling the lower parts of the lungs, which then stimulates the parasympa-thetic nervous system—the part that helps make you calm.

◆ *Drink water.* I know this sounds too simple, but if you have chronic dry mouth, eight glasses of water daily isn't enough; you need twelve. Keep a water bottle with you at all times to help you reach this goal. Sip, don't gulp. Your goal should be about one cup of water every hour.

◆ *Coenzyme* Q_{10} improves circulation, which can help prevent the symptoms that can accompany chronic dry mouth.

Other Options

◆ A mouthwash prepared from the herb goldenseal can keep your mouth moist and relieve tender gums. Prepare a cup of goldenseal tea according to package directions and allow it to cool. Stir in 1 teaspoon baking soda and use this mixture as a mouth rinse every night before retiring.

◆ A homeopathic remedy called natrum muriaticum can relieve cracks in the corners of the mouth. Take one tablet of 30c potency under your tongue daily.

When to See a Doctor

If you have a chronically dry mouth and it does not respond to any of the remedies after several weeks, see your physician. You may have an undiagnosed medical condition. You may also need to see your dentist if the condition is affecting your gums or teeth as well.

EAR INFECTIONS

Ear infections: they're not just for kids. If you're reading this, you may be one of the 3 million American adults who each year suffers with an ear infection. Adults typically are prone to two types of ear infections: those of the middle ear and those affecting the outer ear, also called swimmer's ear.

Types of Ear Infections

If you have a middle ear infection (*otitis media*), the area behind your eardrum will be painful and swollen. You can expect an earache and muffled hearing, and possibly a sore throat, fever of 100°F or higher, chills, and a feeling of fullness in the affected ear. Many people who experience recurrent middle ear infections have chronic respiratory allergies, which make them susceptible to ear problems.

Swimmer's ear (*otitis externa*) is characterized by an itchy or blocked feeling in the ear, pain or tenderness when moving your head, a yellow or watery discharge from the ear, short-term hearing loss, and patches of flaky skin around the ear opening. You don't have to be a swimmer to get this type of ear infection, although getting chlorinated or polluted water in your ears is the main cause of this condition. More adults than children get swimmer's ear.

Remedies

Most ear infections go away by themselves in a few days to a week. But why suffer? Here are some suggestions to take away the pain and speed up recovery.

Best Bets

◆ For swimmer's ear, you can kill the bacteria with a few drops of garlic oil. Put a few drops of garlic oil (pierce a garlic oil capsule with a pin) on a cotton ball and put the cotton in your ear. Leave it in all night. Many healthcare practitioners suggest adding a few drops each of St. John's wort oil and mullein oil to the cotton ball as well.

KID VS. ADULT EARS

Why are children more susceptible to ear infections than adults? The Eustachian tube, which connects the nasal cavity and the inner ear, is much shorter, straighter, and more horizontal in children than in adults. This makes it much easier for bacteria to travel to the inner ear and take up residence. The opening to the tube is also smaller, which means it is easier to block. Young children also have a less developed immune system, which does not allow them to fight off colds and infections quickly, so bacteria attack the inner ear.

◆ Attack the infection from the inside out: take two 500 mg capsules garlic oil daily. Garlic is an effective natural antibiotic.

◆ Boosting your immune system can hasten the departure of a mild ear infection. At the first sign of infection take the following: 25,000 IU vitamin A twice daily for five days, then reduce to 5,000 IU daily; 500 mg vitamin C three times daily for five days, then once daily; 15 mg zinc daily before a meal (good for treatment and prevention); 400 IU vitamin E daily (for prevention); and one capsule of a vitamin B complex that contains at least 50 mg of most of the B vitamins (for prevention).

Other Options

◆ The herbs goldenseal and echinacea can eliminate an ear infection. Goldenseal has a drying effect, and echinacea is a natural antibiotic. These herbs can be purchased in a combination form. Take according to the directions on the package.

◆ Essential oils can relieve the pain caused by ear infections. Add 3 drops each lavender and chamomile oil to a bowl containing 1 pint of boiling water. Lean over the bowl with your face about 12 inches from the water. Make a tent over your head with a towel and breathe in the vapors for five to ten minutes.

When to See a Doctor

If your ear is extremely painful, if there is a discharge, or if you have a high fever (greater than 100°F), see your doctor. If you suffer with chronic middle ear infections, they may be caused by a food allergy. Dairy products and wheat are the most common culprits. You may want to consult a physician who is knowledgeable in nutrition to help you identify the allergens.

GLAUCOMA

Glaucoma has been called the "sneak thief of sight" because it usually moves in slowly and quietly. This eye disease, which affects about 3 million Americans and more than 67 million people worldwide, can lead to blindness. The trouble is, about half of the people with glaucoma don't know it because of its sneaky reputation.

Glaucoma Defined

The inside of your eye contains a gelatinous substance called aqueous humor. This fluid circulates around your eye and then flows through a structure called the drainage angle. From there it enters a tiny tube and drains out into your bloodstream. In some people, the fluid stops draining and causes a buildup of pressure in the eye. The intraocular pressure (IOP) gradually destroys the optic nerve, which is the structure responsible for sending visual signals to your brain. As the pressure increases, your vision decreases.

About 90 percent of people with glaucoma have the open-angle type. This means the tube becomes blocked, which allows pressure to build up slowly.

Your peripheral vision (your ability to see to either side) is affected first, which makes it easier to not notice the loss of sight. As the disease progresses, other symptoms include difficulty focusing on objects that are close, headache, eye pain, and seeing colored halos around lights.

Most of the remaining 10 percent of people with glaucoma experience the closed-angle type, in which the drainage angle becomes blocked. This type of glaucoma comes on quickly and is a medical emergency that requires immediate treatment if you want to save your vision. Symptoms include blurred vision, seeing halos around lights, and a red eye.

At one time, IOP was believed to be the only cause of glaucoma. However, some people have normal IOP and still get glaucoma. So although raised IOP is a major factor in the disease, it is not the only one.

Risk Factors for Glaucoma

People of any age can get glaucoma, including infants, who in rare cases are born with congenital glaucoma. However, you are most likely to get the disease if you are older than sixty years of age (forty years of age if you are African American). Regardless of race, your chances of getting glaucoma are greater if you have relatives with the disease, if you have diabetes, or if you are very nearsighted. Glaucoma may also be caused by certain medications, such as those prescribed for asthma or irritable bowel syndrome, and antidepressants.

Remedies

One reason half the people who have glaucoma don't know they have the disease is because many people fail to get regular eye examinations. Generally, you should be checked every three to five years if you are thirty-nine years of age or older. If you have a family history of glaucoma or severe nearsightedness, are African American, take antidepressants or drugs for asthma or irritable bowel syndrome, or have ever had a serious eye injury you should be checked every one to two years. If you are diagnosed with glaucoma, the sooner you get treatment the better, as delay could mean loss of vision. Although medication is critical, there are some things you can do to help ensure successful treatment.

Best Bets

◆ The over-the-counter herb ginkgo biloba can increase blood flow to the eye and prevent cell death in the optic nerve. The suggested dose is 120 mg twice daily for two months, then reduce to 60 mg twice daily. Check with your doctor first, however, if you are taking prescription medications, especially blood thinners like warfarin or monoamine oxidase inhibitors; or if you are taking any nonsteroidal anti-inflammatory medications or aspirin.

♦ Bilberry extract contains substances called anthocyanosides that improve eyesight. Some experts recommend taking 80–160 mg of the extract three times daily.

♦ Vitamin C helps lower fluid pressure in the eye. A dose of 2,000 mg vitamin C daily is suggested by some doctors. If you are not already taking vitamin C, begin by taking 500 mg, then increasing it by 500 mg every other day until you reach 2,000 mg. If the 2,000 mg dose causes loose stools, cut back to the dose that doesn't cause this symptom.

Other Options

♦ A Chinese herbal formula called *Huang Lian Yang Gan Wan* contains herbs that work together to lower IOP. You can get this formula from practitioners of oriental medicine.

♦ Hydrotherapy can stimulate circulation in the eye. Soak a washcloth in hot water, wring it out, and place it on your eyes for two to three minutes. Then do the same thing with a cold compress. Alternate several times. Do this routine several times a day.

When to See a Doctor

If you have not had an eye exam and you experience the symptoms explained above, see your ophthalmologist or optometrist as soon as possible. If you have symptoms of closed-angle glaucoma, see your ophthalmologist immediately. If you have diabetes or high blood pressure, you are at a higher risk of developing glaucoma; therefore, if you sense that your eyesight is worsening, see your ophthalmologist immediately.

HAIR LOSS

At first you may notice there is extra hair in your comb or brush. Then the shower drain keeps getting clogged with hair—your hair. When you run your fingers through your hair, they make the trip much quicker than they used to. It doesn't matter whether you are a man or a woman, hair loss can happen to you.

It is normal to lose hair. Each strand of hair goes through a two- to six-year growth cycle, after which it is shed and a new one grows in its place. In this way, people normally lose about fifty to a hundred hairs per day.

But at some point for many men and women, hair loss exceeds the norm. The term for both male- and female-pattern hair loss is androgenetic alopecia. "Andro" refers to androgens, the hormones that control masculine characteristics such as testosterone; "genetic" refers to the inheritance of genes for this trait from either side of the family; and "alopecia" means hair loss. Put them all together and you usually have some fairly upset people.

Male Hair Loss

The primary source of hair loss in men is genetic male-pattern baldness. The culprit is a hormone called dihydrotestosterone (DHT), a by-product of the male hormone testosterone. The process goes like this: An enzyme called 5-alpha-reductase converts testosterone into DHT. The DHT shrinks and kills hair follicles, resulting in what is commonly referred to as male-pattern baldness. An effective remedy should in some way reduce the amount of DHT that reaches the hair follicles (see "Remedies" on page 62).

Women Lose Hair, Too

In women, hair loss is generally more complex. Although it can be triggered by DHT (yes, women do have some testosterone), women are much more likely to lose their hair because of other causes, including the following:

- ◆ Significant stress, either physical (illness, rapid weight loss, surgery, anemia) or emotional

- ◆ Thyroid disorders

- ◆ Chemotherapy

- ◆ Poor nutrition (protein or amino acid deficiency)

- ◆ Hair treatments, including dyes and perms

- ◆ Intestinal parasites

- ◆ Hormone changes (due to menopause, birth control pills, pregnancy)

- ◆ Medications, including those for high blood pressure or gout; or high doses of vitamin A (more than 50,000 IU daily)

The good news is that in most cases, if women reverse, correct, or treat these conditions, their hair will usually begin to grow back, although it may take three to six months or longer. If, however, a woman has inherited hair loss from her family (either from the mother's or father's side), then she is in the same situation as men.

Remedies

The remedies listed here can be used by either men or women. However, if you are a woman who is experiencing hair loss, you should first determine whether any of the factors listed under "Women Lose Hair, Too" applies to you. Stopping hair loss may be as simple as changing your diet, a medication, or your lifestyle. Although there are currently no known remedies to reverse natural balding, you can protect your hair from damage that may cause it to fall out or become thinner.

Best Bets

◆ An over-the-counter product for both men and women is minoxidil (Rogaine). The women's form is less potent than the men's. Side effects include chest pain, weight gain, swollen hands or feet, and scalp irritation. It costs about half the price of Propecia (the only FDA-approved drug for male-pattern hair loss on top of the head) but must be applied continuously to be effective.

◆ The herb saw palmetto prevents DHT molecules from attaching themselves to hair follicles and thus can stop hair loss. The suggested dose is 160 mg twice daily. The product should contain 85 to 95 percent fatty acids and sterols and be "concentrated and purified" to be effective.

◆ Massage stimulates blood circulation to the scalp, which helps nourish the hair. Make the massage special by adding a few drops of vitamin E oil. The oil helps prevent dry, flaky skin and strengthens fragile hair.

Other Options

◆ If your hair loss is related to stress, then relaxation techniques may help stop your hair from jumping ship. Yoga, deep breathing exercises, guided imagery, meditation, and tai chi are some proven relaxation methods.

◆ The herbs pygeum and nettle work together to inhibit the production of 5-alpha-reductase. The pygeum should be standardized for 13 percent beta-sterols. The recommended dose is 50–100 mg nettle and 60–500 mg pygeum daily.

HAIR LOSS MYTHS

According to the American Hair Loss Council, the following statements are myths about hair loss. Perhaps the most important one to remember is that if someone claims to have a cure for male- or female-pattern hair loss, they are not telling you the truth. Currently there is no cure for androgenetic alopecia.

◆ Washing your hair every day contributes to hair loss.

◆ Brushing your hair 100 strokes a day will make your hair healthier.

◆ Permanents, coloring, and other cosmetic treatments can cause permanent hair loss (but they *can* cause temporary hair loss).

◆ There are products on the market that will make your hair grow thicker and faster.

◆ Dandruff causes permanent hair loss.

◆ Wearing a hat or wig causes hair loss.

◆ Standing on your head stimulates hair growth because of the increased circulation to your head.

When to See a Doctor

If your hair is coming out in patches or clumps, see a dermatologist who is knowledgeable about hair loss. You may have alopecia areata, an autoimmune disorder, in which the body attacks its own cells. More than 2.5 million men, women, and children in the United States have alopecia areata. If you are interested in trying the prescription drug Propecia, you must see your doctor. At the March 2001 American Academy of Dermatology annual meeting, researchers reported that after five years of use, 65 percent of users reported no further hair loss and 35 percent continued to have hair loss. Propecia inhibits the production of 5-alpha-reductase and so prevents the conversion of testosterone into DHT. Propecia is costly: it averages more than $600 per year and it is only effective if you use it regularly. It causes sexual side effects (loss of sex drive, impotence) in about 2 percent of users.

LARYNGITIS

You had a great time at the game. You cheered on your kids, yelled at the umpires, shouted greetings to friends across the parking lot. And now when you open your mouth, nothing comes out but a squeak. You've irritated your voice box (larynx) and caused it to swell. You've lost your voice.

Laryngitis caused by overuse is called chronic laryngitis. Overuse can mean too much talking, shouting, smoking, or drinking alcohol. Symptoms include hoarseness or temporary loss of your voice, and it may be difficult to swallow.

Laryngitis caused by a viral or bacterial infection is called acute laryngitis. This type of laryngitis often follows a bout of pneumonia, flu, tonsillitis, or bronchitis. It causes the same symptoms as chronic laryngitis, and can also be accompanied by a cough and a roughness or tickling in the throat. Acute laryngitis is most common in late fall, winter, or early spring.

Remedies

With or without treatment, acute laryngitis usually clears up completely within seven to fourteen days. The chronic form can take shorter or longer, depending on whether you continue the activity that caused it.

Best Bets

◆ For acute laryngitis, rest your voice as much as possible and drink plenty of fluids. Medicated throat lozenges may help soothe the irritation.

◆ For chronic laryngitis, rest your voice completely or as much as possible and avoid irritants such as alcohol, smoke, and air pollution.

◆ Use a cool-mist steam vaporizer (humidifier) in your room at night, or breathe the steam from a bowl of boiling water. Hold your head about 12 inches above the bowl and make a tent with a towel over your head. Breathe in the steam for five to ten minutes.

Other Options

◆ Drink a mixture of warm lemon juice and honey to soothe your throat.

◆ Check your medications. Some drugs can cause hoarseness, especially steroids like prednisone and flunisolide. Ask your doctor or pharmacist about the possible side effects of drugs you may be taking, and ask to switch to another medication.

When to See a Doctor

If you have tried one or more remedies and your voice does not begin to return after four or five days, you should see your doctor. Other signs and symptoms that should be checked by a doctor include high temperature, bleeding in your throat, hoarseness or frequent loss of your voice, difficulty swallowing or breathing, or the presence of large, tender lumps in your neck.

LICE (HEAD)

There was a time when lice were seen only in poorer neighborhoods and schools. Today they cross all economic and social barriers. As one mother put it, "Those bloodsuckers don't discriminate anymore."

Approximately 10 percent of elementary school children will get head lice some time during the school year. The first indication is usually intense itching of the scalp. If you notice your child scratching, examine his or her hair for lice using a flashlight and a magnifying glass. Although adult lice are about the size of a sesame seed and visible without magnification, using the glass makes it much easier to find them and especially their smaller eggs, or nits.

What to Look For

Adult lice are grayish brown, wingless insects that are about an eighth of an inch long. After they lay their eggs, they can often be found behind the ears, at the nape of the neck, or feeding on blood throughout the scalp. Their nits are grayish white and oval and cling to the hairs at the scalp.

Remedies

Head lice can be easily spread among school mates or family members by sharing combs, hats, clothing, and bedding. The first step in getting rid of lice is to use a good-quality treatment on the hair and remove the nits with a special comb. Then you need to ensure you've gotten rid of the lice on clothing, hair accessories, and furniture and bedding.

Best Bets

♦ Use a head lice shampoo that contains 1 percent permethrin or pyrethrin and follow the package directions exactly. This should be used not only on the affected child but on any other family members who may have become infested.

◆ Remove all nits using a special fine-toothed comb while the hair is wet. Do this in a well-lit area so you can see the eggs. You must remove all the nits; otherwise, any that remain that are still alive will hatch in about a week and a reinfestation will occur.

◆ Wash all clothing, bedding, and towels that were in contact with anyone who is infested. Use hot water and the hot setting on the dryer. Stuffed animals and pillows should be placed in a tightly sealed plastic bag and left for twenty days to kill any nits. Areas of the house in which any infested person has been in contact must be cleaned and vacuumed.

Other Options

◆ An alternative to pyrethrin shampoos is a mixture of 50 drops tea tree oil in 2 ounces of warm olive oil. Apply the mixture to the hair and scalp and cover the head with a shower cap and a hot, moist towel for two hours. Then rinse out the hair, and comb for nits.

◆ HairClean 1-2-3 is a natural product that is sold as a head hygiene product.

When to See a Doctor

Most lice infestations can be eliminated with a thorough home treatment. However, call the doctor if scratching leads to bleeding and infection, if a rash or seizures develop after using the medicated shampoo, or if lice appear on the eyelashes, as the doctor will need to remove them.

MACULAR DEGENERATION

If telephone poles look bent, door frames look wavy, the white line down the middle of the road no longer looks straight to you, or if you notice a blurry spot in the center of your vision, you could have had too much to drink last night. Or you could have macular degeneration.

Macular degeneration works like this: In the back of your eye is the retina, a light-sensitive area that translates light into images. These images are sent as signals along the optic nerve to the brain. In the center of the retina is the macula, a highly sensitive spot that enables you to see fine detail and color. When this area becomes damaged, objects in the center of your vision look crooked or wavy and colors are replaced by black and white. Eventually your ability to see things that are straight ahead vanishes, and you are left with peripheral vision in the affected eye.

Causes of Macular Degeneration

Molecules called free radicals are naturally produced as by-products of various bodily functions. Low numbers of free radicals are helpful, but when their numbers rise, as they do when certain lifestyle and environmental factors are involved, they begin to damage cells throughout the body through a process called oxidation. A high-fat diet, smoking, exposure to chemicals, food additives, radiation, and air pollution are just a few of the factors that can stimulate free-radical production. When these radicals affect the macula, the result is macular degeneration.

Age is also a deciding factor. Macular degeneration is most common in older individuals. Twenty-five percent of people aged sixty-five to seventy-five have the vision disorder, and one in three people older than seventy-five have the disease. It is rare in people fifty years and younger. Other contributing factors include smoking and excessive exposure to ultraviolet light.

Types of Macular Degeneration

Between 80 and 90 percent of all cases of macular degeneration are the dry form. This type develops slowly and painlessly as tiny yellow spots called drusen form on the macula. Eventually central vision is affected. In the wet form, destruction of central vision is rapid. Abnormal blood vessels grow under the macula and displace it, and the resulting scar tissue affects vision. The wet form is more serious than the dry and usually requires surgery. Dry macular degeneration can be treated in various ways (see "Remedies" below).

Remedies

Conventional and alternative health practitioners don't always see eye-to-eye when it comes to treatment of macular degeneration. Alternative health practitioners tend to believe there are things people can do to stop or even reverse the disease; conventional doctors don't. Regardless of their feelings on that topic, nearly all agree that some lifestyle changes are helpful. They include stopping smoking, wearing sunglasses to protect your retina from further damage, and avoiding alcohol as it can harm the macula. The following are some treatment approaches.

LIVING WITH MACULAR DEGENERATION

If you have macular degeneration, you can made some adjustments to your life so you can continue with as normal a lifestyle as possible. Here's what you can do:

◆ Get large-print books, a telephone and clock with large numbers, and other oversized products. Ask your ophthalmologist about where to get such items, or contact Lighthouse International, a nonprofit group for people who are blind or have partial vision.

◆ If reading is a problem, you can get audiobooks. Most libraries have many you can borrow, or they can be purchased from bookstores.

◆ Move closer to your television. Some people find that sitting as close as 3 feet away allows them to see most of the screen.

◆ Get a high-quality magnifying glass. There are handheld varieties and those that attach to a gooseneck or swing arm that you can attach to your desk, table, or nightstand.

◆ Keep your living space well lit. Use 100 watt soft lightbulbs, but first make sure the lamps you want to put them in can handle this high wattage.

Best Bets

◆ Since macular degeneration is caused by free radicals and oxidation, taking antioxidant supplements can be helpful. Joseph Pizzorno Jr., N.D., recommends the following regimen. Talk with your doctor before starting this program. Take 1,000 mg vitamin C three times daily; 600 to 800 IU vitamin E, 400 mcg selenium, and 45 mg zinc daily.

◆ Take lutein supplements. Although many conventional doctors insist nothing can stop or reverse macular degeneration, many alternative health practitioners believe that lutein, a pigment found in leafy green vegetables, can prevent and treat the disease. Experts suggest 6 mg daily of lutein.

Other Options

◆ The herb bilberry improves circulation to the retina. Some experts recommend taking bilberry along with lutein. This duo is available in combination products. Take 180 mg bilberry along with the lutein.

♦ Ginkgo biloba improves circulation to the eye and brain. The recommended dose is 80 mg twice daily for six months.

When to See a Doctor

If you have macular degeneration, you need to be under the care of qualified healthcare practitioners. If you wish to use alternative treatment approaches, make sure your ophthalmologist is knowledgeable; or if you are also using an alternative health practitioner, make sure that both professionals are fully informed of the treatments you are using.

NOSEBLEED

A nosebleed can result from a variety of situations—from a blow to the nose to blowing your nose too hard to living in a very dry environment. Rarely is a nosebleed a sign of something serious (see "When to See a Doctor" on page 70).

Periodic nosebleeds become more common as we mature, because the moisture in the nose tends to dry up faster. Medications can contribute to nosebleeds. Any drug that thins the blood can make nosebleeds occur more frequently and also make it more difficult to stop a nosebleed. Medications such as aspirin, anticoagulants (warfarin), and nonsteroidal anti-inflammatory drugs (ibuprofen), fall into this category.

Remedies

The following suggestions are for dealing with and preventing nosebleeds.

♦ If your nose starts to bleed, don't panic. Instead, follow these steps:

1. Sit up straight with your head tilted slightly forward. This prevents the blood from running down your throat.

2. *Gently* blow your nose to eliminate any clots that could prevent the blood vessels from sealing.

3. Pinch the soft part of your nose between your thumb and forefinger. Hold this position for ten minutes. Some blood may drip from between your fingers. That's normal; just place a tissue under your nose while you're holding the pinch. Resist the temptation to let go sooner, as the bleeding may start up again.

♦ If the above method doesn't work, use a nasal spray such as Neo-Synephrine.

This over-the-counter drug constricts blood vessels and therefore can stop blood flow. Four or five squirts into the bleeding nostril should do the trick. Pinch your nose for ten minutes immediately after spraying.

◆ Keep the humidity up. Many heating and cooling systems can dry out the mucous membranes in the nose.

Other Option

◆ If nosebleeds are a frequent problem for you, increase your intake of vitamin C with bioflavonoids. Vitamin C helps maintain blood vessels, and bioflavonoids help clot the blood and maintain healthy tissues. One 200 or 500 mg tablet immediately before bedtime should be sufficient.

When to See a Doctor

If your nosebleed does not stop bleeding after you have applied pressure for twenty minutes, go to the emergency room. You should also seek immediate medical attention if blood is running down your throat when you are standing or sitting or after you have already applied pressure to the nostrils. This could mean that the blood vessels behind your nose are affected (posterior bleeding). Bleeding from these vessels, which is seen more often in older people, can cause significant blood loss.

TINNITUS

Ringing. Clanging. Roaring. Buzzing. Hissing. If you're hearing these sounds and they're coming from inside your head, then you have tinnitus, a condition typically referred to as "ringing in the ears." As many as forty-five percent of American adults and ninety percent of people who have hearing loss experience tinnitus at least occasionally. However, according to the American Tinnitus Association, about twelve percent of Americans have "problematic" tinnitus, that is, tinnitus that causes significant discomfort or hearing distortion.

Tinnitus Defined

Tinnitus is defined as the perceived sensation of sound in the absence of auditory stimulation. That means the sound is literally "all in your head," but it doesn't mean it isn't real. The sounds can change; they can be loud or soft, constant or intermittent. Tinnitus usually affects people between forty and eighty years of age, but it is more common among older individuals.

A wide range of factors have been associated with tinnitus, including:

- Moderate to high doses of aspirin and high doses of some antibiotics
- Use of antidepressants, antihypertensives, nonsteroidal anti-inflammatory drugs, atropine ergotamines, chloroquine, and quinine
- Food sensitivities, usually in people who have a family history of allergies or food cravings
- High cholesterol
- Prolonged exposure to loud noise
- Hypertension
- Ear infections
- Temporomandibular joint (TMJ) problems
- Chronic stress

No objective tests exist that can detect tinnitus. The only people who can hear the noises are those who are affected, so doctors, spouses, and friends can find it difficult to understand the frustration tinnitus can cause.

Remedies

Although tinnitus is not a typical indicator of serious illness and may disappear on its own, it can be very distracting. Tinnitus can make it difficult to sleep, work, and concentrate. If you are taking any of the drugs mentioned above, ask your doctor if you can switch to an alternative and see if the tinnitus goes away. Here are some other ways to deal with the noise.

Best Bets

- B vitamin supplements can eliminate tinnitus in people who may have deficiencies of these nutrients. With the high levels of stress in today's society, a deficiency of B vitamins is not unusual, as stress strips them from the body. A high-potency B vitamin supplement that contains 50 mg of most of the B vitamins is a good start. Some healthcare practitioners also suggest taking higher levels of three B vitamins—niacin, thiamine, and vitamin B_{12}—with your physician's approval. Recommended dosages are 50 mg of niacin twice daily; 100–500 mg of thiamine daily; and 1,000 mcg of vitamin B_{12} daily for six months, then 100 mcg daily.

◆ Ginkgo biloba increases circulation to brain, and to the inner ear as well. The recommended dosage is 120–240 mg twice daily.

◆ For chronic tinnitus, try a tinnitus masker. This electronic device is worn in the ear like a hearing aid and produces a pleasant sound that competes with the tinnitus. Some people find it helpful to use a portable music player and listen on earphones to soothing background music, like environmental sounds, at a volume a little softer than the tinnitus.

Other Options

◆ Biofeedback (a behavior modification technique) and relaxation training can be helpful for tinnitus that is associated with stress. One study showed a 50 percent improvement in people who used biofeedback.

◆ Magnesium (400 mg daily) can reduce symptoms of tinnitus.

When to See a Doctor

If you experience a sudden or total hearing loss, feel dizzy, have pain or pus in your ear, or if tinnitus is interfering with your daily activities, call your physician. In very rare (less than 1 percent) cases, tinnitus is caused by a brain tumor. You may want to have your hearing tested by an audiologist, who can determine whether you have damage to your inner ear, which can occur from use of some medications (see the list of factors associated with tinnitus on page 71).

YELLOW TEETH

You want your teeth to sparkle and to send out a message that welcomes people, not put up a "yield" warning. Yet yellow teeth can do just that. When you want to put your best foot forward, it's a good idea not to follow up with yellow or discolored teeth.

Smile Me a Rainbow

Staining occurs on the outer surface, or enamel, of the teeth. Several factors can affect the color of the enamel. One is baseline tooth color. People can have a wide range of shades of white as their baseline tooth color, and some people have a "whiter white" than do others. Things that can stain the enamel include coffee, tea, tobacco, marijuana, certain prescription drugs, poor oral hygiene, aging, dental fillings, tooth trauma, and fluoride.

Yellow is not the only color your teeth can be. Coffee, tea, and red wine can cause dark brown stains, which are difficult to remove. Tobacco, depending on whether you smoke or chew it, can turn your teeth yellow-brown to black. Marijuana use causes dark brown to black stains, usually appearing as dark rings near the gum line.

Orange or green stains can occur from poor oral hygiene and are actually the result of bacterial growth. Exposure to too much fluoride (more than 2 parts fluoride per million parts water) during childhood years when teeth are developing can cause mottled teeth, in which part of each tooth is white opaque compared with the normal hard, glossy enamel. Sometimes mottled teeth become brownish. Children who are on long-term treatment with drugs like tetracycline during tooth development typically have yellow, brown, gray, or black stained teeth. For that reason, tetracycline should not be given to infants, children, or pregnant women unless the medical condition is life threatening.

Both types of dental fillings—composite resin fillings and amalgam fillings—can stain the teeth, and so can cavities. If there is trauma to the teeth that causes blood vessels to break, the broken vessels may be seen through the enamel and give the tooth a gray, brown, or black color. Teeth that have undergone root canal also sometimes darken.

SWIMMING STAINS TEETH?

If you swim more than six hours a week and you've noticed hard, brown deposits on your front teeth, you probably have "swimmer's calculus." According to the Academy of General Dentistry, this problem occurs because avid swimmers continually expose their teeth to chemically treated water, which contains additives that raise the pH level. Because the resulting pH level is higher than that of saliva, the salivary proteins break down and form deposits on the teeth. Unfortunately, brushing doesn't seem to help remove this tartar, but professional dental cleaning does. The Academy suggests that high-volume swimmers visit their dentists and hygienists regularly.

Remedies

Routine cleanings by your dentist or hygienist are recommended, but many people neglect this part of their dental care. Professional cleanings can usually remove most stains caused by food and tobacco, and bleaching can be used for more resistant stains. Techniques such as bonding and porcelain veneers are options if you have more difficult stains.

But there are several things you can do at home to get rid of a rainbow smile and make it shine like a sunny day.

HOME TEETH-WHITENING KITS: WHAT'S THE STORY?

You want a whiter, brighter smile, but how safe are the whitening products on the market? Home whitening kits contain whitening solutions (usually hydrogen peroxide or hydrochloric acid) that are weaker than those used in a dentist's office, but they are less expensive. They can lighten most stains that are caused by coffee, tea, tobacco, and age, while those caused by tetracycline or fluoride are less responsive. There are two main types: those that come with the materials to make your own custom tray into which you place the bleaching agent; and those in which you send the manufacturer an impression made from materials in the kit and a custom tray will be sent back to you. Generally, the instructions are to place the whitening solution in the tray, which you wear over your teeth for up to several hours each day. These solutions do not lighten crowns, bridges, bonding, or fillings.

Most people report good to excellent results when using home teeth-whitening kits, but there can be some side effects. Hydrogen peroxide can increase the temperature sensitivity of your teeth (this is temporary), and the use of the trays can cause gum irritation in some people. The cost of kits can range from a little less than $100 to about $300. The trays can be reused again and again, although you will need to purchase additional bleaching agents. Home teeth-whitening kits are available at some pharmacies and over the Internet. Talk to your dentist before using such kits.

Best Bets

◆ Whitening take-home trays from your dentist can help. These are home bleaching kits that your dentist prepares for you. Your dentist makes a mold of your teeth and makes a flexible tray that holds the bleaching gel (usually carbamide peroxide) that you fit on your teeth. You will need to wear the tray overnight for about one week or up to ninety minutes daily for two weeks. The results can last years.

◆ Whitening toothpastes can help remove stains from teeth and may help maintain their appearance after you've had your teeth cleaned professionally or at home with a whitening product. Some are more abrasive than others.

◆ Whitening strips, which contain peroxide, can be placed over your teeth for a short period of time and then removed. That typically means thirty minutes twice a day for two weeks.

When to See a Doctor

Consult your dentist before using a home bleaching kit. If your efforts to whiten your teeth have not produced the results for which you had hoped, see your dentist about having your teeth whitened professionally. If you have difficult stains, you may need bonding or veneers.

◆ CHAPTER 4 ◆

Aches and Pains

Pain is a bitter-sweet phenomenon: it's the body's way of letting us know that something is causing it harm—a burn, a broken bone, a nail in the foot, a sprained back muscle—and that treatment, caution, or management is needed. Often, pain is also accompanied by inconvenience or potentially lengthy disruptions to our lives. However, if we didn't feel pain, we wouldn't survive very long on this planet.

That doesn't mean we have to *like* pain or tolerate it any longer than we need to. So in this chapter we discuss how you can cope with and manage some common painful conditions so you can get back to living pain-free.

BACK PAIN

When your mother used to tell you to sit up straight, she was giving you some good advice. Poor posture is one cause of back pain, a condition that affects about 80 percent of Americans at some point during their lives. In most cases, the problem is the lower back, because it is under a lot of stress from sitting, leaning back, and lifting.

About 45 percent of people with back pain have chronic pain. According to the National Center for Health Statistics, back pain is the fourth most common chronic complaint in the United States, and Americans lose 60 million work days per year because of an aching back. Our pain in the back costs the economy about $20 to $50 billion yearly in medical treatments and disability payments.

Welcome, Back

The spinal column consists of a series of bones (vertebrae) separated by disks, which act as shock absorbers. Ligaments and muscles surround the spinal column and help support it. The slight "S" shape of the spinal column gives it strength and allows us to walk upright. For a back to be healthy and pain-free, it's important for all these structures to be in optimal shape. Unfortunately, that's often not the case, as you'll see below.

Causes of Back Pain

Back pain can be caused by more than one factor. Many people suffer from back pain due to a combination of weak abdominal and back muscles, and a lack of flexibility. The abdominal muscles (flexors) help support the lower back and are instrumental in bending forward and in lifting. Back muscles (extensors) help in maintaining posture, bending, lifting, and turning from side to side. Erector spinae run alongside the spinal column and help support it. Weakness and lack of flexibility in any of these muscle groups can contribute to and cause back pain.

When it comes to sitting, it's not *because* you sit but *how* you sit that matters most. If you lean back while sitting, the lower area of your back is flattened. This position pulls down on your lower vertebrae and places undue stress on the ligaments and disks in your back. You want to sit with your lower back well supported.

Incorrect lifting—particularly bending from the waist—sends many people crawling to the doctor or chiropractor. Lifting and twisting at the same time is another sure move toward trouble. About 20 percent of people with back pain have spinal injuries, such as a ruptured disk (disks are the gel-filled structures between the vertebrae that absorb shock).

Several diseases and medical conditions are also associated with back pain. Osteoarthritis, osteoporosis, scoliosis (curvature of the spine), kyphosis (hunchback), fibromyalgia, kidney disease, obesity, rheumatoid arthritis, and pregnancy can all have back pain as a symptom.

Remedies

For many years, doctors used to prescribe bed rest for people who had back pain. Today, we know that in the majority of cases, inactivity can cause more harm than good. With that in mind, here are some remedies that are definitely beneficial.

Best Bets

✦ Do exercises that strengthen your abdominal muscles and incorporate stretching exercises to increase flexibility. Nearly everyone can benefit from this suggestion, as strong, flexible muscles counteract stress to the back and can prevent pain from occurring. Ask your doctor or chiropractor for instructions on back exercises, or consult one of the many books on back pain (see Resources and Further Reading on page 289). If you choose exercises on your own, get clearance from your doctor before doing them.

◆ Apply ice, five to ten minutes at a time, to the painful area for the first few days after back pain begins. After two days, apply heat from a heating pad, hot shower, or hot-water bottle.

◆ Back, side, or stomach? The debate about how best to sleep to prevent or ease back pain goes on. Here's what seems to work best, depending on your situation. If you sleep on your back and back pain disturbs your sleep, put a pillow under your knees. If you sleep on your side, bend your knees and place a pillow between them to ease the stress on your lower back. Only sleep on your stomach if you have sciatica; this position can help relax the muscles and ligaments and allow the sciatic nerve to heal.

Other Options

◆ If you have chronic back pain and taking anti-inflammatory drugs—and coping with their side effects—does not appeal to you, try methylsulfonylmethane (MSM). MSM reportedly is effective for back pain secondary to arthritis, accidents, and disk breakdown. Stanley W. Jacob, M.D., professor of surgery at Oregon Health Sciences University in Portland, recommends taking up to 8 grams of MSM daily in divided doses with food. Because MSM can cause loose stools, start with 2 grams daily and slowly increase up to 8 grams, if needed.

◆ Press away your pain with acupressure. This treatment, which you can perform on yourself or with help from a partner, is based on the principle of restoring energy flow—and thus relieving pain—by applying pressure and stimulation to specific points on the body. Acupressure can be learned from a book, but it is recommended that you get instructions from a professional acupressure therapist so you can better understand the technique when you treat yourself. For lower back pain, the most commonly treated points are the bladder points 23 and 47 (located waist level on your back), 48 (middle of the buttocks), and 57 (middle back of the knee). See pages 28–29 for the acupressure chart and instructions.

When to See a Doctor

Call your doctor immediately if you experience intense pain that travels down your leg or radiates to your spine, sudden weakness in your foot or leg, or a loss of control of your bladder or bowels. These symptoms suggest a ruptured disk or other spinal problem. Back pain that is the result of an accident or any type of physical trauma should be investigated by your physician.

HEADACHE

Do you know anyone who has never had a headache? He or she would be an unusually lucky individual, as the vast majority of people have at least one headache during their lives, and most people experience them periodically. When you consider that there are 129 different types of headache (according to the International Headache Society), it's hard to imagine anyone escaping them all.

By far the most common types of head pain are tension headache and migraine. The first is explored here; migraine is discussed under "Migraine," which directly follows this section.

Tension Headache

Your kids are fighting. Your boss wants you to work overtime again. You're stuck in traffic for the umpteenth time. These are all opportunities for the muscles in your neck, scalp, jaw, and face to contract. The pain of a tension headache is believed to come from prolonged muscle contractions, which trap pain-producing chemicals in your muscles. The pain is typically constant, can be dull or intense, and feels like pressure is being applied to your entire head. Your upper back and neck muscles may be tender as well. Tension headache may also be triggered by menstruation (both before and during menses), insufficient sleep, depression, grinding your teeth, use of artificial sweeteners, poor posture, eyestrain, and exposure to carbon monoxide.

Rebound Headache

We have a natural tendency to reach for the first thing that relieves headache pain, especially when it's chronic pain. And with a wide variety of over-the-counter products on the market, it's easy to do. But for many people, habitual use of these drugs leads to a tolerance for the drugs, and the result is that you get a headache whenever you don't take the drugs. This phenomenon is called rebound headache, and it affects millions of Americans.

Remedies

For a mild, occasional headache, two aspirin eliminate the pain for most people. Aspirin is an herb-based medication with more than 100 years of proven effectiveness. The pain-relieving ability of aspirin actually derives from salicin, an extract from the bark and leaves of the willow tree. Scientists then converted salicin into salicylic acid, which is the form aspirin takes today. In more recent times we've added acetaminophen, ibuprofen, and naproxen to the headache-treatment list. But there are other options, especially if you are experiencing chronic tension headache and don't want to rely on drugs—or risk rebound headache. Although medications can control pain, lifestyle changes can reduce or eliminate the need for drugs altogether.

Best Bets

◆ Because many chronic tension headaches are caused by stress, replacing the vitamins that are depleted from the body during stress can both prevent and relieve headache pain. Take a high-potency B vitamin complex plus a high-potency multivitamin and mineral supplement.

◆ Exercise relieves tension, thus it can also relieve tension headache. Include twenty to thirty minutes of aerobic activity (walking, jogging, biking) in your schedule four to five days a week. Also take mini breaks during the day: two to five minutes of stretching, running in place, stair climbing, or deep breathing to help release built-up tension.

◆ According to the National Institutes of Health, in eight out of nine studies acupuncture relieved headache pain significantly better than placebo (sugar pill) treatment. You must see a professional acupuncturist for treatments, but if you suffer with chronic headache, it may well be worth the effort.

Other Options

◆ For non-chronic headache, try acupressure (see page 28). Using your thumb, apply steady, focused pressure on each of the following points for three minutes each.

  • Governing vessel 24.5—between your eyebrows where the bridge of your nose meets your forehead

- Governing vessel 16—center of the back of your head, in the hollow at the base of your skull

- Large intestine 4—back of your hand where the bones of your index finger and thumb meet

- Bladder 2—on both sides of your nose, where the bridge meets the ridge of your eyebrows

- Stomach 3—at the base of the cheekbone, directly below your pupil

- Liver 3—on top of your foot in the webbing between your second and big toes

◆ Ice works nice: two-thirds of people with tension headaches report some relief when applying ice to the forehead. Wrap ice cubes or an ice pack in a towel and apply it to your forehead for ten to fifteen minutes. Remove the ice for ten minutes and then reapply.

When to See a Doctor

Consult your doctor or a headache specialist if you have severe or frequent headaches; if your headache is accompanied by changes in memory, vision, behavior, or ability to walk; if you have a stiff neck, rash, and fever with the head pain; if the head pain is sudden and excruciating; if you've never had headaches and they've started suddenly; or if the headache gets progressively worse over days or weeks.

MIGRAINE

About 24 million Americans—18 million women and 6 million men—know what it's like to experience head pain that can knock them off their feet for hours or even days. About 20 percent of women and 7 percent of men get migraines. Migraine is classified as a vascular headache, which means it is caused by changes to the blood vessels. In this case, it involves vessels at the base of the brain, which constrict and restrict blood flow to the brain; and then relax and dilate, sending a surge of blood to the brain, resulting in intense pain.

Scientists have noted that the platelets (a component of blood) of people who suffer with migraines behave differently than those found in healthy individuals. A substance called serotonin, which helps blood vessels relax, among many other functions, is found in platelets. The platelets of people with migraines stick together easily, causing high levels of serotonin to be released. These high serotonin levels cause blood vessels to constrict.

Types of Migraines

Migraines appear in two main forms: classic and common. The only significant difference between the two is the presence of an aura stage in the classic form. Between 20 and 30 percent of all people who get migraines experience the classic variety. The aura stage begins about sixty minutes before the head pain starts and is characterized by visual disturbances, such as spots or wavy lines before the eyes; and a pins-and-needles sensation somewhere in the body.

The head pain for both the classic and common forms of migraine is similar. The pain usually begins as throbbing on one side of the head and moves to the forehead, temples, top of the head, jaw, or one nostril. The migraine is typically accompanied by other symptoms, such as oversensitivity to light or sounds, constipation or diarrhea, paleness, nausea and/or vomiting, muscle aches, chills and/or fever, muscle spasms in the neck and back, or oversensitivity to touch on the face, neck, and scalp.

Migraine Triggers

Some people know that if they allow themselves to get overtired, they run the risk of getting a migraine. Others steer clear of strawberries, because just a few bites of the ruby red fruit can set their head pounding. Fatigue and food sensitivities are just two of the many risk factors and triggers of migraine. Here are a few more:

- *Heredity.* About 50 percent of people who get migraines have a family history of the problem.

- *Hormonal changes.* Migraines are more common before and during a menstrual period and in women who take birth control pills.

- *Sleep.* Too much or too little sleep.

- *Weather.* Weather changes, including fluctuations in both temperature and humidity.

- *Chemicals.* Exposure to chemicals (for example, monosodium glutamate, aspartame, nitrates, nitroglycerin).

- *Foods.* Foods that contain or release histamines, such as cheeses, fermented meats, red wine, sherry, pickled herring, and overripe avocados and fruits.

- *Smoking.*
- *Eyestrain and glare.*
- *Stress and intense emotions.*
- *Magnesium deficiency.*

Remedies

Conventional doctors have about 200 different drugs at their disposal to treat migraine. Many migraine sufferers find that combining conventional and alternative treatments can provide them with better relief than if they use just one approach. Naturally, you should do your best to avoid those things in your diet or your environment that you know or suspect will trigger an episode. An ounce of prevention, after all, is worth a pound of cure—and may avoid a pounding head.

Best Bets

- The herb feverfew (*Tanacetum parthenium*), 125 mg of dried herb daily, standardized at 0.25 to 0.5 percent parthenolide, is very effective against migraines and can be taken as a preventive measure. To offset an acute attack, a suggested dose is three 125 mg capsules as soon as you feel symptoms coming on, then take the same dose every four hours. Do not exceed twelve capsules within a twenty-four-hour period.

- Taking 400–600 mg magnesium daily can help prevent migraines in individuals who have low magnesium levels. Magnesium helps reduce the expansion and contraction of blood vessels.

- The following supplements taken daily can greatly reduce the intensity and frequency of migraines: 2,000 mg vitamin C, 400–600 IU vitamin E, 100 mg vitamin B_6, 600 mg 5-hydroxytryptophan (5-HTP), and 1,400 mg omega-3 oils.

Other Options

- You can learn to use your mind to rid yourself of migraine. In thermal biofeedback, you are taught to redirect some of the blood flow in your head to your hands, which relieves the pressure in your head. To initially learn this technique, you can consult with a biofeedback specialist, who will train you on a biofeedback machine, or you can purchase a biofeedback machine of your own. After several sessions, many people learn how to redirect the blood flow without the help of the machine, and so can use the technique whenever they feel a migraine coming on.

♦ If you typically experience classic migraine, you can take 100 mg niacin (nicotinic acid) during the aura period to cause a quick dilation of the constricted blood vessels and hopefully abort a migraine attack.

When to See a Doctor

If you experience any of the following situations with your migraine, call your doctor immediately: unusually severe head pain, a migraine that does not respond to home treatment and lasts longer than three days, migraine accompanied by a fever of 102°F or higher, head pain accompanied by slurred speech, blurred vision, numbness, weakness, or head pain that worsens when you bend your chin to your chest.

Several prescription drugs (for example, sumatriptan [Imitrex], naratriptan [Amerge], and zolmitriptan [Zomig]) offer relief from both head pain and also reduce nausea, vomiting, and sensitivity to light. For about 75 percent of users, relief comes within one hour, and in as little as fifteen minutes. One drawback, however, is that long-term treatment (about sixty days) is needed for potential results to appear.

OSTEOARTHRITIS

It happens to machines, most animals, and people: their moving parts break down from daily use. Our joints degenerate—from normal and not-so-normal wear and tear—and the result can be osteoarthritis. The word "arthritis" means "joint inflammation." In osteoarthritis, the cartilage (the tough, shock-absorbing material that secretes a thick clear fluid and prevents your bones from grinding together) wears down, allowing the bones to rub against each other. Tiny bone spurs develop and cause pain. Some joints may have an insufficient amount of fluid, causing stiffness, while others may have an excess, which causes swelling. In addition to these symptoms, people often experience limited movement and flexibility.

About 40 million Americans of all ages have osteoarthritis, but it mostly affects people forty years of age and older. Most people who have osteoarthritis have mild to moderate symptoms and typically self-treat. But about 16 million Americans have symptoms that grow progressively worse and eventually become disabling.

Causes and Risk Factors for Osteoarthritis

Osteoarthritis is not an inevitable part of aging, although an estimated 80 percent of people age sixty-five and older have some degree of the disorder. The Centers for Disease Control and Prevention (CDC) estimates that nearly 60 million Americans will have arthritis in the year 2020, when the youngest baby boomers will be sixty years old. Risk factors and causes for osteoarthritis include heredity, a severe or recurrent joint injury, obesity (especially of weight-bearing joints like the knee), living in a cold climate, and prolonged exercise (joint-pounding activities, such as long-distance running can predispose some people to osteoarthritis).

Remedies

Many people who have osteoarthritis use a combination of conventional and alternative treatments for relief. If you choose that path, make sure you inform each of your healthcare practitioners about any and all remedies you are using, and do not start or stop any treatments without telling them.

Best Bets

◆ Glucosamine sulfate is a natural remedy that is proving to be very effective. Not only does it reduce inflammation, it also may build cartilage and slow the progression of the disease. This is unlike the action of conventional anti-inflammatory remedies, such as ibuprofen or indomethacin, which may worsen or speed up joint destruction by preventing the formation of new, healthy connective tissue in the joints. The suggested dose of glucosamine sulfate is 500 mg three times daily before meals. Take this dosage for up to six months, then reduce it to between 500 and 1,000 mg daily as a maintenance dose. If this lower dose doesn't provide enough relief, you can increase it to 1,500 mg daily. Many doctors recommend taking chondroitin sulfate along with glucosamine sulfate. Chondroitin helps bring fluid into cartilage, reducing pain and wear and tear. If you take both remedies, the ratio should be 5:4; that is, for each 500 mg glucosamine, take 400 mg chondroitin.

◆ Help prevent cartilage loss by including lots of antioxidant-rich foods in your diet, especially those containing vitamins A, C, and E. Excellent candidates include broccoli, bell peppers, citrus fruits, cabbage, cauliflower, strawberries, and spinach. Because it is difficult to get enough vitamin E in a healthy diet, a supplement that gives you 400–600 IU daily is recommended. Antioxidants help prevent cell damage that leads to cartilage loss.

♦ Oil your joints with omega-3 fatty acids. This type of healthy fat eases the swelling and pain of arthritic joints. Visit your health food store or pharmacy and look for any of the following: evening primrose oil (often abbreviated as EPO), flaxseed oil, borage oil, black currant oil, and fish oil. All are available either as an oil or in capsules. If you take the oil, 1–2 tablespoons daily is recommended; take capsules according to package directions. Flaxseed oil is recommended by many experts, as it contains about twice the omega-3 fatty acids as fish oil. Also, flaxseed oil can easily be included in your diet, so you don't need to take capsules (see "Flaxseed Dressing" below).

Other Options

♦ Exercise. Regular, low-impact movement helps reduce pain, reduces swelling, strengthens the muscles around the joints, releases pain-killing endorphins, and keeps your joints supple. The secret is to be gentle: running or football are not good choices, while swimming, walking, tai chi, yoga, and cycling are.

♦ If you're looking for pain relief, try pepper—red pepper, that is. The capsaicin in red pepper has unique pain-relieving abilities. Creams containing 0.025 and 0.075 percent capsaicin are available over-the-counter. When rubbed into the skin, the capsaicin intercepts the pain signals that travel through your nerves.

FLAXSEED DRESSING

YIELD: 2 SERVINGS

3 tablespoons red wine	2 cloves minced garlic
1$^1/_2$ tablespoons extra-virgin olive oil	2 tablespoons minced fresh parsley
1$^1/_2$ tablespoons flaxseed oil	$^1/_2$ teaspoon sea salt
2 tablespoons red wine vinegar (optional)	2 tablespoons finely ground flaxseeds
	1 tablespoon Dijon mustard

Directions: Combine all ingredients and shake well.

When to See a Doctor

Seek professional help if your joint pain is accompanied by fever, a loss of appetite, or an overall sick feeling; if you experience numbness, burning, tingling, or weakness; or if you have a single joint that is painful, warm, and swollen. You may have an infection or a problem with your nervous system.

REPETITIVE STRAIN INJURY

Do you use a keyboard for several hours a day? Play video games for long periods of time? Cut hair for a living? Work at a checkout counter in a grocery store? Play a musical instrument? All of these activities, and many more, involve repetitive motions of the upper extremities, which include the hands, fingers, wrists, elbows, forearms, or shoulders. Millions of Americans experience inflammation, tingling, numbness, and pain in these body sites because of repetitive movements and have what has been termed repetitive strain injury (RSI). Carpal tunnel syndrome is a type of repetitive strain injury.

Risk Factors for Repetitive Strain Injury

Repetitive strain injury is nothing new. For years, meat and fish packers, and people who use vibrating tools like chain saws and jackhammers have complained of pain and disability in their hands. A high risk for RSI is found in assembly-line workers, cake decorators, postal workers, dentists, and dental technicians. But with the advent of computers and video games and their keyboards, mice, and joysticks, RSI has not only come to the forefront, but it is also now affecting younger and younger people, including children who are "hooked" on computer games.

More Than Repetitive Movements

Repetitive strain injuries can be caused not only by repetitive movements, but by poor posture and stress (which causes muscles to tighten). In fact, all three contribute to RSI in many cases. If these factors continue to be a part of your life, then the condition will get progressively worse. Taking painkillers will only mask the problem, not solve it. Therefore, the best approach is to go directly to the core of the problem.

Remedies

Early treatment is crucial, because healing can be a very slow process. Also, once repetitive strain injuries become too serious, they are often impossible to cure. That's why it's important to recognize the early warning signs (inflammation, tingling, numbness, and pain) so you can take steps to prevent additional damage and heal whatever harm has already occurred. The most obvious solution is to stop whatever activity is causing the injury, but if the repetitive movements are part of your job, that may be easier said than done. In some cases, people work with their employers to find new ways to perform old tasks, or they wear supportive devices, such as wrist supports, to relieve the strain. Working with your employer to eliminate or reduce repetitive strain injuries should be your first step.

Here are additional ways to tackle RSI.

Best Bets

◆ Heal while you sleep. Every night, you spend at least six hours or more sleeping, and the posture you have during that long period can have a big impact on the pain you experience with repetitive strain injuries. The preferred way to sleep when you have RSI is to lie on your unaffected side (the side that is not painful) with a pillow under your head. Place your affected arm on another pillow that you put in front of you. If you prefer to sleep on your back, you'll need three pillows: one for under your head, and one under each of your arms, starting under your shoulders.

◆ Stretch periodically. In many cases, repetitive strain injuries are successfully treated by doing routine stretches, which exercise the nerves and remove stress and tension on muscles. A physical therapist can show you which stretching exercises will best help your particular situation. Don't be surprised if you are given exercises for your back and neck if your wrist and hands are bothering you. Very often, tension in the back and neck contributes to pain in the hands and arms, even though you don't realize it.

◆ Practice RICE. This stands for *rest* (stop or reduce the amount of time you do the offending movements); *ice* (which can reduce swelling and pain); *compression* (use of elastic bandages, along with ice, can reduce swelling); and *elevation* (elevate the injured area above the heart to help reduce swelling).

Other Options

◆ Massage can improve blood flow, release tension, and help eliminate toxins that build up in stressed muscles. Massage works best if done daily. Learn how to self-massage the affected areas, or ask your partner to do a quick massage after work each day.

◆ Improve blood flow. The herb ginkgo biloba can improve blood circulation in your hands and arms, which can reduce symptoms. The recommended dose is 60 mg capsule once daily taken with water.

When to See a Doctor

If you've tried various remedies and you're still experiencing symptoms; or if you are experiencing numbness, clumsiness, or tingling that wakes you up at night, consult with your doctor.

RESTLESS LEGS SYNDROME

You're lying in bed, the blanket is tucked comfortably under your chin, and you're just drifting off to sleep when it starts—a crawling, tingling, fidgety, itchy feeling in your legs. Your legs begin to kick and jerk, and not because you're trying to chase creatures out of bed. Your legs are moving involuntarily. If you don't sleep alone, your partner is probably awake now, too, but not because he or she has felt the creepy crawly sensations. Only you've felt them, because you have restless legs syndrome.

About 12 million Americans have this movement disorder, which is characterized by the above symptoms, as well as by pins and needles and sometimes pain. The sensations are usually accompanied by an overwhelming urge to move the legs or by sudden muscle jerks. In rare cases, the arms are affected as well. The sensations are worse during inactivity, such as sleep, sitting, or lying down.

Symptoms can begin at any age, although it is more common as people get older. Often symptoms get worse with age and can cause severe insomnia in some people.

Causes of Restless Legs Syndrome

Scientists have several theories about why some people have this syndrome. Poor circulation in the legs is one; stress is another. And although it's not hereditary, restless legs syndrome does run in families in about 33 percent of cases.

Various medical conditions and substances seem to exacerbate restless legs symptoms, although the connections are not well understood. They include iron deficiency, pregnancy (19 percent of pregnant women experience this syndrome), vertebral disk disease, end-stage renal disease (up to 50 percent of patients), spinal lesions, and use of caffeine or tricyclic antidepressants, lithium, dopamine antagonists, and selective serotonin reuptake inhibitors.

Remedies

So far no one has a cure for restless legs syndrome, but there are steps you can take to relieve or reduce the symptoms.

Best Bets

♦ Massage your legs before you retire every night. Using the palm and heel of your hand, apply long, firm, downward strokes on your legs, followed by gentle kneading of your calf muscles.

♦ Take magnesium supplements. Taking 400 mg daily, can help keep your legs from kicking. If you have heart or kidney problems, talk to your doctor before taking magnesium supplements.

♦ Manage your stress. If you think stress is the culprit, try relaxation techniques every day. Meditation, yoga, biofeedback, visualization, and tai chi are just a few suggestions.

Other Options

♦ Heat up your legs. The American Sleep Disorders Association recommends taking a hot bath, followed by placing a heating pad on your legs, before going to bed. Do not take the heating pad to bed, however, because you could burn yourself.

♦ Exercise your restlessness away. Choose activities that stretch the leg muscles, such as walking, yoga, dancing, and biking. Gentle stretching exercises are also recommended. Exercise not only improves circulation but helps tone the muscles, which may reduce symptoms.

When to See a Doctor

See your doctor if none of the suggestions bring any significant relief, or if restless legs syndrome is causing you (or your partner!) to lose sleep. Prescription medications such as levodopa/carbidopa, bromocriptine, and pergolide mesylate, which are used to treat Parkinson's disease, are effective, but they have side effects.

RHEUMATOID ARTHRITIS

When the doctor told Dolores that she had arthritis, she found it hard to believe. "But I'm only thirty-two years old," she said. "I'm too young to get arthritis." If the doctor were talking about osteoarthritis (see OSTEOARTHRITIS on page 84), Dolores's statement would be more believable: osteoarthritis rarely strikes people younger than forty. But Dolores has rheumatoid arthritis, a degenerative, autoimmune condition that typically first affects people between the ages of thirty and forty, although it can happen at any age.

Rheumatoid Arthritis Defined

Rheumatoid arthritis is a condition in which the body, for reasons unknown, attacks itself, specifically joint tissue, and surrounding muscle and skin. The membranes in the damaged joints become inflamed, and white blood cells accumulate. These cells release enzymes and other substances that damage the cartilage, bones, tendons, and ligaments within the joint area. The result is pain, limited mobility, swelling, and stiff joints.

Because rheumatoid arthritis is a systemic condition—one that affects the entire body—you can expect to experience more than joint problems. During the early course of the disease, it is common to have fatigue, low-grade fever, a feeling of malaise (feeling ill), inflamed eyes, and loss of appetite. These symptoms may occur even before your joints become painful.

Most people who have rheumatoid arthritis experience a series of ups and downs: sometimes they feel much better, other times they feel much worse. This rollercoaster ride of symptoms often continues for the rest of their lives. For about 20 percent of people with the disease, damage to the joints is significant and leads to serious disability.

Criteria for a Diagnosis of Rheumatoid Arthritis

The Arthritis Foundation has named the following symptoms as the criteria for a definitive diagnosis of rheumatoid arthritis. Seven of the items must be present, and the first five must occur for at least six weeks.

◆ Morning stiffness that lasts for one hour or longer

◆ Swelling in at least one joint

◆ Swelling of at least one other joint

◆ Symmetrical joint swelling, but not including the joint closest to the fingertips

◆ Pain on motion in at least one joint

◆ Presence of nodules (tiny bumps, each about the size of a pea) beneath the skin, usually on the forearm below the elbow

◆ X-ray evidence of rheumatoid arthritis

◆ Presence of rheumatoid factor (an antibody seen on a blood test)

DRUGS FOR RHEUMATOID ARTHRITIS: MORE HARM THAN GOOD?

For many years, the backbone of drug therapy for rheumatoid arthritis has been nonsteroidal anti-inflammatory drugs (NSAIDs)—aspirin, ibuprofen, naproxen, indomethacin, and others. That's because they provide fast relief from pain and inflammation. But in the long run, they also speed up the destruction of the very joint tissues they are supposed to help. These drugs also irritate the digestive system and can cause stomach bleeding. A newer addition to the NSAID family—the COX-2 inhibitor celecoxib—is less likely to cause gastrointestinal bleeding. However, celecoxib should be used with caution as other COX-2 drugs have been withdrawn because of increased heart-related risks.

Another class of drug used to treat rheumatoid arthritis is disease-modifying antirheumatic drugs. One of them, Arava (leflunomide) is a relatively new drug that suppresses the immune system, thereby reducing the body's attack on the joints. So far Arava appears to help inhibit the progression of the disease, but it is not without side effects. They include diarrhea, hair loss, rash, and an increase in liver enzyme levels. Because of the risk of liver damage, liver tests should be done before and for a few months after taking Arava.

Remedies

Researchers now know that early intervention is the best way to limit damage to the joints. That intervention can take the form of a combination of drugs, lifestyle changes, and supplements, depending on the severity of your symptoms. Because it is virtually impossible to avoid experiencing side effects from the many medications available to treat rheumatoid arthritis, many healthcare practitioners suggest making lifestyle modifications and taking nutritional supplements before resorting to drug treatment if possible. Here are some of those alternatives to drug treatment.

Best Bets

◆ Eat a (mostly) plant-based diet. Many doctors believe that food allergies and sensitivities play a significant role in causing inflammation in people who have rheumatoid arthritis. Several studies have shown (and many anecdotal stories report) that eliminating all animal products (including meat and dairy products), except cold-water fish such as herring, tuna, sardines, and salmon, can dramatically reduce pain and inflammation. Because of high mercury levels found in many fish, however, some doctors are recommending that patients avoid fish and instead take 1–2 tablespoons of flaxseed oil daily (which supplies the essential fatty acids like those in fish).

◆ Do periodic juice fasts. For more than fifty years, people in Europe have had excellent results in relieving rheumatoid arthritis symptoms using periodic juice fasting. Fasting promotes elimination of toxins from the body, such as excess calcium, minerals, and acids that are deposited in the joints, and allows the digestive system to rest. Juice fasts, which involve drinking fresh, highly nutritious vegetable juices, should be supervised by your doctor. They typically last three to seven days and can be done several times a year.

◆ Clean up your act. Eliminate alcohol, coffee, sugar, saturated fat, hydrogenated fat, excess salt, and smoking from your life.

Other Options

◆ Practice hydrotherapy. Water has the power to ease pain and improve mobility. When you immerse yourself in a warm pool and perform underwater exercises or swim, you strengthen the muscles around the affected joints without causing injury and pain. You also increase blood circulation and, some scientists believe, slow tissue deterioration. Try to exercise several times a week for about thirty minutes each.

◆ Wax yourself. An at-home hot wax or paraffin treatment kit can provide relief for hands affected by arthritis. Orthopedic supply stores and mail-order companies carry these items. The procedure is simple: you heat the wax in the heating unit, apply it to your hands, and then wrap them in plastic gloves for about ten minutes.

When to See a Doctor

If you are having trouble controlling your symptoms, your joints become inflamed and infected, or you are experiencing side effects from medications (NSAIDs or disease-modifying antirheumatic drugs) such as abdominal pain, gastric distress, or ringing in the ears, contact your doctor. NSAIDs especially are associated with stomach problems, including bleeding and ulcers that can be life threatening.

SHINGLES

Now that you're an adult, do you think your chicken pox days are well behind you? Think again. If you had chicken pox as a child, you may get the "grown-up" version known as shingles, a blistering, painful version of the childhood disease. Both conditions are caused by the same herpes virus, known as varicella zoster virus, or herpes zoster. Instead of the virus going away after a bout of chicken pox, it hides in the nerve cells near the spine, waiting to re-emerge. Twenty percent of people who had chicken pox as children develop shingles as adults.

Shingles Triggers

Stress and a weakened immune system are the main triggers of shingles. Emotional stress, such as the death of a spouse, especially among older people, can set off an outbreak. The good news is that most people who get shingles once don't get it again. If you have AIDS or another disease that impairs the immune system, however, shingles can recur.

Even though shingles is caused by a virus, it is not contagious. However, people with shingles can cause chicken pox in some people who never had chicken pox or the vaccine. Scientists believe that with widespread use of the chicken pox vaccine and with so few people now getting the childhood disease, shingles will eventually become rare.

Signs and Symptoms of Shingles

The virus must be very patient, because in most cases, shingles waits to strike people older than fifty, and about 50 percent of people older than eighty-five get the disorder. When it does appear, it is characterized by moderate to severe pain that pulsates, itches, or tingles, or causes extreme sensitivity in an area of the skin on only one side of the face or body. Usually one to three days after the pain begins, a blistering rash forms on one side of the body. The blisters become filled with fluid and usually scab over in two to three weeks. Headache and fever typically accompany the rash and pain. In 10 to 15 percent of people with shingles, severe pain and sensitivity continues for a month or longer even after the blisters disappear. This condition is called postherpetic neuralgia.

Remedies

The sooner you begin treating shingles, the better your chances of avoiding the pain. Once the blisters appear, remember the warning you gave to your kids if they had chicken pox (or the warning your mother gave to you): don't scratch them, because they can become infected and leave scars. Once treatment begins, the rash and pain usually go away within three to five weeks. Even if you decide to take a prescription medication for shingles (see "When to See a Doctor" below), the following remedies can be used along with the drug.

Best Bets

* Although you have to let the rash run its course, an application of calamine lotion or Burrow's solution (made from Domeboro tablets; available in drugstores) dries out the oozing blisters.

* Capsaicin cream, which contains a pain-relieving substance found in chili peppers, can reduce the severe pain associated with postherpetic neuralgia. Use as directed on the package.

* Squeeze the milky liquid from the inside leaves of an aloe vera plant and apply it to the affected areas several times daily. This herbal remedy soothes blisters.

Other Options

* Place cold compresses or ice packs on painful areas several times daily.

* Adding a supplement of the amino acid lysine could shorten your bout with shingles. During an outbreak, a suggested dose is 500–1,000 mg three times a day. Consult with your doctor before taking this dosage.

When to See a Doctor

In rare cases, blisters appear on the face, putting you at risk of getting herpes in your eyes and causing blindness. If you do have facial blisters, or you experience eye pain, see your doctor immediately. Less serious but still worth a doctor visit as soon as possible is the presence of a fever higher than 101°F or swelling, pus, and redness in the affected areas, as it may indicate a bacterial infection. A doctor can also prescribe any of the drugs available to treat shingles, including acyclovir (Zovirax), famciclovir (Famvir), and valacyclovir (Valtrex). Side effects of these drugs can include nausea, headache, and vomiting.

SORE NIPPLES

Before Rhonda gave birth to her daughter, Chloe, she had decided she would breast-feed for at least six months, perhaps a year. Rhonda's first attempt was awkward and somewhat painful, but she had expected that. After all, nipples are very sensitive, and infants have an amazingly strong suck for such tiny persons. After the first three to four days, Rhonda had expected the pain to go away, but it didn't. In fact, her nipples were very tender and cracked. She was ready to quit breast-feeding until a lactation specialist gave her some advice.

Breast-feeding is the most common cause of sore nipples, and sore nipples are the main reason new mothers stop breast-feeding prematurely. In the vast majority of cases, sore nipples can be remedied very quickly; and new mothers may need to be a bit patient until the soreness subsides.

NATURE MADE

Women in primitive societies have little or no problem with sore nipples associated with breast-feeding, because their breasts are exposed to the air and sunlight, which make them less sensitive. Our ancient ancestors likely had no problems either. But in modern society, women's breasts are covered and protected, so they don't have a chance to "toughen up." So when that eager tiny mouth latches on and sucks every few hours around the clock, your nipples can take a beating.

Nipple soreness usually begins during the first two days of breast-feeding and gets progressively worse until day four or five, and then it begins to go away. By the time the infant is two weeks old, breast-feeding should be pain-free.

Causes of Sore Nipples

The most common cause of nipple soreness is improper latch on and positioning during breast-feeding. "Latch on" is the way the infant places his or her mouth on the nipple. An infant is latched on correctly if his lips are flanged out and the nipple is far back in his mouth. His tongue should be extended over his gums and under the nipple. If his lips are sucked in, you can gently pull them out with your finger. Even a slight improper movement of the infant's lips, tongue, or gums can irritate the nipple tissue and cause soreness. Remember: cats and rats are born knowing how to nurse; humans are not. An infant needs a little practice before he or she gets the hang of it. Most infants learn how to latch on within a few days.

Other causes of nipple soreness may not be as common, but that doesn't mean your nipples will hurt any less. One cause is engorgement, which is when the breasts become overly full of milk. An engorged breast is hard and tight, and the nipple often flattens out, making it difficult for the infant to latch on. Another cause is referred to as nipple switching. Some infants can switch back and forth from breast-feeding to a bottle without any problems. However, because infants use their tongue to press against the hard artificial nipples of bottles, they may do the same thing when breast-feeding, causing the mother's nipple to get sore. If you are breast-feeding it is recommended that you avoid using bottle nipples or pacifiers for at least three to four weeks, until your infant has become more practiced at breast-feeding.

Beware of how you remove your infant from your breast. An infant should never be pulled away from the breast. Instead, pull down on his or her chin, press down on your breast near his mouth, or put your finger in the corner of his or her mouth to break the suction.

In some cases, there are medical reasons for sore nipples, including the presence of thrush, yeast infection, eczema, herpes, impetigo, allergies, and staph infections. If you have any of these conditions, nipple soreness will be only one of the symptoms you'll experience. Treating the underlying condition should remedy the nipple soreness.

Remedies

To stop nipple soreness, you need to know what is causing it. The explanations given here may help you, or you may want to consult with a nurse or lactation specialist. In either case, here are some proven ways to manage sore nipples.

Best Bets

- For dry, cracked nipples, apply hydrogen peroxide onto the crack with a cotton swab. This will kill the bacteria from your baby's mouth, which can get into the crack and cause an infection of your breast.

- Apply anhydrous lanolin to your nipples after you nurse to help prevent cracking, or to help heal cracks if you have them. This is available over-the-counter at drugstores.

◆ Express some colostrum or milk onto your nipples after you nurse and allow it to dry. Human milk helps kill bacteria.

Other Options

◆ Vary breast-feeding positions to relieve some of the pressure on any one part of the nipple.

◆ If your breasts are engorged, massage them, apply heat using hot compresses or a hot-water bottle, and express a small amount of milk before you offer your breast to your infant. You can use this approach even if your breasts are not engorged, as your infant will not have to suck as vigorously until your milk lets down.

When to See a Lactation Specialist

If you're having any of the following problems, contact a lactation specialist: cracked or bleeding nipples, persistent nipple or breast pain during or between feedings, a burning sensation, or pain that lasts for more than one week.

TEMPOROMANDIBULAR DISORDER

Temporomandibular disorder (TMD)—that's a mouthful for a painful condition that, well, affects the mouth and jaw. The pain originates in the temporomandibular joints, the ones that make it possible for us to talk, chew, laugh, and yawn, and which connect the lower jaw to a bone on each side of the head. Unfortunately, these same joints also allow us to grind our teeth and clench our jaw, two causes of TMD usually associated with emotional stress or anxiety. Other causes include arthritis, poorly fitted dentures, and a jaw injury. A family history of TMD also increases your chances of getting the condition.

Symptoms of TMD

People may have been suffering with TMD as far back as ancient times, when Hippocrates described "a group of patients whose teeth are disposed irregularly, crowding one on the other and they are molested by headaches." Some medical historians believe that the painter Van Gogh cut off his ear because of pain associated with TMD. About two-thirds of Americans develop TMD occasionally, and women are four times more likely to get it than men. So what do these people experience?

People with TMD typically have pain in the jaw joint or their chewing muscles on either side of the head, or the pain may radiate to the face, neck, or shoulders. The pain may make it difficult for them to open their mouths, and when they do, they may experience a clicking, popping, or grating sound in the jaw joints. Recurring earaches or headaches are common, and about 20 percent of people who have TMD experience dizziness as well.

Remedies

Because stress, tension, and anxiety are usually at the core of TMD, taking steps to reduce these emotional triggers in your life is critical. Here are some ways to do that, plus other ways to deal with TMD.

Best Bets

◆ Identify the situations that cause you to tense your muscles, clench your jaw, or grind your teeth, and learn to relax. There are dozens of methods you can use to relieve tension; make one or more of them part of your lifestyle. Such methods include yoga, meditation, jogging, visualization, hypnosis, tai chi, progressive relaxation, biofeedback, deep breathing, and journaling.

◆ Press the pain away. If you apply pressure to a special acupressure point on your forearm, you may get significant relief from pain in your cheek muscles. The point is located on the outer forearm, three finger widths below the elbow crease. To find it, place your forearm and hand palm down on a table. Place three fingers at the elbow fold and search for a painful point in that area. Once you find it (and it may be very painful), use your index finger or knuckle on the point and press down using a circular motion with as much pressure as you can tolerate. Keep pressing for thirty to forty seconds. Repeat on your other forearm. If the point is extremely painful, rub the area with ice before you apply pressure.

◆ Apply heat, using a heating pad, a warm washcloth, or a hot-water bottle. Place the heated item on the jaw for fifteen minutes every two hours.

Other Options

◆ Until your pain disappears, eat soft foods, such as cooked rice or potatoes, gelatin, yogurt, soups, bananas, applesauce, cooked cereal, and pasta. Avoid chewy or crunchy foods.

◆ Exercise your face. Because misaligned jaw muscles are a big contributor to TMD pain, balancing these muscles can provide much relief. A quick and easy resistance exercise can help. Place your elbows on a table, bend your arms, and place your chin in your palms, with your fingers on either side of your face. As you gently try to open your mouth, resist with your hands so you can't open it. Then, with your left hand, press on your chin and try to move your jaw sideways. Resist the pressure with your jaw muscles and keep your jaw in line. Repeat on the right side. This entire cycle takes about one minute; repeat the cycle four or five times throughout the day.

When to See a Dentist

In most cases, TMD resolves itself in a week or two with treatment. But it's time to see your dentist if you still have pain after trying various remedies or after taking pain medication; if you have new or unusual symptoms, such as dizziness; or if you have trouble chewing or opening your mouth. You may also want to seek professional help from an osteopath who knows cranial manipulation, a technique that realigns bones in the skull; or a chiropractor, who can correct imbalances in the spine that can affect the jaw. Acupuncturists can also provide pain relief.

TENDINITIS AND BURSITIS

If you're a weekend warrior, or if you have a tendency to "overdo it" at work or at play, tendinitis and bursitis may be familiar to you. That's because both of these conditions are usually caused by overuse or injury, especially in people who may be a bit out of shape, or in those who have bad posture. Occasionally, they are caused by an infection.

Tendinitis and bursitis are characterized by inflammation, irritation, and pain. In tendinitis, the affected part is a tendon, a thick, fibrous cord that attaches to muscles and bones. In bursitis it's a bursa, a small sac located between bone and a moving structure such as a muscle or tendon. Both conditions can occur in people of any age, although they are most common among active adults.

Tendinitis and bursitis are often mistaken for arthritis, because the inflamed tendons and bursae are located near joints, the affected body parts in arthritis. However, unlike arthritis, tendinitis and bursitis are usually temporary, and they do not cause deformity. Tennis elbow and golfer's shoulder are two common types of tendinitis. People who do heavy lifting or repetitive motions, like hammering, tend to get bursitis.

Diagnosing Tendinitis and Bursitis

Because tendons and bursae are usually not visible on x-rays, doctors need to conduct a careful medical history and physical examination to diagnose tendinitis and bursitis. For suspected bursitis, a doctor may inject a needle into the swollen bursa to rule out infection or gout (a metabolic disease characterized by painful inflammation of joints).

Remedies

Although tendinitis and bursitis are not the same ailment, they have very similar symptoms: pain and swelling in or near a joint that may limit motion. Both conditions usually improve significantly or disappear in one to two weeks if they are treated promptly and wisely. Here are some ways to do just that.

Best Bets

◆ Rest the affected area and stop the activity that causes the pain and inflammation. Both these conditions can become worse and chronic if this advice is not followed.

◆ When the pain starts, apply an ice pack to the affected area for twenty minutes three to four times a day for two days. This will help reduce swelling. Then, for the next two days, apply heat for fifteen to twenty minutes, three to four times a day, to relieve pain.

◆ Over-the-counter anti-inflammatory drugs can reduce inflammation. Ibuprofen and aspirin are the most commonly used and most effective. Avoid long-term use of these drugs, however, as they can cause gastrointestinal upset and bleeding.

Other Options

◆ For tendinitis, you may want to wear a splint or strap-support device, depending on the area affected. For tennis elbow, for example, some players wear a Velcro tennis-elbow strap, available in sporting goods stores.

◆ If you prefer natural supplements, try one of the following:

  • *Methylsulfonylmethane (MSM),* a form of organic sulfur, is very effective at relieving pain and inflammation, says Stanley W. Jacob, M.D., professor of surgery at Oregon Health Sciences University in Portland and coauthor of *The Miracle of MSM.* Dosages vary, but start with 2 grams daily (divided and taken with meals). After seven days, increase by another 2 grams if you have not had relief. You can increase the dosage an additional 2 grams if necessary. Increase your dosage gradually, as high doses of MSM can cause loose stools in some people.

- *Turmeric extract* ($\frac{1}{4}$ to $\frac{1}{2}$ teaspoon three times daily) is rich in a substance called curcumin, which is a powerful anti-inflammatory agent. You may opt to take curcumin instead: the suggested dose is one 200 mg capsule or tablet two or three times daily until the pain disappears. Do not take turmeric or curcumin if you are taking nonsteroidal anti-inflammatory drugs, and vice versa, as they can cause a reaction when taken together.

- *Bromelain*, an enzyme found in pineapple, improves blood flow to painful, injured muscles and is also an anti-inflammatory agent. The recommended dosage is 250–500 mg three times daily before meals.

When to See a Doctor

Call your doctor if your bursitis is accompanied by a high fever (more than 101°F) or if the skin around the affected area turns swollen and red. These symptoms indicate an infection of the bursa. If you have tendinitis and the area around the joint appears deformed or discolored, or if the pain and swelling have lasted more than two weeks even though you have been resting the area and you have taken anti-inflammatory drugs, call your doctor.

◆ CHAPTER 5 ◆

The Nether Regions

S ome health problems, even though they affect tens of millions of people and everyone has heard of them, are usually discussed in hushed tones. These health issues are of a more sensitive nature, because they involve the organs of either reproduction or elimination. We've labeled these areas the "nether regions," and we turn to them now to learn how we can treat the annoying ailments that affect them.

ERECTILE DYSFUNCTION

Erectile dysfunction (ED), or impotence, used to be a condition people didn't talk about, even between sexual partners. Now there are TV commercials about ED during prime time. Magazine advertisements boldly offer treatment solutions. Impotence has come out of the closet, so to speak, and into our living rooms.

But that still doesn't mean men are comfortable talking about it. And some doctors still don't like to talk about it with their patients. So what's a man (and his partner) to do? First, it helps to understand a little about impotence.

Erectile Dysfunction Defined

ED is an inability to attain and maintain an erection that is sufficient for satisfactory sexual activity. Up to 30 million men are believed to experience this problem, with prevalence increasing with age. Thus, while about 5 percent of men have ED at age forty, up to 25 percent—with some studies showing 50 percent or higher—experience it at age sixty-five and older.

Although ED can cause significant stress in a man's—and his partner's—life, the underlying cause of ED is medical or physical in up to 90 percent of cases. That statistic offers a lot of hope, because once men identify the cause, they can often treat it and thus eliminate the ED.

Physical and Medical Causes of Erectile Dysfunction

To get and maintain an erection, the penis must receive an adequate blood supply. Therefore, it comes as no surprise that most of the medical problems associated with ED are those that somehow hinder blood flow. They include diabetes (which also affects the nerves), hypertension, high cholesterol, cardiovascular disease, low levels of high-density lipoprotein, stroke, and renal failure. Men who have a neurological condition, such as Parkinson's disease, spinal cord injury, or multiple sclerosis also may experience ED. Trauma to the pelvic region, radiation, and prior pelvic surgery also are associated with this problem.

Several drugs have been identified as causing ED. Antidepressants (including monoamine oxidase inhibitors and tricyclics), most antihypertensive drugs, cimetidine (for duodenal ulcers), finasteride (taken for prostate enlargement or baldness), calcium channel blockers, and ACE inhibitors are all associated with impotence. Physicians sometimes neglect to mention this side effect when prescribing these drugs, so many men don't realize that merely changing their medication could eliminate their ED. (*Note:* never change your medication without your doctor's supervision.)

Psychological Causes of Erectile Dysfunction

In about 10 percent of cases, psychological difficulties are the cause behind erectile dysfunction. The psychological causes can be classified as (1) related to conditions such as psychotic disorders, obsessive-compulsive personality disorder, and sexual deviation; (2) intense fear of failure; (3) a strained relationship with the sexual partner; (4) ignorance about normal sexual function and anatomy; and (5) depression.

Even though a physical problem is usually at the core of a man's ED, psychological factors can soon creep into the picture and compound the situation. You may ask yourself, "Will I be able to get an erection this time?" before every sexual encounter, and the anxiety created can actually hinder blood flow.

Little-Known Contributors to Erectile Dysfunction

Often it's the little things in life that make a big difference. If you smoke, for example, the nicotine constricts the blood vessels and restricts blood flow to the penis. If you are a dedicated bicyclist and have ED, the constant pressure against the main artery that supplies blood to the penis may be damaged. It may be time to take up jogging or swimming.

You may not think that what you have for dinner could have an effect on your sex life, but foods such as hot dogs, smoked sausages, cold cuts, and other packaged meats that contain preservatives called nitrates can hinder sexual function. Even small amounts of alcohol can cause temporary impotence, while excessive use can cause permanent ED. Recreational drugs such as marijuana and cocaine are also known to cause impotence.

Remedies

Although millions of men experience ED and it is a problem that the media has catapulted into the mainstream, many men still don't seek treatment. That is unfortunate, because there are many different approaches to this problem. Several require that you get a prescription from your doctor; those are mentioned under "When to See a Doctor." However, there are some nondrug methods you can try first. Perhaps one will work for you. First, however, if you are taking any of the medications mentioned above and are experiencing ED, please talk to your doctor about taking an alternative drug. Second, consider psychotherapy with a sex therapist even if the cause of your ED is physical and you and your partner are experiencing some psychological difficulties.

Best Bets

◆ Use a vacuum device. Although the thought of using a pump may mar a romantic mood, these devices are effective. A cylinder, with an attached pump that can be hand- or battery-operated, is placed over the penis. When the pump is activated it creates a vacuum, which draws blood into the penis. Once an erection is achieved, a constriction ring is placed at the base of the penis and the cylinder is removed. The ring maintains the erection, usually for about thirty minutes. Occasionally the vacuum can cause some bruising, but no other side effects have been reported.

◆ Take the amino acid arginine. According to Jonathan Wright, M.D., director of the Tahoma Clinic in Kent, Washington, arginine can improve a man's ability to attain an erection. He even suggests that men who are considering Viagra (see "When to See a Doctor" on page 106) should try arginine first. The suggested dosage is 3,000 mg daily; you should expect results after about three to four weeks. Talk to your doctor about arginine before you take it, and don't use it if you have genital herpes or if you are taking lysine supplements.

Other Options

◆ The herb ginkgo biloba improves blood circulation. The suggested dosage is

60 mg daily, but don't expect an erection to happen overnight: it takes about two to six months for results.

◆ Ginseng (*Panax ginseng*) has long been considered to be an aphrodisiac by the Chinese. Studies in animals show that the herb does increase sexual activity and increases testosterone (male hormone) levels. Scientists in Russia have shown ginseng to be useful in treating ED in men. This may be because the herb increases a process called nitric oxide synthesis, which increases blood flow. A suggested dose is 500 mg one to three times daily of a standardized ginseng powder that contains 5 percent ginsenosides (the active ingredients). If the ginsenoside content is 18 percent, take 150 mg one to three times daily.

When to See a Doctor

If none of the home remedies have worked or if you have a total or inconsistent inability to achieve an erection, you may have an undetected medical problem. See a urologist and tell him what measures you have tried and about any medications you are taking. There are several medical approaches, including a prescription for sildenafil citrate (Viagra), tadalafil (Cialis), vardenafil (Levitra), or alprostadil (injectable or pellet), or a surgical procedure in which an implant is placed into the penis.

GENITAL HERPES

It's an epidemic: genital herpes is a sexually transmitted disease that affects 67 million Americans, and the number continues to grow. One reason for the rising numbers is that the virus that causes this infection is easily spread, sometimes by people who don't know they have the virus.

Genital herpes is caused by the herpes simplex virus, or HSV. There are two types of HSV: type 1, which most commonly affects the lips and causes fever blisters or cold sores; and type 2, which typically causes genital herpes. Occasionally, however, HSV type 1 can infect the genitals, and HSV type 2 can infect the mouth. HSV is a sneaky virus, because it hides in certain nerve cells of the body for life and can cause symptoms off and on in some people.

The virus is transmitted from an infected person who is having an outbreak (active disease) to another person during sexual activity. When the disease is active, sores can be visible in the genital region. These sores shed the viruses, which then infect the other person. Often, however, people have an outbreak without any visible sores and unknowingly pass along the disease. Genital herpes can be spread through vaginal, anal, and oral sex.

Symptoms of Genital Herpes

Unfortunately, most people who have genital herpes don't know they have the disease because they either never have symptoms, or they don't recognize them. That's because symptoms can differ among people. The first time someone becomes infected, symptoms usually appear within two to ten days and last two to three weeks. The first symptoms to appear usually include pain in the buttocks, genital area, or legs, along with itching or burning in the genital or anal region. You may feel pressure in the abdomen, and women often experience a fluid or sticky discharge from the vagina.

After a few days, small red sores appear near where the virus entered the body, which may be the penis, vagina, or mouth. Sometimes the sores develop inside the vagina or on the cervix in women, or in the urinary tract of men and women. The sores turn into blisters and become painful open lesions, which crust over and heal without leaving scars. Some people also experience fever, headache, painful urination, swollen glands in the groin area, and muscle aches during their first episode of genital herpes.

HSV: A Frequent Visitor

Once you've been infected by HSV, you can expect to have recurrent outbreaks. After the virus has been active, it retreats and hides in the nerves at the end of the spine. Then, perhaps once a year, perhaps more, the virus can become active again. Scientists don't know why this reactivation, called a recurrence, happens. Some people say that stress, illness, or having a menstrual period triggers an outbreak. However, outbreaks often are not predictable. Recurrences typically are shorter—about one week—than the first episode. Sometimes a recurrence doesn't produce any visible sores or pain, but the disease can still be spread during sexual contact.

Some people who know they have genital herpes learn to recognize the signs that an outbreak is about to happen. Those symptoms—tingling or itching in the genital region, pain in the buttocks or in the leg—let them know to avoid sexual contact until the recurrence runs its course.

Remedies

Scientists are exploring several ways to prevent the spread of HSV. A few different vaccines are in development, but whether they will work, and when they might reach the market, is uncertain. Another approach is a topical microbicide, a substance that kills microbes, such as viruses. The idea is for women to insert the gel or cream into the vagina before intercourse to prevent spread of the infection. This product will probably be available before we see a vaccine.

For now, here are a few ways to treat and deal with genital herpes. There is no cure.

Best Bets

◆ The amino acid lysine can both help prevent outbreaks and speed up the healing process when an outbreak occurs. Although lysine is found in some foods, such as milk, fish, and cheese, taking a supplement is a sure way to get what you need. To prevent outbreaks, take one 500 mg capsule daily. As soon as you notice symptoms, take 1,000 mg daily during the outbreak, then reduce to 500 mg daily once healing has occurred.

◆ Lemon balm (*Melissa officinalis*) cream, made from the herb, "can actually fight herpes," says Varro E. Tyler, Ph.D., Sc.D., author of *The Honest Herbal.* A placebo-controlled, double-blind study found that lemon balm prevents spread of infection, shortens healing time, reduces pain, and may increase the time between recurrences.

◆ Boost the immune system and help control outbreaks. Michael Murray and Joseph Pizzorno, authors of *Encyclopedia of Natural Medicine,* along with other healthcare practitioners, recommend daily doses of vitamin C (2,000+ mg), vitamin E (400–800 IU), zinc (30–60 mg), bioflavonoids (1,000 mg), and copper (1 mg for every 10 mg of zinc).

Other Options

◆ Help dry up the sores by applying any one of the following: diluted lemon juice, vitamin E (squeeze the oil from capsules), or tea tree oil. Use a cotton swab to apply these healing substances.

◆ Apply topical zinc oxide, which can reduce pain and healing time. But this treatment is for men only, as it can irritate vaginal tissue. Women can try topical licorice (as glycyrrhetinic acid) for the same results.

When to See a Doctor

Genital herpes usually doesn't cause major problems in otherwise healthy adults, but if your immune system is compromised, an outbreak of herpes can last many weeks and be severe. Call your doctor if an outbreak is unusually long or troublesome. There are several prescription medications available: acyclovir (Zovirax), which is for first and subsequent episodes; famciclovir (Famvir), for later episodes and prevention of future outbreaks; and valacyclovir (Valtrex), for later episodes. Also, if you are pregnant and have genital herpes, you need to be monitored closely by your doctor before, during, and after the baby is born. A woman can pass the virus to her unborn child, and about 50 percent of infants infected with herpes die or have nerve damage.

HEMORRHOIDS

Two friends meet on the street and they stop for a moment to talk. "Say, Barb, how's your tendinitis? Still acting up?" "No, Sue, it's not bad. I'll be back playing tennis in a few days. How have you been? Did you try that new migraine medication your doctor prescribed?"

That's a believable conversation. Now, substitute the word "hemorrhoids" for "tendinitis" or "migraines." Suddenly the conversation becomes unreal. People don't stop in the middle of the street and chat about their hemorrhoids. Yet hemorrhoids are a big problem in America. About 50 percent of adults have hemorrhoids by the time they reach fifty years of age.

Hemorrhoids are swollen blood vessels in and around the anus and lower rectum. They are usually the result of repeated straining to move stool through the bowel, although they can also result from chronic diarrhea or constipation, pregnancy, or heredity.

Symptoms of hemorrhoids include bright red blood covering the stool, in the toilet, or on toilet paper, pain during bowel movements, itching in or around the anus, and mucus discharge from the anus. Sometimes external hemorrhoids show as a painful swelling or hard lump around the anus. This type of hemorrhoid is known as a thrombosed external hemorrhoid. When an internal hemorrhoid extends through the anus outside the body, it is known as a protruding hemorrhoid, and it is usually very painful and irritated.

Remedies

Obviously hemorrhoids involve some very unpleasant symptoms, but what can you do about them?

Best Bets

◆ Sitz baths have been used for centuries and really work to relieve the pain. To take a sitz bath, sit in warm water (not hot) for ten to fifteen minutes several times a day, especially after a bowel movement.

◆ For external hemorrhoids, apply witch hazel or a cold compress to the affected area several times a day.

◆ Gently apply a dab of petroleum jelly just inside the anus to help make bowel movements less painful.

Other Options

◆ Modify your diet. Eat plenty of vegetables, fruit, bran cereals, whole-grain products, and drink at least eight glasses of water daily. Avoid meat, animal fat, and alcohol.

◆ Be kind to your bottom: dampen your toilet paper with water before using it, or use cotton balls or alcohol-free baby wipes.

When to See a Doctor

If bleeding lasts for more than a few days, you may have a more serious problem, such as colon cancer. Or, if the pain is severe or persistent, you may need to have the hemorrhoids removed by a doctor, which often can be done on an outpatient basis.

JOCK ITCH

You don't have to be a jock or an athlete to experience jock itch, an itchy, uncomfortable feeling in the groin, anal, and inner thigh areas. You don't even have to be a male (yes, females can get this condition, too). Jock itch is an equal opportunity infection that is caused by a fungus (called tinea cruris), which thrives in dark, damp places, such as the genital area.

The name jock itch comes from jock strap, a male athletic supporter, which when worn during a workout, stored in a poorly ventilated locker, and then worn again before being washed creates a perfect environment in which tinea crusis can grow. Women's clothing such as panties and panty hose, under similar conditions, can host the same fungus.

Signs and Symptoms of Jock Itch

In both men and women, jock itch causes chafed, irritated, and itchy skin in the groin, inner thighs, and anal or pubic areas. Sometimes the skin becomes scaly. Jock itch commonly occurs during hot, humid weather and among people who perspire heavily or who are overweight. It is possible for the fungus to be transmitted from the groin to the feet, as the same fungus is responsible for athlete's foot. The fungus can also be transmitted on towels or clothing, so don't share these items.

Remedies

Prevention is key. Even if you use one of the over-the-counter products discussed below, jock itch will come back if you don't practice preventive measures. So here are ways to both treat and prevent jock itch.

Best Bets

◆ Over-the-counter cream products that contain miconazole or clotrimazole are effective against jock itch. Another is a product called Zeasorb-AF, a superabsorbant powder with an antifungal ingredient. Apply these products as directed. Use these products for a month to make sure the fungus has been killed. Even though jock itch and athlete's foot are caused by the same fungus, don't use products specified for athlete's foot on the groin area, as they may contain ingredients that can irritate that sensitive area. Preventive measures (see "Other Options" below) must be taken at the same time you use miconazole or clotrimazole if you want results.

◆ Tea tree oil (*Melaleuca alternifolia*) is an excellent natural antibacterial product. Dilute 2 to 3 drops of tea tree oil with 5 to 6 drops of a carrier oil, such as almond oil, and apply the mixture to the affected area several times a day.

Other Options (Preventive Measures)

◆ Change your underwear. Men, if you're wearing tight briefs, switch to boxers. Tight underwear helps create a perfect environment in which the fungus can thrive. Your underwear should be 100 percent cotton instead of synthetic fabrics, because cotton allows for air circulation.

◆ Watch how you wash. Use antibacterial soap; never use perfumed soaps to wash your groin or anal areas. After bathing or swimming, always dry yourself carefully and apply a light dusting of baby powder to your genital area.

◆ Care for your clothes. Don't store damp clothing in a locker or gym bag. Change your athletic supporter and underwear every day and wash them in hot water.

When to See a Doctor

With treatment, most cases of jock itch clear up within a few weeks. However, if your symptoms are still significant after two weeks of self-care, consult your doctor. You should also call your doctor if the rash gets worse or spreads, or if the condition becomes chronic.

MENOPAUSE

Unlike the majority of conditions discussed in this book, menopause is *not* a medical problem—it is a natural change in a woman's life cycle. It can, however, cause a variety of symptoms that can range from barely noticeable to unbearable.

Menopause is the end of menstruation and a woman's reproductive period. For most women, this change of life occurs naturally between the ages of forty-five and sixty years as their sex hormone levels gradually decline. Menopause can occur earlier, however, as a result of a hysterectomy (removal of the uterus or ovaries—or both), illness such as anorexia or bulimia, or severe stress.

Perimenopause

Menopause doesn't happen suddenly—it is a gradual process that typically takes several years and generally starts when a woman is between forty-two and fifty-five. This period is called perimenopause, a time when the ovaries become less and less sensitive to signals to produce estrogen and progesterone. As a result, the ovaries become less likely to release a mature egg each month. The menstrual cycle becomes irregular, and eventually it stops completely. Usually, doctors declare that a woman has entered menopause if she has not had a menstrual period for at least twelve consecutive months and blood tests show she has low levels of estrogen and high levels of follicle-stimulating hormone.

Common Symptoms of Perimenopause and Menopause

Perhaps the most common symptom of perimenopause and menopause is the hot flash. Like a news flash, a hot flash comes on unexpectedly and usually with a bang. About 50 percent or more of women experience these episodes. During a hot flash, you feel unbearably hot and your face and sometimes other parts of your body perspire a great deal. The sensation usually lasts two to three minutes and can recur at any time. Hot flashes tend to be most intense during the first few years of perimenopause.

Other symptoms of menopause can include headache, fatigue, nervousness, irritability, insomnia, heart palpitations, aches and pains, vaginal dryness, and emotional stress. Sex drive may change: for some women it increases, for others it decreases.

Most if not all of the symptoms associated with menopause are linked to the decline in estrogen levels. Estrogen plays a key role in maintaining cardiovascular health and in helping bones retain their calcium. Therefore, the sharp decline in this hormone needs to be addressed by women who are in their perimenopausal and menopausal years to prevent osteoporosis and heart disease.

Remedies

Although menopause is associated with many different symptoms, addressing the root cause of those complaints—the decline in estrogen levels—is one of the best ways to tackle them. Throw in a few lifestyle modifications, like those below, and you can sail through menopause.

Best Bets

◆ Increase your consumption of foods that are rich in plant estrogens (phytoestrogens). Soybeans and foods made from them—tofu, soy milk, soy yogurt, miso, aburage, koridofu, tempeh, and textured vegetable protein—are the best sources. As little as 2 ounces of soy products each day may be sufficient to reduce your symptoms. Soy also reduces the risk of heart disease and cancer. Phytoestrogens are also found in apples, barley, cabbage, flaxseeds, oats, olive oil, pumpkin, rice, sesame seeds, split peas, and yams.

◆ Soy supplements can be taken instead of or in addition to adding soy products to your diet. Soy isoflavones are phytochemicals derived from soybeans and available in supplement form. If you haven't added soy foods to your diet, take 250 mg of soy isoflavones up to three times daily. If you eat some soy, take 250–500 mg daily.

◆ The herb black cohosh boosts production of estrogen and helps eliminate hot flashes. Look for an extract standardized to contain 2.5 percent triterpenes per tablet and take 20–40 mg twice daily.

Other Options

◆ Follow the WED—water, exercise, and diet—rule. Water: Drink eight 8-ounce glasses of pure water daily to help reduce menopausal symptoms and prevent dehydration, which can occur with hot flashes. Exercise: Regular weight-bearing exercise (walking, low-impact aerobics, jogging, dancing) for at least thirty minutes four to five times a week helps prevent osteoporosis, helps heart health, and relieves stress and pain. Diet: Avoid sugar, alcohol, chocolate, caffeine, and red meat, all of which worsen menopausal symptoms. Increase intake of fresh fruits and vegetables, soy foods, and whole grains.

◆ Take gamma-linolenic acid (GLA), an important and powerful essential fatty acid. GLA is necessary for the production of prostaglandins, hormonelike chemicals that are critical for bone formation and that also relieve menopausal symptoms. Take 1 tablespoon (or 500–1,000 mg) flaxseed oil twice daily, plus 500–1,000 mg black currant seed, borage, or evening primrose oil two to three times daily.

When to See a Doctor

Menopause is a natural event, thus a healthcare practitioner who is willing to explore alternative remedies, including lifestyle modifications and natural hormones, can usually make the transition easier for you. If you are experiencing severe symptoms of menopause and you are not getting relief from various remedies, you may want to talk to a doctor about hormone replacement therapy (HRT).

PREMENSTRUAL SYNDROME

In England in the 1980s, Sandie Craddock was tried for stabbing and killing a fellow employee. Her defense counsel argued that Craddock suffered from premenstrual syndrome (PMS) and therefore had diminished responsibility for the crime. When the verdict came down, it was decided that Craddock had stabbed the woman in a fit of rage and her murder charge was reduced to manslaughter.

Before Craddock was sentenced, she was treated with the hormone progesterone for three months to see if she would respond to treatment. She calmed down significantly, so the court decided that PMS was a mitigating factor in the crime and sentenced Craddock to probation only, as long as she continued to receive progesterone treatment.

Beware: PMS Ahead

Fortunately, Sandie Craddock's case is the exception rather than the rule. Although there have been a few other PMS-defense cases since that time, the medical phenomenon known as premenstrual syndrome does not drive the vast majority of women to commit violent crimes. It can, however, cause a wide variety of symptoms, ranging from mild to severe, in an estimated 90 percent or more of women.

Premenstrual syndrome is a condition in which various physical and emotional symptoms surface the week or two before menstruation begins. Symptoms may last a few hours, a day or two, or up to two weeks. The symptom list is long, but the most common ones include anxiety, crying spells, depression, mood swings, food cravings, swelling of the fingers and ankles, abdominal bloating, breast pain or tenderness, headache, backache, and weight gain.

Cause of PMS

The treatment ordered for Sandie Craddock gives you a hint as to the cause of PMS: hormone changes. Dramatic hormonal changes occur in a woman's body during the seven to fourteen days before menstruation. For some women, the fluctuations in estrogen and progesterone throw body and mind into temporary turmoil. Therefore, taming those hormonal swings can provide much relief.

Remedies

There are nearly as many ways to treat PMS symptoms as there are symptoms. Women need to try several different approaches to find which ones work best for them. Here are a few of the ones many women find effective.

Best Bets

◆ Natural progesterone (as opposed to the synthetic drug, progestin) is highly effective in treating PMS symptoms, especially breast tenderness and pain and fluid retention. Dosages can range from 50–400 mg daily for twenty-one days, used topically (in a cream), orally, or vaginally. Natural progesterone is available over-the-counter and from compounding pharmacies and should be used according to package directions. Micronized progesterone USP is the form that is best absorbed by the body. You may wish to discuss the use of natural progesterone with your healthcare practitioner.

◆ Modify your diet. Food has a significant impact on PMS symptoms. Increase your consumption of vegetable protein (such as legumes, soy foods), fish, and vegetables (especially leafy green ones). Reduce your consumption of dairy products (linked with irritability and mood swings), salt and salty foods (fluid retention), alcohol (dehydration), and refined carbohydrates, including sugar, corn sweeteners, white-flour foods, and fruit juice. Eliminate meat, as it promotes the absorption of estrogen from the intestinal tract, which then leads to a hormone imbalance.

◆ A high-potency multivitamin and mineral supplement can often relieve many PMS symptoms, because nutritional deficiencies contribute to hormone imbalance. If the supplement you chose does not contain the recommended amounts of the following B vitamins, you will need to take a vitamin B complex supplement: 25 mg of each of the B vitamins, two to three times daily, plus 50–100 mg of vitamin B_6. Also, you should add a magnesium supplement (250–500 mg daily), as this mineral helps relieve menstrual cramps.

Other Options

◆ The herb chaste berry (*Vitex agnus castus*) relieves PMS symptoms. Take 200 mg of standardized extract three times daily during the two weeks before the anticipated start of your period. You should notice significant improvement after one month.

◆ Exercise. You are much less likely to experience PMS symptoms if you walk briskly for thirty to forty-five minutes five days a week. Other types of aerobic exercise, such as dancing, handball, bicycling, and jogging are excellent as well.

When to See a Doctor

It usually takes a month or two of trying different approaches before you will notice an improvement in symptoms. Dietary changes, herbs, and supplements do not work overnight. However, if you have tried various remedies and your symptoms are not improving or are unbearable, see your healthcare practitioner.

PROSTATE PROBLEMS

Women are not the only ones who experience unpleasant symptoms caused by a shift in their hormone levels. Around age forty, the prostate gland in men begins to undergo changes that are related to shifts in hormone levels. In men, the hormones in question are testosterone and, to a lesser degree, prolactin and a few others as well.

As a man's testosterone levels begin to decline, there is a parallel increase in the amount of a metabolic by-product of testosterone called dihydrotestosterone. This increase, along with a rise in the amount of prolactin and varying levels of other hormones, prompts the body to produce too many prostate cells. The result is an enlarged prostate, known as benign prostatic hyperplasia or benign prostatic hypertrophy (BPH).

In some men, an enlarged prostate can eventually lead to another condition known as prostatitis, an infection of the prostate gland. We discuss both BPH and prostatitis below.

Benign Prostatic Hyperplasia

At least 50 percent of men forty-five years of age or older have some degree of prostate enlargement. Because there are rarely any symptoms during the early stages, most men who have BPH don't realize anything is wrong until they notice they are having difficulties with urination. The most common symptoms include partially obstructed flow of urine, reduced force of the urine stream, dribbling after urination, an inability to completely empty the bladder, and having to urinate frequently, but with little flow.

These symptoms are the result of the enlarged prostate squeezing or pressing against the urethra, the tube through which urine and semen flows. As the prostate grows larger, the urine flow is affected more and more. Fortunately, growth is usually very slow; however, it is not so slow that men should not take treatment steps immediately.

Prostatitis

If urine is not completely emptied from the bladder, it can stagnate in the bladder and lead to an infection. Urine can remain in the bladder even if you don't have any other symptoms of BPH. As the infection sets in, however, the prostate becomes tender and inflamed. Symptoms then appear, including difficulty urinating, fever, back pain, blood in the urine, pain during urination, chills, and pain in the area between the genitals and the anus.

How to Prevent Prostate Problems

Prevention should always be your number-one priority, and there are steps you can take to prevent prostate problems.

◆ Include lots of tomatoes and tomato products in your diet. Tomatoes contain phytochemicals, including lycopene, that promote and improve prostate health.

◆ Eat a low-fat diet and eliminate saturated fat (meat, butter, cheese) from your diet. A low-fat diet significantly reduces your risk of developing prostate problems.

- Reduce and manage stress. Both emotional and physical stress affect hormone levels and can lead to prostate enlargement.

- Avoid alcohol and caffeine, both of which are associated with urinary problems.

- If you notice any signs or symptoms of prostate problems, see your doctor for an examination to identify the condition and to rule out prostate cancer. BPH caught in the early stages can be treated effectively at home.

Remedies

When treated in the early stages, it is possible to treat BPH on your own and avoid medication. Do consult with your healthcare practitioner. Prostatitis, however, generally requires antibiotic treatment. You can enhance your treatment with the suggestions below under "Other Options."

Best Bets

- Saw palmetto is an herb with a proven track record for fighting prostate enlargement. The herb works because it is a 5-alpha reductase inhibitor, which means it reduces the amount of testosterone that is converted into dihydrotestosterone. Saw palmetto can increase the urinary flow rate by more than 50 percent and reduce retention of urine in the bladder by about 40 percent. The recommended dosage is 150–250 mg twice daily of an extract standardized to contain 85 to 95 percent essential fatty acids and plant sterols.

- Zinc provides several essential benefits. One, it reduces the levels of prolactin. Two, like saw palmetto, it suppresses the activity of 5-alpha reductase, thus reducing the production of prostate cells. Zinc should be taken with food to prevent stomach upset. The suggested dosage is 15–60 mg daily of zinc oxide or zinc picolinate. (Some healthcare practitioners recommend even higher amounts. However, high doses of zinc can compromise the immune system if taken for long periods of time. If you want to take a higher dosage, consult a physician first.) When taking zinc, also take 2–4 mg copper, as these two minerals compete for absorption by the intestinal tract.

- To promote absorption of zinc and reduce levels of prolactin, take 50–100 mg vitamin B_6 daily, between meals. Also take a vitamin B complex supplement once daily, but not at the same time as the B_6 dose.

Other Options

- If you are taking antibiotics for prostatitis, also take probiotic supplements during and for two weeks after the treatment course. Antibiotics destroy the beneficial bacteria in your intestinal tract, and probiotics can restore them. Take acidophilus or bifidobacteria (or a mixture) according to package directions.

✦ The herb oregano has antibacterial powers. For prostatitis, take 75 mg of standardized extract three times daily. Another botanical product, Cernilton (an extract of flower pollen), has been used to treat prostatitis and BPH for more than forty years in Europe. The recommended dosage is 63–126 mg two to three times daily.

When to See a Doctor

Because the symptoms of BPH and prostate cancer can be similar, you should see your doctor for tests to identify the cause of your difficulties. If prostate cancer has been ruled out and you experience a worsening of symptoms during self-treatment, or if you develop new ones, consult your physician. The National Cancer Institute recommends that all men older than fifty have a yearly blood test for the prostate-specific antigen (PSA) for cancer.

STRESS INCONTINENCE

Have you ever laughed, coughed, or sneezed so hard that you wet yourself? It's a common occurrence, especially if you get a case of the giggles or you're laughing uncontrollably. Typically a few drops or a dribble of urine escape involuntarily, and after perhaps a few moments of embarrassment (even though no one else probably noticed the "problem"), you go about your business.

But for millions of women in America, stress incontinence—leaking of urine due to sudden or sustained exertion, such as coughing, bending over, jogging, or jumping—is a chronic problem. Although stress incontinence can happen to anyone at any age, it is most common in women, especially those forty-five years and older.

Causes of Stress Incontinence

In women, the bladder is sandwiched between the uterus and pelvic floor muscle. The bladder walls are composed of muscle that stretches to accommodate the influx of urine from the kidneys. A normal adult bladder can hold about 16 ounces of urine, but the "urge" to urinate usually comes when there are 4 to

6 ounces in the bladder. At the neck of the bladder is a ring of muscle that acts like a door, allowing urine out, but also keeping it in. In people who have stress incontinence, the muscles in the bladder neck aren't strong enough to hold in the urine when pressure from the abdomen increases.

Experts say that pregnancy and menopause are two reasons why the pelvic floor muscles lose their strength. Compounding the loss of muscle strength is movement. Many women who engage in exercise or sports notice some urine leakage, especially as they get older. In fact, up to 47 percent of healthy middle-aged women who exercise regularly have some stress incontinence. But it need not be a source of embarrassment.

Remedies

Because the majority of people who experience stress incontinence are mature women, the remedies discussed are targeted for them. If you are experiencing incontinence unrelated to stress, please consult with your physician.

Best Bets

- Drug-free, painless, and free—could you ask for a better remedy? Kegel exercises are a highly effective way to strengthen your pelvic floor muscles and thus minimize or even eliminate stress incontinence. You can do them while sitting or lying down; while watching television or sitting at a red light. Here's all you need to do:

  - Firmly tense the muscles around your vagina and anus by inwardly lifting and squeezing them. Pretend you are stopping the flow of urine. (However, do not practice Kegel exercises when you are urinating.)

  - Hold the contraction for a count of five, then relax.

  - Repeat the exercise ten times, two to three times a day. Eventually work up to holding the contractions for a count of ten and repeating the exercise twenty times, three to four times a day.

  - Do not hold your breath or strain while doing these exercises.

  - Be patient. It takes about six weeks to see a definite improvement. You will need to do these exercises daily and probably indefinitely.

- Avoid sports and exercises that weaken the pelvic floor muscles. These include activities like running, high-impact aerobics, tennis, skiing, and horseback riding. Low-risk activities include swimming, bicycling, walking, and low-impact aerobics.

◆ Limit intake of foods and beverages that can irritate the bladder, such as carbonated drinks, tea, chocolate, citrus fruits, tomatoes, apple juice, alcohol, spicy foods, and foods that contain caffeine or the sweetener aspartame.

Other Options

◆ If you are overweight, lose weight. Extra pounds are a contributing factor in incontinence.

◆ If you are taking any type of over-the-counter or prescription medication, check with your doctor or pharmacist to see if it has incontinence as a side effect. You may need to switch to another drug. Never, however, stop taking prescription medication without your doctor's approval.

When to See a Doctor

See your doctor if you are experiencing incontinence that is unrelated to stress; the stress incontinence is not responding to Kegel exercises or is getting worse despite the exercises; you have a urinary tract infection along with incontinence; you've had prior radical pelvic surgery or radiation treatment; or you have a history of recurrent urinary incontinence.

URINARY TRACT INFECTIONS

Christine came back from her honeymoon in Bermuda with a tan, a suitcase full of beach wear, and a case of honeymoon cystitis. Cystitis, the most common type of urinary tract infection, can be triggered by sexual intercourse. Not all cases of urinary tract infections are caused by sexual activity, however. Improper hygiene is a major cause of infection.

A urinary tract infection is an inflammation and/or infection of the lower part of the urinary tract, which includes the bladder and urethra (the tube that transports urine in women, and urine and sperm in men). While cystitis refers to a bladder infection, urethritis is an infection of the urethra. If the infection travels up to the kidneys, which is a more serious problem, it is called pyelonephritis.

Most urinary tract infections are caused by bacteria, *Escherichia coli,* which are normally found in the large intestine. Sometimes, however, these bacteria travel from the anus to the urethral opening and move up to the bladder. This can occur if, after using the toilet, you wipe from back to front instead of the reverse, allowing bacteria to be introduced to the urethra. If the conditions are right—for example, if urination does not remove the bacteria in a timely manner or if the lining of the bladder is unable to resist the bacterial invasion—an infection occurs.

Symptoms of a Urinary Tract Infection

If your bladder or urethra is infected or inflamed, you may experience lower abdominal pain (which indicates that the bladder is involved), along with burning or stinging before, during, or immediately after urination. You may have a frequent urge to urinate but only release a small amount each time. There may be pus or blood in the urine, and the urine may have a strong smell, perhaps like fish. Pain in the back above the waist (indicating involvement of the kidneys) also occurs, as does fever.

Women Beware

Women are much more likely to experience a urinary tract infection than men, largely because of their anatomy. In fact, 20 percent of women experience a urinary tract infection each year. The main reason is that women have a shorter urethra than men, which gives bacteria an easier and quicker journey to the bladder. Another reason is that bacteria can be pushed into the urethra during intercourse. Use of tampons or a diaphragm can also irritate the base of the bladder.

Urinary tract infections are common during pregnancy, because the pressure of the enlarged uterus against the bladder can make completely emptying the bladder difficult. When small amounts of urine remain in the bladder, infection can occur. After menopause women can become more susceptible to urinary tract infections because the lining of the urinary tract may become thinner, making it more vulnerable to irritation.

How to Prevent Urinary Tract Infections

To help prevent urinary tract infections, and to ease the discomfort they can cause, consider the following tips:

◆ Reduce or eliminate your intake of caffeine, nicotine, citrus fruits, and alcohol, all of which can irritate the urinary tract.

◆ Avoid refined sugar, because bacteria thrive on sugar.

◆ Never delay urinating unnecessarily. Retaining urine in the bladder can lead to infection.

◆ Don't wear tight underwear or pants.

- Avoid using bubble bath, bath salts, feminine hygiene products, and scented soaps, which can irritate the urethra.
- Urinate before and after sexual intercourse to help flush out bacteria. Also, drink 8 ounces of pure water before and after intercourse.

Remedies

You may decide to self-treat after seeing your doctor, who will do a urine analysis and urine culture to identify the bacteria that are causing your problem. The typical treatment for urinary tract infections is a course of antibiotics. However, if promptly treated, mild cases can be effectively eliminated using self-treatment. Here are the steps you need to take.

Best Bets

- Drink lots of pure water, and often, to flush the bacteria out of your bladder. The longer bacteria stay in your bladder, the more they will multiply, and the more pain they will cause. You are drinking enough water if your urine is clear. It usually takes at least six glasses of water per day to achieve this goal.
- Take 1,000 mg of vitamin C two to three times daily. Vitamin C can acidify the urine, which helps kill the bacteria. If you are also taking antibiotics, discuss the use of vitamin C with your doctor. Some antibiotics are not effective in acidic urine. (Also, if you are taking antibiotics, be sure to take a probiotic agent such as acidophilus or bifidobacteria to restore the healthy bacteria in your urinary tract. Follow package directions, and take the probiotics during and for two weeks after antibiotic therapy.)
- Drink cranberry or blueberry juice. These fruits contain quinolic acid, which causes an acidic reaction that helps eliminate the infection. Drink at least three 8 ounce glasses of pure unsweetened juice daily. If you cannot tolerate cranberry juice, you can take cranberry extract, 500 mg two or three times daily, until the infection clears.

Other Options

- The herb uva ursi has been used for centuries to treat urinary problems. Take 100 mg of standardized extract two or three times daily for three to four days. Although this herb is effective, it causes mild irritation in some people. Therefore, drink several cups of soothing corn silk tea each day you take the extract.

❖ The recommended homeopathic remedy is cantharis, which relieves the burning pain associated with urination. Take one dose 12x or 6c three to four times daily for two to three days.

When to See a Doctor

Generally, anyone who has symptoms of urinary tract infection should see a doctor before attempting self-treatment. This is especially important if your urine is bloody or contains pus, or if you have back pain as one of your symptoms. It's also important to consult a physician if you experience urinary tract infections frequently, say two or three within a few months' time. This may indicate an anatomical abnormality or another underlying problem.

VAGINITIS

When Brenda experienced a bout of vaginal itching, she believed she knew what to do. Yet after treating herself with an over-the-counter remedy and following the directions explicitly, her condition got worse. Confused, she went to her gynecologist, who took a culture and told Brenda that she had bacterial vaginitis. Brenda had purchased a product that treats yeast vaginitis, but which is ineffective against bacteria. "I never knew there was more than one kind of vaginitis," she said. "Now I do."

Brenda is not alone. Although 95 percent of women questioned in a Gallup survey had heard of yeast vaginal infections, only 36 percent had ever heard of bacterial vaginitis, which is actually more common than the yeast variety. Perhaps because of the widespread availability of over-the-counter treatments for yeast vaginitis and advertisements for them, women are not aware that there are other types, which will not respond to these medications.

Vaginitis is a general term for various types of vaginal infections, each of which is caused by different organisms. The most common types are caused by yeast (monilia), bacteria (*Gardnerella vaginalis*), and protozoa (*Trichomonas vaginalis*).

Each type of vaginitis must be treated differently, therefore an accurate diagnosis is important. The test can be done in just a few minutes in a doctor's office or clinic using pH paper and a microscope. Both bacterial and protozoan vaginitis must be treated by a physician, so here we focus on yeast vaginitis. All three forms, if left untreated, can travel up the genital tract and cause pelvic inflammatory disease, infection of the fallopian tubes, or other complications, so if you have yeast vaginitis, it is important that you treat it promptly.

Yeast Vaginitis

Yeast vaginitis, often referred to as candida, affects most women at least once in their lives. It is caused by one of many types of fungi called *Candida* and other organisms normally found in the vagina, mouth, and digestive tract. These fungi/yeasts live in a delicately balanced environment that, when disrupted by use of antibiotics, birth control pills or steroids, stress, pregnancy, warm weather, a compromised immune system, or diabetes, can result in an infection. Obesity, prolonged exposure to moisture, and poor feminine hygiene may also cause yeast vaginitis.

The telltale signs of yeast infections usually include an itchy red vulva and vagina, and an odorless, white, cottage-cheese-like discharge. Burning and pain with urination are common as well. One hint that a vaginal infection may not be caused by yeast is that bacterial and protozoan vaginitis are accompanied by a gray or yellow-green discharge that has an odor.

How to Prevent Yeast Vaginitis

Whether you already have a yeast infection or you want to ward one off, there are several preventive measures you can take, beginning with your choice of clothing—here my motto is "think cotton." Cotton breathes and prevents moisture buildup, so wear 100 percent cotton underwear. If you must wear panty hose, only wear those that have a cotton crotch. Although panty hose can be quite confining, you want to wear loose-fitting clothing whenever possible. Tight jeans and underwear promote infection.

When it comes to the laundry, avoid enzyme-containing laundry detergents. It is also best to wash your underwear in hot water with chlorine bleach, as this kills any microorganisms that can cause vaginitis. To prevent any intestinal microorganisms from entering the vagina, always remember to wipe from front to back after using the toilet. And although we all like to smell nice, avoid use of bath oils, scented soaps, bubble bath, feminine deodorants, and douches, unless your doctor specifically prescribes them or they are herbal.

Remedies

Once you have been properly diagnosed as having yeast vaginitis by a healthcare practitioner, you can choose to treat yourself. Do it promptly, however, as the infection can make its way into your genital tract and cause more serious infections.

Best Bets

♦ Over-the-counter products include antifungal creams and vaginal suppositories, including Femstat, Monistat, and Gyne-Lotrimin, among others. Follow the directions; do not stop treatment before the recommended time, even if you feel better.

♦ An herbal douche can be very effective against yeast infections. Try one of the following, douching once or twice a day for five days, then once a day for five more days.

   • Combine 20 drops of an echinacea and goldenseal formula extract, 6 drops of tea tree oil, and 1 tablespoon of liquid calendula extract in 2 cups of water.

   • Mix 40 drops each of liquid extract of goldenseal and calendula and 2 tablespoons of aloe vera gel in 2 cups of water.

   • Mix 4 tablespoons of white or apple cider vinegar in 1 cup of water.

♦ A boric acid douche also can be effective. Dilute 1 teaspoon of boric acid in 32 ounces of tepid water. Douche once or twice daily until the infection clears.

Other Options

♦ Help maintain a healthy balance of microorganisms in your vagina and intestinal tract by taking *Lactobacillus acidophilus* supplements every day (according to package directions) or by eating yogurt that contains live acidophilus cultures every day.

♦ Garlic has good antifungal properties. Take 500 mg of aged garlic extract three times daily for seven to ten days.

When to See a Doctor

You should see your doctor if any of the following occur: if your infection has not improved significantly after several days of self-treatment; if you develop a mouth infection (commonly known as thrush); if you are or might be pregnant; or if you are experiencing pelvic or abdominal pain.

✦ CHAPTER 6 ✦

Tummy Troubles

f you stop to consider the number and variety of substances you consume daily, it's no wonder you occasionally, or perhaps often, experience some kind of gastrointestinal distress. In fact, we've become so accepting of tummy troubles that there are several drugs on the market that people are urged to take *before* they eat certain foods in anticipation of problems. Thus, if you can't tolerate milk products, or beans, or spicy foods, there are medications you can take before eating these foods that will allow you to enjoy them with little or no problems.

In this chapter we explore the range of stomach (and intestinal) troubles that may plague you and how you can avoid them or treat them naturally.

BELCHING

It happens quickly. You feel the pressure rising in your throat. You put your hand to your mouth to muffle the sound, but some still escapes. You burp, and the people sitting next to you in your office or restaurant or train pretend they didn't hear it. But you know they did. And you're embarrassed.

But all you did was belch. Or, according to the dictionary, you "voided" a small quantity of gas, a process known as eructation. Doesn't that definition make a burp sound a bit more sophisticated? In fact, in some cultures, belching after a good meal is considered good manners and a compliment to the chef.

Causes of Belching

Normally, the air in your stomach travels down into the intestinal tract. If, however, the valve between the esophagus and stomach (called the lower esophageal sphincter, or LES) relaxes and allows air from the stomach to go up into the esophagus, it is released through the mouth and makes a sound.

Air gets into the stomach in a process called aerophagia (swallowing air), which occurs during eating, drinking, smoking, chewing gum, and even seemingly harmless activities like sucking on pen caps or toothpicks. People who are very nervous or anxious tend to swallow more air than other people, because they take it into both the windpipe and food pipe during anxious moments.

Belching after eating is common, and occurs for several reasons. One is the fact that you swallow air while eating; another is that the air already in the stomach is displaced by the food in the stomach, forcing the air to move. Certain foods help the LES relax, especially alcohol, mints, onions, carbonated beverages, and tomatoes. So if you're eating a pizza with onions and washing it down with a beer or soda, beware! However, even the mere act of eating can cause you to belch.

Remedies

For the most common causes of belching—those we've talked about—the remedies listed here will probably resolve your problem. If, however, you don't get relief, you may want to see a doctor to determine if your belching is caused by a medical condition.

Best Bets

♦ Relax. Chronic belching is often caused by anxiety and stress. Make a note of when you experience belching episodes and see if they are associated with stressful or anxious situations. Many people find that once they learn to relax (using meditation, yoga, deep breathing, visualization, or relaxation exercises) and think about the air they are swallowing, they can stop swallowing excess air and eliminate their belching problem.

♦ Ginger (two 550 mg capsules of powdered herb or 30 drops of tincture) before eating helps prevent and relieve belching. A cup of ginger tea before eating is also effective.

♦ Avoid foods known to relax the LES, such as alcohol, chocolate, mints, onions, carbonated beverages, and tomatoes.

Other Options

♦ Eat slowly and chew your food well. People tend to swallow much more air when they gulp down their food.

♦ Don't use a straw or chew gum. Both activities can cause you to swallow excess air.

When to See a Doctor

If you've tried different remedies and you are still experiencing chronic belching, you may want to see a gastroenterologist (a doctor who specializes in disorders of the digestive tract) because your belching may be caused by a medical problem such as hiatal hernia, peptic ulcer, gastroesophageal reflux disease, or another gastrointestinal problem.

CONSTIPATION

Most of us live such busy lives that we often find ourselves rushing from place to place, appointment to appointment. We often drive too fast, eat too fast, and fill our calendars with activities day after day, rarely stopping to relax. But sometimes, something in our lives may not move as fast—or as often—as we wish it would. Sometimes we get constipation.

At one time, medical professionals thought that everyone needed to have one to three bowel movements a day in order to stay healthy. Now they realize that everyone is unique and that being "regular" can mean anything from two or three bowel movements a day to one every three days. The deciding factor is the stools themselves: "normal" stools, regardless of how often they are passed, should be neither abnormally soft or hard, and you should not have to strain to pass them. If you do, then you likely have constipation.

Causes of Constipation

How often have you said (or overheard someone else say) the following:

- "I'm too busy to stop and eat; I'll just grab some fast food later."
- "I always forget to drink enough water."
- "I'm so busy I barely have time to go to the bathroom."
- "Exercise? Who has time to exercise?"

Most cases of constipation are preventable because they have to do with lifestyle. We are a nation of fast-food lovers. If it can be shoved into a bag and handed to us through a drive-in window, we'll eat it. If it can be microwaved or delivered to our door in a pizza box, we'll buy it. The problem is, the vast majority of fast food is not nutritionally sound. It lacks sufficient fiber, which is essential for keeping stools normal and moving through the intestines. A healthy diet must include fresh fruits and vegetables, whole grains, legumes, seeds, and nuts to keep the intestinal tract healthy.

Water and exercise are also essential to healthy stools. Fiber needs water to help move it through the digestive tract, so everyone should drink at least 48 to 64 ounces (six to eight 8-ounce glasses) of water every day. Regular exercise helps move waste material through the body. And when nature calls, don't ignore it. Many people "put off" going to the bathroom when they feel the urge to go. The longer stool remains in the colon, the harder it becomes and the more difficult it will be to pass it later on.

Other causes of constipation include:

◆ *Pregnancy.* More than half of pregnant women experience constipation. Although no one is sure exactly why this is true, the changes in hormones that occur during pregnancy likely play a big role. .

◆ *Medications.* Some drugs, such as opiates (morphine, codeine), antacids that contain aluminum salts, certain antihistamines, diuretics, antidepressants, antipsychotics, and blood-pressure medications cause constipation.

◆ *Emotional problems.* People who are experiencing major stress or depression sometimes have bouts of constipation.

◆ *Medical conditions.* Conditions associated with constipation include irritable bowel syndrome, diabetes, Parkinson's disease, multiple sclerosis, and colorectal cancer (see "When to See a Doctor" on page 131).

Remedies

Often, a few modifications to your lifestyle are all you need to get rid of annoying bouts of constipation. If they fail, you may want to consider some of the over-the-counter medications. Here are some options for you to consider.

Best Bets

◆ Add fiber to your diet. Most Americans eat only half of the 30 grams of fiber that the American Dietetic Association recommends per day. (You'll want to add fiber gradually to avoid experiencing gas.) Fiber increases the bulk and frequency of bowel movements. Take a look at your diet and see where you can add some nutritious, fiber-rich foods (see "Fiber-Rich Foods" on page 132). Have a cup of bran cereal for breakfast, an apple or raw vegetables for a snack, or cooked beans or legumes for dinner.

◆ Establish regular bowel movements. This may take a few weeks or even months, but it is a habit worth forming. Choose a time—after a meal is good because having food in the stomach stimulates the colon—and sit on the toilet for ten minutes. It doesn't matter if you feel the urge to move your bowels; you are trying to establish a habit. (This is an excellent opportunity to practice deep breathing, which will help you relax and thus facilitate elimination. You can also use the palm of one hand to firmly massage your colon—the area below your belly button—in a clockwise motion to help move things along.)

◆ Try psyllium (*Plantago psyllium*), a natural fiber supplement. Add 1 rounded teaspoon of powdered psyllium to a glass of water or juice and stir well. Drink it down immediately, as it becomes gelatinous when combined with water. After drinking the psyllium mixture, drink another glass of plain water. Psyllium usually works within two days, and it is safe to take every day if needed.

Other Options

◆ A yoga position called "cobra" is excellent for toning the abdominal region. The motion stimulates the abdominal organs and also relieves gas. To perform cobra:

1. Lie on your stomach with your forehead resting on the floor. Keep your legs together. Place your hands, palms down, just beneath your shoulders. Keep your elbows close to your body.

2. Inhale and lift your head and chest off the floor. Keep your head aligned with your spine.

3. Hold this position for fifteen to twenty seconds.

4. Exhale and slowly return your torso and head to the floor. Repeat this exercise three to four times.

◆ Take acidophilus for thirty days. Acidophilus is a type of good bacteria that helps break down food and keeps the intestinal tract healthy. Acidophilus supplements are available in capsules and tablets. Take 2 to 4 billion units in two doses (1 to 2 billion units per dose).

When to See a Doctor

Constipation can be a sign of something more serious. If constipation is accompanied by fever and lower abdominal pain, and your stools are loose or thin, you may have a condition called diverticulitis. You should also contact your doctor if there is blood in your stools. If you have been constipated for a week or more, you may have fecal impaction, in which stool has hardened in the rectum and colon. This is common among the elderly and disabled individuals. If an enema does not relieve this problem or if you are unable to perform one, you should see your doctor.

FIBER-RICH FOODS

Here are some common foods and their fiber contents. Remember: 30 grams of fiber per day is recommended. It won't take long to reach that goal if you add a few high-fiber foods to your daily fare.

Food	Fiber (grams)
Apple, whole with skin	2.8
Black beans, cooked, $^1/_2$ cup	4.4
Blueberries, 1 cup	3.3
Bran cereals, 100% bran, $^1/_3$ cup	3.0–10.0
Corn, cooked, $^1/_2$ cup	3.0
Dates, 10 raw	7.0
Kidney beans, cooked, $^1/_2$ cup	4.6
Lentils, cooked, $^1/_2$ cup	2.7
Navy beans, cooked, $^1/_2$ cup	4.9
Oatmeal, cooked, $^3/_4$ cup	3.9
Orange	3.0
Pasta (spaghetti), cooked, 1 cup	3.1
Peas, cooked, $^1/_2$ cup	3.0
Pear	4.2
Potato, baked with skin (7 oz)	2.2

DIARRHEA

None of us like having diarrhea. It can be embarrassing, it's usually inconvenient, and it doesn't make the stomach or intestines feel very good. But there is one good thing about diarrhea: in many cases it allows the body to get rid of something that is irritating it. That "something" could be a virus or bacteria, a food or substance your digestive system cannot process or that it is allergic to, or a medication your body cannot tolerate (see "Drugs and Diarrhea" below). Diarrhea also can be caused by stress, which can be just as potent as any of the other possible causes. In the case of stress-related diarrhea, your body is trying to tell you that you need to relax.

There's more good news about diarrhea: it usually resolves within seven days, sometimes sooner. That may sound like a long time, but if your body needs to eliminate a problem, it can take that long for that "something" to be completely gone.

DRUGS AND DIARRHEA

Drugs known to cause diarrhea include those in the following list. If you get diarrhea soon after starting a new medication that is not on this list, check with your doctor or pharmacist, as the medication could be causing the problem.

◆ Antibiotics such as amoxicillin (Amoxil) and azithromycin (Zithromax)

◆ Antacids (over-the-counter) such as Maalox and Mylanta, or others that contain magnesium

◆ Anti-inflammatory drugs, including naproxen (Naprosyn) and indomethacin (Indocin)

◆ Drugs used to treat constipation, especially those that contain senna or bisacodyl (for example, Senokot, Ex-Lax, Correctol) or those that contain mineral oil or castor oil

◆ Antihypertensive drugs, such as enalapril (Vasotec)

Dehydration Alert

Along with the loss of the "something" that you want to eliminate, diarrhea also causes you to lose essential body fluids and minerals called electrolytes. Your body needs both water and these minerals—potassium, sodium, glucose, chloride, magnesium, and phosphorus—to function properly. Although you've probably heard that you need to drink lots of water when you have diarrhea to prevent dehydration, you also need to replace the lost minerals. That's why many healthcare professionals recommend downing sports drinks that contain electrolytes, fruit juices, herbal teas, or vegetable broth. An old naturopathic replacement drink consists of equal parts of sauerkraut juice and tomato juice.

Remedies

When you have diarrhea, if the first thing you reach for is an over-the-counter antidiarrheal drug, stop. Think again about why diarrhea is a *good* thing. If you take something to stop the diarrhea, the offensive "something" will not be eliminated. Therefore, you should be reaching for remedies that can help soothe your stomach and intestines while letting nature take its course. So, here are some ways to make the whole experience easier to live with.

Best Bets

◆ Try some carob. This natural remedy can significantly reduce the symptoms of diarrhea. Andrew Weil, M.D., director of the program in integrative medicine at the University of Arizona College of Medicine in Tucson, suggests mixing 1 tablespoon carob powder (available in health food stores) with a little bit of applesauce and honey to make it go down easier and taste better. You can use this remedy up to three times a day for up to three days. Take the carob on an empty stomach.

◆ Bring back the good bacteria. Diarrhea eliminates a lot of substances from the body, and among them are the healthy bacteria in the intestinal tract. Taking a supplement of acidophilus ("friendly bacteria") helps the intestinal tract heal during the turmoil of a bout of diarrhea. The suggested dose is 2 to 3 billion units daily, or follow the package directions. Some experts suggest taking acidophilus along with the carob mixture mentioned above.

◆ Be kind to your tummy. During a bout of diarrhea, it is best to eat only foods that are very easy to digest and that will not irritate the stomach. Recommended foods include bananas, rice, applesauce, toast, mashed potatoes, and tea (preferably herbal or decaffeinated).

Other Options

◆ Make a few cups of garlic tea. This old Chinese medicine remedy works because garlic is an antimicrobial, which means it kills bacteria and viruses. To make the tea, bake six unpeeled garlic cloves in foil for ten minutes at

350°F. Then boil the cloves in 30 ounces of water for seven to eight minutes. Strain and drink 10 ounces every three hours until the diarrhea stops. You may need to repeat the recipe if the diarrhea hasn't disappeared after the third dose.

◆ Porridge is like chicken soup: it has healing powers. To get rid of diarrhea, make a 10 ounce bowl of white rice or Cream of Rice until it is very soupy and add 1 teaspoon of ginger and $\frac{1}{2}$ teaspoon of black pepper. Eat a bowl of porridge every four hours until the diarrhea improves. The ginger soothes the gastrointestinal tract, the pepper helps slow down bowel movements, and the porridge gets liquid and nourishment back into your body.

When to See a Doctor

Sometimes diarrhea is a signal that something more serious is happening behind the scenes. If diarrhea is accompanied by blood in the stool, constant pain (instead of just having cramps before or during a bowel movement), dizziness, fever, or vomiting (for more than twenty-four hours), then call your doctor immediately. You should also call your doctor if your diarrhea has lasted more than two weeks despite your attempts to treat it.

PREVENTING TRAVELERS' DIARRHEA

When you're traveling outside the United States, you want to see the sights, not the inside of a toilet. And you want to come home with souvenirs, not diarrhea. But every year, tens of thousands of people become infected with bacteria that causes travelers' diarrhea. Here are some tips on how to prevent this stowaway.

◆ Drink bottled water. Do not drink tap water or use it to brush your teeth, make ice cubes, or make coffee or tea.

◆ Do not eat raw or fresh fruits and vegetables. Everything you eat should be cooked thoroughly.

◆ If you do eat fruit or vegetables, peel them first. Avoid those that cannot be peeled (for example, lettuce, cabbage, and other greens).

◆ Travel with water-purifying tablets just in case you get into a situation in which you must drink the local water.

FLATULENCE

Believe it or not, there was a study that determined the average number of times per day that gas (flatus) builds up in the lower bowel and is released through the anus. If you're sitting around some day with little else to do, you may want to count the number of times you make such a release to the world.

But, please, don't invite your friends to join you.

Flatulence: Everybody Has It

Releasing intestinal gas, or flatulence, is a common and necessary bodily function. It is a by-product of the body's digestive process, which goes something like this: After food enters the stomach, it is processed by stomach acid and digestive enzymes. The partially digested food particles are then passed into the small intestine, where the particles are broken down further into absorbable parts (nutrients) that are transported through the intestinal wall into the bloodstream. The remaining particles are passed along to the large intestine, where the final phase of digestion takes place.

A by-product of the digestive process is the production of gas, which gathers in the lower portion of the large intestine and waits to be released to the world. According to the study that we mentioned above, the average number of times people experience flatulence each day is fourteen, with a range of six to twenty times daily.

Gas Producers—Carbohydrates

Of the three main nutrients—protein, fats, and carbohydrates—the latter wins first prize in the gas-producing department. If you have a healthy digestive system—adequate stomach acid and digestive enzymes, and a healthy population of good bacteria in your intestines—you probably have no trouble digesting carbohydrates. You can expect the "normal" amount of flatulence.

If, however, you are among the estimated 50 percent of Americans who have trouble digesting carbohydrates, you may be experiencing more than the normal amount of gas and the discomfort—and red face—that can go with it. That's because your stomach and small intestine are not breaking down your food completely, which allows food to find its way into the large intestine in an undigested state.

For example, if you are lactose intolerant, you lack a sufficient amount of the enzyme lactase in your intestinal tract. Lactase breaks down lactose—found in dairy foods such as milk and cheese—into nutrients that then enter the bloodstream. But without lactase, the lactose escapes and enters the large intestine undigested. The lactose is then attacked by bacteria, which digest it and produce a lot of gas, such as hydrogen, carbon dioxide, methane, and hydrogen sulfide. The latter two gases are responsible for the "aroma" of flatulence. Not all flatulence has an odor, however.

More Gas Producers

When people think of gas-producing foods, beans are usually the first that come to mind. Beans have a reputation for causing flatulence, but there are ways you can change that (see "Gas-Free Beans" on page 139). Other foods that may produce excessive gas are cabbage, broccoli, raisins, carrots, spinach, cauliflower, onions, prune juice, bran, and celery.

Are you fond of diet or low-calorie foods? The bad news is that foods that contain the no-calorie sugar substitutes sorbitol and xylitol contribute to flatulence. The body cannot digest these substances very well, leaving them for the gas-producing bacteria in the large intestine.

If you've taken an antibiotic for an infection, it could have contributed to your gas problems as well. Although antibiotics can kill bacteria that cause infections, they also destroy the good bacteria that live in the body, including those that are needed in the large intestine to break down food. When the good bacteria are killed, unfriendly bacteria and other harmful organisms move in and produce toxins that can lead to flatulence, bloating, and diarrhea. Unfortunately, even one course of antibiotic treatment can result in days, months, or years of problems with flatulence unless you restore the population of good bacteria (see "Best Bets" below).

Remedies

Except in rare cases, flatulence can be managed or prevented easily with a change in lifestyle. Here are some things you can do to put a cap on your gas production.

Best Bets

◆ Adjust your eating habits. If you're not sure which foods are causing you to produce excess gas, use a trial-and-error approach. Make a list of the possible suspects and then eat only one of them at a time, waiting a day or two in between to see how you react. (Also see "Gas-Free Beans" on page 139.)

◆ Restore the population of good bacteria. If you've ever taken antibiotics—and most Americans have—chances are the number of good bacteria in your body has been negatively affected. Help restore a healthy balance of good and bad bacteria by taking probiotics—supplements that contain helpful bacteria. Health food stores and pharmacies carry items such as acidophilus and bifidobacteria, live bacteria that you can take in the form of a tablet, powder, or capsule. The recommended dosage is 2 to 3 billion units per day. Probiotics should always be taken during antibiotic therapy and for at least two weeks after you finish taking the drugs. Even if you haven't taken antibiotics for some time, take probiotics for several weeks to see if your flatulence improves. Probiotics are completely safe.

◆ Take digestive enzymes. It's possible you are not producing enough digestive enzymes to help break down your food. This is especially common among people who are older than fifty, because the amount of digestive enzymes we produce declines as we age. Digestive enzyme supplements can be purchased as single products or combinations. Popular natural plant enzymes include papaya and bromelain (derived from pineapple). Other enzymes to look for are protease (helps digest proteins), lipase (digests fats), amylase (digests carbohydrates), cellulase, lactase, and maltase. Combination enzyme supplements often contain all these enzymes and more. Take the supplement according to directions on the label. Many people say they get even better results if they take the enzymes along with probiotics.

Other Options

◆ Take activated charcoal. If you're getting ready to meet your future in-laws or are about to give a speech and you're having a gas attack, you need quick relief. Just pop one or two 200–500 mg tablets of activated charcoal into your mouth and wait thirty minutes. That's how long it takes for the charcoal to attach itself to the gas producers in your digestive tract and eliminate them quietly out of the body. Do not, however, take these pills if you are on other medications or nutritional supplements, because they will inhibit the body's ability to absorb those necessary items. If you're in a pinch and don't have any activated charcoal handy, eat a piece of burnt toast.

◆ Chew fennel seeds. The oils in this herb help eliminate excess gas. You must chew the seeds completely (take five to ten seeds) and then swallow them to get the most benefit.

When to See a Doctor

Flatulence is rarely related to a medical problem, but if you have chronic flatulence that is causing a problem in your daily life, see your doctor. You may have a digestive disorder, such as lactose intolerance or celiac disease. He or she may also suggest a nonprescription product that contains simethicone, a substance that breaks up gas bubbles in the stomach and intestines.

GAS-FREE BEANS

This recipe for "gas-free beans" comes from the California Dry Bean Advisory Board. Boil 10 cups of water in a large pot. Place 1 pound of raw beans into the water and boil for three minutes. Turn off the heat, cover the pot with a lid, and allow the beans to soak overnight (about eight hours). In the morning, drain off the water. Between 75 and 90 percent of the indigestible sugars that are responsible for beans' gas power just went down your drain. Rinse the beans and then cook them in fresh water. If you are using canned beans, drain off the fluid and rinse the beans before using them.

FOOD POISONING

You love Aunt Helen's potato salad, so when you see there's still a little left in the bottom of the bowl during the family picnic, you scoop it up. You don't think about the fact that it's been sitting out on the picnic table, unrefrigerated, for several hours. After all, it tastes fine. But later that night, after a few bouts of vomiting and a lot of stomach cramps, you vow never to eat her potato salad again.

But it's not Aunt Helen's fault. You've been a victim of food poisoning, likely caused by microorganisms such as staphylococcus or salmonella. These microscopic critters typically cause symptoms of food poisoning—nausea, vomiting, diarrhea, stomach cramps, and headache—within one to six hours after eating contaminated food.

According to the Centers for Disease Control and Prevention (CDC), foodborne diseases cause up to 81 million illnesses each year in the United States. Up to 9,000 people die of these diseases, although food poisoning does not normally pose a serious threat to people who are healthy. In fact, most people experience a few hours to a day or two of symptoms. After that they return to normal, except that for a while, they may stay clear of the food that made them feel so bad.

How Food Becomes Contaminated

Gastroenteritis, inflammation of the lining of the stomach and the intestines, occurs when people eat food that has been contaminated in some way, often at a restaurant or an event where food is served. Bacteria are the usual culprits in food poisoning; however, protozoa or toxins (usually present because of improper packaging or preparation, or naturally present in the case of some fish) can also be a cause.

Certain conditions need to be in place to promote food contamination. For example, pay attention to temperature. Food poisoning bacteria grow best when the temperature is between 40 and 125°F. That's why it's important to keep your refrigerator colder than 40°F and to heat food at temperatures greater than 125°F. If food is being served at a buffet, it should be kept in serving containers that maintain safe temperatures.

Bacteria also need some help from nutrients. Bacteria need a food supply in order to grow and multiply, and they grow best in foods that contain eggs, dairy products (milk, cheese, cream), meat, fish, poultry, or shellfish. This also includes foods such as mayonnaise and salad dressings. All of these foods are considered to be high-risk foods. Combination foods, such as Aunt Helen's potato salad (made with eggs and mayonnaise), macaroni salad, deviled eggs, crab salad, egg salad, quiche, meatballs, and chicken salad are also high-risk foods.

Moisture also helps promote food contamination. Without moisture, bacteria cannot grow quickly and may stop. That's why drying food is a safe and effective way to preserve it. And speaking of time: under ideal conditions, one bacterium can multiply more than 2 million times during a seven-hour period. Even in half that time, you are still faced with many bacteria ready to cause you much discomfort.

How you handle your food also plays a big role in food contamination. Food can become contaminated any time during the production or serving process, whether that means food processing equipment is not properly cleaned, items are not stored at safe temperatures (like Aunt Helen's potato salad), or an individual who handles the food is ill and passes along harmful bacteria. One type of contamination to especially watch for is fishy toxins. In contaminated fish, the toxins in the flesh cannot be destroyed by cooking. Some types of fish (and shellfish) are more likely to be contaminated than others, including barracuda, red snapper, grouper, tuna, mackerel, puffer fish, mussels, and various shellfish caught off the coast of Alaska, the Atlantic Coast, the Gulf Coast, or the West Coast during different parts of the year.

PREVENTING FOOD POISONING AT HOME

To prevent food poisoning at home, follow these guidelines:

- Always wash your hands before you prepare any food. If you handle raw meat, fish, or poultry, wash your hands before you handle any other foods.

- Never eat cooked meat or dairy products that have been out of the refrigerator for more than two hours.

- If you use a cutting board or other utensils to cut and prepare raw food, wash them thoroughly with soap and hot water before they touch any other food items. If ready-to-eat or cooked foods come in contact with those unwashed items, those foods could become contaminated with bacteria from raw food.

- Store raw foods and cooked foods away from each other in the refrigerator so there can be no cross-contamination. Each food item should be stored in clean, washable containers with tight covers or lids.

- Throw away any canned foods that have a bulging top, a strange odor or color, or a broken seal. Spoiled canned foods are a source of botulism, an often fatal form of food poisoning.

- Keep meat, fish, poultry, milk, dairy products, and gravies refrigerated until you are ready to cook or serve them.

- Even foods that are typically thought to be safe, such as cooked beans, rice, barley, and pasta, can become contaminated if they are kept at a warm temperature for more than two hours. Refrigerate them after serving.

- Keep the temperature of your refrigerator between 34 and 37°F, never higher.

- Cook all meat and poultry thoroughly. Avoid uncooked marinated food and raw meat, eggs, or fish.

Remedies

Most cases of food poisoning are mild and resolve within a few hours or days. The treatments offered here can help relieve the symptoms and make recovery time a bit shorter. Remember, however, that because you have ingested something the body needs to eliminate, vomiting and diarrhea are usually *good* symptoms. If they are excessive, however, you should see a doctor (see "When to See a Doctor" below).

Best Bets

♦ Calm your stomach with ginger. Take two capsules of powdered ginger or drink a cup of ginger tea every two hours as needed. A tried-and-true remedy is flat ginger ale. It can be cold, but make sure it's flat because the carbonation can upset your already disturbed stomach.

♦ Try one of the following herbs in an infusion: meadowsweet, catnip, or slippery elm. All of these herbs soothe the stomach. Make an infusion by steeping 2 teaspoons of the chosen herb in a cup of boiling water for fifteen minutes. Drink up to three cups per day.

♦ Several homeopathic remedies can be helpful. Try any one of the following over-the-counter remedies in 12c or 30c strength and take it every three to four hours until you feel better: arsenicum album, nux vomica, or podophyllum.

Other Options

♦ If you are experiencing vomiting and/or diarrhea, make sure you stay hydrated. Drink plenty of water or one of the herbal teas mentioned above. Avoid caffeinated or carbonated beverages and alcohol. Better yet, make the following brew, which will help replace the water and minerals your body is losing. In a large pot add 1 cup each finely chopped celery, carrots, parsley, and spinach. Add 4 cups water and bring the mixture to a rolling boil. Drink three to four cups for two to three days during and after symptoms have stopped.

♦ Once your symptoms subside and you feel like eating again, start with mild foods, such as white rice, mashed potatoes (plain), ripe bananas, and cooked vegetables.

When to See a Doctor

If you are experiencing severe vomiting or diarrhea that lasts for more than a day, see a doctor. Also, a rare type of food poisoning called botulism can be fatal.

It is caused by a toxin created by *Clostridium* bacteria and is found in improperly canned foods. Symptoms sometimes take several days to appear and can include nausea, vomiting, blurred vision, dry mouth, constipation, difficulty swallowing, and general weakness followed by progressive paralysis. If you suspect you have botulism, go to an emergency room or your doctor immediately.

HEARTBURN

It's that burning sensation that occurs just behind your breastbone near your heart. Doctors often refer to it as gastroesophageal reflux, but most Americans know it as heartburn or indigestion. Heartburn can be mild to severe and may be accompanied by chest pain, nausea, vomiting, reflux (surges of stomach acid that enter your throat and mouth), and problems with swallowing.

If you suffer with heartburn, you're not alone. More than 60 million American adults experience heartburn at least once a month, and about 25 million deal with it daily. Heartburn occurs when the valve at the juncture between the esophagus (tube through which food travels from the mouth to the stomach) and the stomach becomes weak and allows stomach acid to flow backward through the valve, causing a burning sensation. This is known as reflux, or acid reflux.

Although many people automatically think that heartburn is caused by too much stomach acid, an acid deficiency can cause heartburn symptoms, too. That's because stomach acid is necessary for digestion to take place, and if you have too little acid, the digestive process is hampered, which then causes heartburn, belching, bloating, nausea, and other symptoms. Too much stomach acid may occur naturally or be related to the intake of fatty foods. (See "Too Much or Too Little Acid? How Can I Tell?" on page 144)

How to Prevent Heartburn

Heartburn is often a by-product of a hectic lifestyle and poor eating habits. A few minor adjustments in these areas could very well "cure" you of your heartburn. Here are some tips:

◆ Eat at a leisurely pace. Eating too fast can disrupt the flow of stomach acid.

◆ Eat moderate amounts of food. Eating too much can stimulate reflux.

◆ Reduce or eliminate your intake of fatty foods, as they encourage the production of excess stomach acid.

- If you smoke, stop. Chemicals in tobacco can weaken the valve between the esophagus and the stomach.

- Avoid stress, especially around mealtimes. Stress impairs digestion because it sends blood to the muscles instead of to the stomach, where it is needed for your food to be processed.

- Avoid caffeine and alcohol. Both can increase stomach acid production.

- Don't exercise for more than an hour after you eat, as exercise requires blood to be sent to the muscles rather than be used for the digestive process.

- Eat ginger, apples, dill, or papaya with your meals, as they contain enzymes that help digestion.

TOO MUCH OR TOO LITTLE ACID? HOW CAN I TELL?

If you are experiencing heartburn and don't know if the cause is too much or too little stomach acid (hydrochloric acid), try this experiment: take a supplement that contains hydrochloric acid, such as Gas-X Extra Strength liquid, about ten minutes before a meal. Follow the label directions. If your heartburn symptoms go away, then your heartburn is related to low levels of hydrochloric acid. If, however, you experience a mild burning sensation, then you have excess hydrochloric acid. You can quickly relieve the burning sensation by drinking $1/4$ teaspoon of baking soda in 8 ounces of water.

Remedies

Although there are lots of commercials touting the benefits of antacids, many healthcare practitioners warn that antacids can interfere with the natural digestive process. In fact, people who have heartburn that is associated with a deficiency of stomach acid may experience worse symptoms if they take antacids. Here are some surefire ways to get rid of your heartburn.

Best Bets

- If the problem is too much stomach acid, try licorice tablets. Take one or two chewable tablets three times daily on an empty stomach. Buy deglycyrrhizinated licorice (DGL), which is believed to be more effective than regular licorice and does not cause high blood pressure, a problem associated with regular licorice.

◆ The juice made from the gel of the aloe plant helps protect the stomach lining and stops heartburn quickly. Make sure you buy an aloe juice that is intended for internal use and follow package directions.

◆ MSM (methylsulfonylmethane) is a natural supplement that protects the esophagus from stomach-acid damage. Take one to three 500 mg capsules twice a day with meals as long as you are experiencing symptoms.

Other Options

◆ Drink 4 ounces of raw potato juice immediately before eating a meal. Potatoes are very alkaline, which means they have the ability to neutralize acid in the stomach. Potato juice can be prepared from potatoes, using a juicer or blender. Remember to peel the potatoes first.

◆ The herb slippery elm heals the mucous membranes that are irritated by acid reflux. To prepare a tea, add a heaping tablespoon of powdered slippery elm bark to 1 pint boiling water, steep for one hour, and reheat before drinking. Drink one cup before every meal.

When to See a Doctor

If you have persistent heartburn (several weeks or longer) and/or your symptoms (for example, nausea, vomiting, difficulty swallowing) are severe, you should see your doctor as soon as possible. It may be a symptom of a more serious condition called gastroesophageal reflux disease (GERD), which can cause or contribute to asthma, chronic cough, and ulcers of the esophagus if not treated. If your heartburn is accompanied by chest pain that travels to your arm, jaw, or neck, or symptoms such as nausea, cold sweats, or a squeezing sensation in the chest, get to an emergency room immediately, as you may be having a heart attack.

HICCUPS

Charles Osborne, of Anthon, Iowa, got the hiccups in 1922. Every day for the next sixty-five years, Mr. Osborne was plagued by this malady. During that time he got little sleep and lived on blended foods because he was unable to chew properly.

Wait a minute, you may be thinking. Aren't hiccups annoying and sometimes embarrassing, but they only last maybe a few minutes and then go away once you breathe into a paper bag or drink water real fast? Can the condition really last years and years?

Actually, Mr. Osborne's case is rare. The vast majority of people experience what are called *benign hiccups*—temporary, harmless contractions of the diaphragm (the muscle below the ribs that is involved in breathing). Only infrequently do hiccups last for days, weeks, or even years.

Although seemingly a simple ailment, the hiccups condition is complex. It affects virtually every person at least once during his or her lifetime, yet despite being so common, researchers have been fascinated and puzzled by hiccups for years.

Hiccups: What Are They Good For?

One reason hiccups fascinate us is they seem to serve no practical, physiological purpose. Another is that scientists cannot agree on how they occur. One theory is that they are the result of spasmodic contractions of the diaphragm, which is the muscle right below the rib cage. Another says they are the result of several central and peripheral processes in the body. Yet another is that there is a hiccup reflex center in the upper spinal cord region.

Why hiccups occur can be answered in several ways. Hiccups can result from overeating, drinking too much alcohol or soft drinks, or from gastric distress. Infants get hiccups when they eat too quickly. Some medications, such as corticosteroids and benzodiazepines, can cause hiccups. Often, however, the cause of benign hiccups is unknown.

But infrequently, people get chronic or persistent hiccups. Such hiccups can last days, weeks, or even years. Persistent hiccups can result in weight loss, malnutrition, fatigue, depression, problems with heart rhythm, and esophageal reflux (food coming back up the esophagus). Chronic hiccups can be a sign of alcoholism, nervous system tumors, brain tumors, gastric ulcers, heart attack, kidney failure, liver disease, or even cancer. Pope Pius XII had chronic hiccups as well as what was called a "delicate stomach," or gastritis. About 4,000 people are hospitalized each year for hiccups.

Remedies

Cures for hiccups are creative. If one doesn't work, try another one. Each of the treatments discussed here has worked for many people. Perhaps they'll work for you. Some have much better success rates than others, and a few have even been tested scientifically.

The goal of hiccup cures is to increase the level of carbon dioxide in the blood or to disrupt the nerve impulses that cause the hiccups. Here are the most effective ways to put a hamper on your hiccups. Good luck!

Best Bets

◆ Swallow a teaspoon of dry sugar.

◆ Chew and swallow dry bread.

◆ Gargle with water.

Other Options

◆ Hold your breath for as long as you can, but not so long that you feel faint.

◆ Suck on crushed ice. Don't chew the ice; then you'll likely get a headache.

When to See a Doctor

If you have persistent hiccups (also known as singultus), contact your physician. He or she can try to determine the cause of the hiccups and treat you as needed. There are drugs that can stop chronic hiccups. They include the antipsychotic drugs chlorpromazine and haloperidol; the anticonvulsive drugs phenytoin, valproic acid, and carbamazepine; and various other drugs, including amitriptyline, ephedrine, nifedipine, and metoclopramide.

INFLAMMATORY BOWEL DISEASE

In 1932, an American doctor named Burrill Crohn described an intestinal disorder in which chronic, often severe diarrhea, blood in the stool, and abdominal pain were the classic signs and symptoms. Back in those days, the condition that became known as Crohn's disease wasn't very common, but we can't make that claim today. In the United States, it is estimated that nearly 2 million people suffer with inflammatory bowel disease (IBD), the most common types of which are Crohn's disease and ulcerative colitis. People of any age can get these diseases, although most cases occur in people ages fifteen to forty.

The Difference between Crohn's Disease and Ulcerative Colitis

Most people experience a bout of diarrhea once in a while, but imagine living with it every day. People who have IBD know what it's like. In Crohn's disease, the entire digestive tract—from the mouth to the anus—can be affected with inflammation and sores. Most people, however, have inflamed portions of the intestinal tract, which makes digestion difficult. The result is insufficient absorption of nutrients, diarrhea, weakness, weight loss, and pain.

In ulcerative colitis, the disease is confined to the colon and rectum. Tiny ulcers or lesions in the colon irritate the lining of the intestinal tract and cause bloody stools and painful diarrhea. Like Crohn's disease, you can also experience weakness, weight loss, and fatigue. Arthritis and rashes often accompany both of these conditions as well.

Causes of IBD

Although IBD is a fairly common condition, scientists can't explain exactly why it occurs. Some blame diet, noting that the disease nearly always occurs in people who consume high amounts of animal protein, fat, sugar, and refined foods. Inflammatory bowel disease is virtually nonexistent among primitive people or in cultures that rely on simple, whole foods. Some researchers point to parasites, bacteria, or other microorganisms, which can cause symptoms similar to those of IBD. Yet other experts say that use of antibiotics damages the lining of the intestinal tract and triggers the disease. Perhaps it is a combination of these factors. All of this uncertainty isn't helped by the fact that there is no known cure for the disease.

Remedies

Treating IBD involves a combination of relieving symptoms and trying to prevent them. The following tips on foods and other substances to avoid should help. However, there is no known way to prevent Crohn's disease or ulcerative colitis.

Best Bets

◆ Avoid foods that irritate the intestinal tract. The most common foods in this category are dairy products, eggs, wheat, spicy foods, and high-fiber foods (raw fruits and vegetables, grains, legumes, seeds). Well-cooked fruits and vegetables are okay.

◆ Stay away from alcohol, carbonated drinks, and iced drinks. They will trigger excessive activity in the intestines and stimulate diarrhea.

◆ Eat smaller meals and more frequently. This prevents the bowel from becoming distended and allows more time for it to heal.

Other Options

◆ Take a pectin supplement. Although it is best to avoid high-fiber foods because they can irritate your intestines, avoiding fiber altogether can weaken the intestines. Research shows that taking a pectin supplement (a water-soluble fiber) may help promote good bacterial growth in the intestines without causing fecal bulk other fiber can. Your doctor can determine how much pectin will be helpful for you.

◆ Relax. Although stress doesn't cause IBD, it can aggravate it. Daily relaxation sessions, with meditation, guided imagery, yoga, deep breathing, or other relaxation methods, are recommended.

When to See a Doctor

Call your doctor immediately if you have blood clots in your stool. Also, if you experience a sudden attack of fever, abdominal pain, and the urge to pass gas or to pass stool, call your doctor immediately or go to the emergency room, as you may be in the beginning stages of appendicitis.

IRRITABLE BOWEL SYNDROME

"Which one will it be today?" says Heidi. "Constipation or diarrhea? When you have irritable bowel syndrome, you never know which one is going to hit you." Heidi is among the 10 to 15 percent of the adult American population who suffers with bouts of irritable bowel syndrome (IBS), the most common of all digestive disorders. Twice as many women as men report having this condition, but experts believe that many people simply never seek help for it and so it may be even more common than reported.

Irritable bowel syndrome, also known as spastic colon or spastic colitis, is characterized by bouts of diarrhea and constipation, usually after meals, and is accompanied by gas, bloating, or abdominal cramps. Each bout may last for several days to several weeks, and there may be months or even years between episodes.

Causes of IBS

When food enters your intestinal tract, it moves through your intestines with the help of a series of synchronized, wavelike motions called peristalsis. In people who have IBS, this synchronized motion, suddenly and without warning, becomes irregular. The entire digestive process is affected, and for days or weeks, affected people can expect fluctuating bowel and digestive problems.

Some experts believe IBS is caused by stress, while others say it is related to food sensitivities or allergies. Many different factors appear to aggravate IBS, but whether they actually cause it has not been definitively determined. Those factors related to food include eating too quickly, overeating or binge eating, lactose intolerance, and use of artificial sugar substitutes such as sorbitol and aspartame, which can cause diarrhea. Antibiotics may also play a big role, as they change the bacteria population in the intestines by destroying good bacteria and allowing bad bacteria to cause diarrhea and abdominal pain. Use of tricyclic antidepressants, antihistamines, antipsychotics, morphine, codeine, methotrexate, diuretics, and some mineral supplements can cause constipation. Smoking also irritates the stomach.

The bottom line is, experts don't really know what causes IBS. For some people, it may be a combination of several factors. It is likely that people who get IBS are genetically susceptible to the condition, and all they need is one or more triggers to set off symptoms.

Remedies

The most effective remedies for IBS are those that involve a combination of lifestyle changes and natural therapies. Here are some options.

Best Bets

◆ Track down the trigger foods. Keep a food diary to help identify which foods set off your symptoms. For some people it's foods that are known to cause allergic reactions; these include wheat, dairy, oranges, soy, eggs, and peanuts. For others the culprits may be spicy or fatty foods. As you identify possible trigger foods, eliminate them from your diet for several weeks and see how you feel. Then, reintroduce them one at a time (one every three to four days). If you have a reaction, you'll know to avoid that food.

◆ Reduce stress, and you'll likely reduce IBS symptoms. Yoga, meditation, visualization, progressive relaxation exercises, deep breathing, and tai chi are all excellent relaxation methods. Practice relaxation every day for ten to fifteen minutes; fit in two sessions a day if possible.

◆ Herbal teas can help promote normal digestion. Drink up to three cups per day of chamomile, peppermint, or pau d'arco tea (available in prepackaged tea bags).

Other Options

+ Foot reflexology can treat diarrhea, constipation, stomach cramps, and bloating, and you can do it yourself. See the reflexology discussion in Chapter 2 for instructions on how to do reflexology and to help you locate the treatment areas for the intestines and stomach.

+ To relieve gas and bloating, try charcoal tablets. Take one or two 500 mg tablets and wait about thirty minutes. That's how long it takes for them to work. In addition, avoid foods that promote gas such as beans, cabbage, chocolate, and onions.

When to See a Doctor

It's time to see your doctor if you have blood in your stool, if you have vomiting, dizziness, or fainting along with your abdominal pain, or if diarrhea or abdominal pain is severe enough to wake you from sleep. You should also talk to your doctor if you have unexplained fever or weight loss.

NAUSEA, VOMITING, AND MORNING SICKNESS

Nausea and vomiting are not diseases but symptoms that can be associated with a wide variety of conditions from food poisoning to alcohol overindulgence to stomach flu to riding in a car. Morning sickness, however, is nausea (and vomiting) with a known cause: pregnancy.

Yet while we feel the uneasiness and queasiness in our stomachs, the origins of those feelings may be elsewhere. The inner ear, for example, is the originating point for people who get nauseous while riding in a car, bus, or other moving object. People of any age can suffer with motion sickness, yet most children outgrow the problem by the time they are five or six years old. For "older kids," feeling nauseous while riding roller coasters may be left over from those younger years.

Nausea can also occur in response to a bad odor such as exhaust fumes, excessive stress, or a frightening or disgusting sight, such as a mutilated body. The brain is the starting point for this type of nausea. We can even blame hormones for one type of nausea: morning sickness is believed to be related to the sudden change in hormone levels in women.

Most nausea is related to the gastrointestinal tract. This is nausea caused by overeating, food poisoning, stomach flu, a reaction to medication, or drinking too much alcohol. Vomiting is a well-synchronized reflex in which the muscles that control the esophageal valve (sphincter) relax and the abdominal and diaphragm muscles contract. The windpipe closes, and the lower portion of the stomach contracts and sends the contents of the stomach upward and out through the mouth.

But enough of the gory details. Let's talk about how to feel better.

Remedies

Unless you are also suffering from other symptoms that may indicate you need a doctor's attention (see "When to See a Doctor" on page 153), treatment of nausea and morning sickness involves some simple, natural remedies.

Best Bets

◆ Ginger, either as a tea or in capsules, can soothe the gastrointestinal tract. Try up to three cups daily of ginger tea, or take 250 mg capsules up to four times daily.

◆ Press away nausea and vomiting using acupressure. The pericardium 6 (PC6) point on the inside wrist is the acupressure site to relieve nausea. You can get a wrist band that applies the pressure for you. These bands are available through the Automobile Association of America (AAA) and travel agencies, as they are often used by people who get motion sickness.

◆ Activated charcoal (available in health food stores and most pharmacies) can relieve or eliminate nausea. Take one 500 mg capsule after eating to help absorb digestive gas.

Other Options

◆ Beat it with beet juice. Beet juice helps correct gallbladder and liver congestion, which can cause nausea. Therefore, a refreshing glass of diluted beet juice can chase nausea away. Because beet juice is a very potent liver enzyme stimulant, you must dilute it first. One part beet juice to 2 parts of another vegetable juice (celery, carrot, tomato) will do the trick.

◆ For persistent morning sickness, try ONE of the following for four to five days only: 25–50 mg vitamin B$_6$ three times daily; or try 250 mg ginger capsules four times daily.

When to See a Doctor

Most people, when they become nauseous, know why. But if you experience nausea often and you can't identify the reason, see your doctor. Also, if nausea lasts for a week or more and is accompanied by headache, malaise, fatigue, fever, sore throat, and rash, you may have mononucleosis or strep throat. Severe nausea that occurs along with pain in the upper abdomen that moves to the right shoulder usually indicates a gallstone attack. See a doctor for an evaluation. (However, tiny gallstones can be treated at home; see GALLSTONES on page 263.)

ULCERS

For about 100 years, doctors and researchers blamed the development of ulcers on stress and diet. People who had these erosions of the mucous membrane of the stomach or duodenum (the upper portion of the intestines) would point the finger at their overbearing boss, financial worries, nosy mother-in-law, or too many bowls of hot chili as the cause of their problem. Now we know that, although stress and diet do play a role, a microscopic spiral-shaped organism named *Helicobacter pylori* is the primary cause of ulcers.

Every year, about 4 million Americans are diagnosed with ulcers, and about 20 million Americans can expect to develop one at some point in their lives. Ulcers can develop at any age, but they are rare among teenagers and younger children. Although ulcers are preventable and treatable, about 6,000 Americans die of ulcer-related conditions each year.

Types of Ulcers

Gastrointestinal, or peptic, ulcers come in two types: gastric (stomach) and duodenal (intestinal). It is possible to have both types at the same time. A reason for this unfortunate situation is that both types of ulcers are partly caused by an imbalance between pepsin (an enzyme) and acid. The stomach and duodenal lining are defenseless against this disharmony. Inflammation of the lining may be precipitated by the use of aspirin, nonsteroidal anti-inflammatory drugs, or smoking.

Specific risk factors for gastric ulcers are the presence of chronic gastritis, blood type A, and age older than fifty years. The incidence of gastric ulcers is 8 out of 10,000 people. Risk factors particular to duodenal ulcers are a family history of peptic ulcer, age older than thirty, and group O blood type. The incidence of duodenal ulcers is 7 out of every 1,000 people.

Role of *Helicobactor pylori*

Although three factors—lifestyle (stress, smoking, diet, drug use), pepsin and acid, and *Helicobactor pylori*—play a role in the development of ulcers, *H. pylori* is now considered to be the main cause. *H. pylori,* among the most common bacteria in the world, set up an environment where ulcers can flourish in the human body. According to R. Carter Davis, Jr., M.D., of Atlanta Gastroenterology Associates and Clinical Associate Professor of Medicine and Gastroenterology at Emory University in Atlanta, Georgia, at least 80 to 90 percent of the duodenal ulcers in the United States are caused or made worse by the *H. pylori* microorganism, and at least 40 to 50 percent of gastric ulcers can credit their existence to the microorganism as well.

The discovery that *H. pylori* are at the root of most ulcers explains why, in the past, when doctors were able to heal ulcers with treatment, the ulcers usually came back. That's because treatment hadn't eliminated the bacteria. However, because the stomach is an acidic environment where bacteria are not supposed to grow, bacteria were not high on the suspect list.

Unfortunately, *H. pylori* do well in the acid setting of the stomach. The bacteria can survive because they produce an enzyme called urease, which neutralizes stomach acid. The bacteria then wiggle their way into the stomach's lining and produce substances that weaken the protective mucus coating, making the stomach cells susceptible to damage from pepsin and acid.

Symptoms of Ulcers

The most common and typically the earliest symptom of peptic ulcers is a gnawing or burning sensation that usually occurs shortly before a meal, about an hour after eating, or during the night. The pain usually occurs in the stomach, although some people experience back or chest pain as well. Sometimes the pain is accompanied by nausea, and if vomiting occurs it usually relieves the pain, but only temporarily.

How to Prevent Ulcers

Don't think you can just point the finger at *H. pylori* as the cause of your peptic ulcers and then continue to live recklessly. Stress, smoking, certain drugs, and diet contribute to ulcer development and pain. Appropriate stress reduction, such as meditation, yoga, exercise, or breathing exercises, can be helpful, and if you smoke, stop. Avoid using medications that contain aspirin, ibuprofen, or other nonsteroidal anti-inflammatory drugs, all of which reduce the stomach's ability to produce its protective coating of mucus and hinder cell repair.

An old-fashioned remedy for ulcers was a tall glass of milk, but we now know that milk stimulates the production of gastric acid. Also avoid coffee, citrus fruits and drinks, animal fats, sugar, fried foods, alcohol, and hot, spicy foods, all of which can irritate the stomach lining.

Remedies

Only a blood test can determine if you have *H. pylori*. If you try various conventional treatments, for example, over-the-counter antacids and prescription drugs such as cimetidine (Tagamet) and famotidine (Pepcid) and your symptoms remain, chances are you have *H. pylori* and may need antibiotics. Here are some approaches you can take to treat peptic ulcers and perhaps avoid antibiotics.

Best Bets

◆ Take probiotic supplements, such as acidophilus and/or bifidobacteria (probiotics are often available in combination formulas). Probiotics provide healthy bacteria for the gastrointestinal tract and may help eliminate the harmful *H. pylori*. Probiotics are especially important if you are taking antibiotics, because antibiotics destroy both good and bad bacteria. If you are taking antibiotics, continue to take probiotics for about two weeks after you complete your drug course. Regular daily supplementation with probiotics is also an effective way to prevent the development of peptic ulcers.

◆ Drink fresh cabbage juice. A controlled study showed that people with ulcers who drank 32 ounces of fresh cabbage juice (in divided doses) every day were healed within ten days. If drinking that much cabbage juice sounds like more than you can handle, there is an alternative: a Chinese patent medicine composed of dried cabbage juice called Fare You. The usual dose is two tablets twice a day.

◆ Goldenseal, an herb with antibiotic powers, can be effective against *H. pylori*. Take 300–500 mg of a standardized extract containing 8 to 10 percent total alkaloids three times a day for five days.

Other Options

◆ Aloe vera juice provides effective relief against stomach acidity. Drink $\frac{1}{4}$ cup two to three times daily. Aloe vera juice is available in health food stores.

◆ The amino acid glutamine soothes stomach irritation. Begin by taking 1,000 mg three times daily for two weeks, then decrease to 1,000 mg twice daily for two weeks, and finally take 500 mg daily for two months.

When to See a Doctor

Consult your doctor if the pain occurs often or is chronic, or if it is accompanied by nausea that doesn't go away in a day or two. A serious sign is the presence of blood in stools or when vomiting, and you should see your doctor immediately.

◆ **CHAPTER 7** ◆

Itchy, Bumpy, Flaky All Over

he skin is our largest organ: an average adult has 2,000 to 3,000 square inches of this wondrous covering that provides protection to the internal organs, helps cool body temperature, creates vitamin D from sunlight, protects us from infection and injury, reflects our emotions, and responds to touch. It is constantly exposed to the environment around us, and so is susceptible to a variety of influences, such as temperature changes, humidity, and light. It is also influenced by our internal environment, including what we eat, and bacteria and other disease-causing organisms. This chapter looks at some of the itchy, bumpy, and flaky responses our skin has to our internal and external environments.

ABSCESSES

An abscess is a small area of infected tissue that the body attempts to isolate and thus prevent the spread of infection. This happens when white blood cells, which help defend the body against various infections, travel to the infected area and gather within the damaged tissue. The result is the formation of pus, which is an accumulation of bacteria and other infectious organisms, living and dead white blood cells, and dead tissue that is walled off from the surrounding healthy tissue.

Like boils (see BOILS on page 161), abscesses can be caused by the bacteria *Staphylococcus,* but they may also be the result of other types of bacteria, viruses, parasites, fungi, or amoebas. In some cases, the cause is unknown.

Types of Abscesses

There are many different kinds of abscesses, depending on where they develop. Abscesses can form in the brain, gums, abdominal wall, ears, tonsils, sinuses, kidneys, prostate gland, breasts, or almost any other body part. Skin abscesses are the most common type.

Skin abscesses are red, raised, and painful. They can affect people of any age, and usually develop after a bacterial infection, a minor injury or wound, or as a complication of boils. Abscesses should be treated promptly to help prevent spread of infection. If the infection spreads, chills, fever, drainage of pus, and localized swelling may occur (see "When to See a Doctor" on page 159).

Remedies

Even small, localized abscesses should be treated rather than be left to heal on their own. Treatment reduces the chance the infection will spread and is less stressful on the immune system. If there are any signs of infection, you should see your doctor so the abscess can be incised, drained, and treated with antibiotics. If you decide to treat a small abscess on your own, here are some recommendations.

Best Bets

- The herbs echinacea and goldenseal have antibacterial properties and also enhance the immune system. They are available in a combination supplement. Take a formula that supplies 250–500 mg echinacea and 150–300 mg goldenseal per dose, and take three to four doses per day for up to seven days.

- The herb cat's claw also has antibacterial properties and can boost the immune system response. Take 500 mg of standardized extract three times a day until the abscess disappears. Do not take cat's claw if you are pregnant or breastfeeding, or if you are taking an anticoagulant (blood thinner).

- Oregano is another herb with antibacterial properties. Take 75 mg of standardized extract three times daily until the abscess clears.

- If you must take antibiotics, also take probiotics to help restore the supply of friendly bacteria in your system. Probiotics such as acidophilus or bifidobacteria help replace the bacteria that are destroyed by antibiotics. Take these according to package directions.

Other Options

- Zinc is a powerful antioxidant and helps the immune system fight infection. Take 80 mg daily in divided doses. The lozenge form provides the best absorption. Do not continue taking this dosage of zinc once the abscess has cleared, as extended use of high doses of this mineral can eventually suppress the immune system.

◆ To help the abscess drain, apply a hot compress. Dip a clean, soft cloth (flannel is good) in hot water, wring it out until it's damp, and place it on the abscess until the cloth cools. Repeat this every two to three hours to promote healing and to help the abscess drain.

When to See a Doctor

Call your doctor if signs of infection occur, such as fever, localized swelling, or drainage of pus, especially if it contains blood. An abscess that has burrowed deep into the skin can cause fever, loss of appetite, and fatigue and should be treated immediately.

ATHLETE'S FOOT

Tinea pedis is the exotic-sounding name for an itchy, irritating fungal infection known commonly as athlete's foot. Yet even the most unathletic among us can get this condition, which is caused by fungi such as *Epidermophyton floccosum* and *Trichophyton* spp.

Causes and Symptoms of Athlete's Foot

All it takes for the fungi to feel welcome between your toes is prolonged exposure to a warm, moist environment. If you walk barefoot in showers and busy locker rooms, have sweaty feet that leave your socks damp, and are predisposed to fungal infections, you are likely to get athlete's foot.

At first, although your feet may not itch, you may notice white, scaly patches between your toes and on the bottom and sides of your feet. Then the symptoms arise: burning, itching, swelling, redness, cracking, and the emergence of tiny blisters and sores.

"Don't Scratch" and Other Tips

Not scratching an itch is difficult, but scratching athlete's foot breaks the sores and blisters, which can spread the fungus and cause a bacterial infection. Because athlete's foot is contagious, scratching can not only make your infection worse, but it can also make it much more likely that you will spread it to other people. If you use a shower or locker room at a health club or gym, or if you share a bathroom with other people in your home, there are precautions you need to take to protect yourself and others.

♦ When in a locker room or shower, wear shower shoes or slippers. Socks do not provide enough protection.

♦ If your socks become damp, change them. You may need to change them several times a day, depending on your activity and perspiration level.

♦ Use an antifungal spray or chlorine bleach in your shower at home.

♦ Expose your feet to the air as much as possible. When circumstances permit, wear sandals, open-toed shoes, or flip-flops.

♦ White cotton socks allow your feet to breathe. Avoid wearing socks made of synthetic materials and those that contain dyes. To kill the fungus and prevent reinfection, wash your socks in chlorine bleach.

♦ Keep your feet dry. After a shower, swimming, or when changing your socks because they are damp, dry your feet thoroughly, especially between your toes.

Remedies

Despite your best efforts, you've got the "crud." Now how do you get rid of it? First, follow the guidelines we've already discussed. Then, select one or more of the following at-home solutions.

Best Bets

♦ Various over-the-counter antifungal creams have been proven to be effective. However, you need to use them for at least three to four weeks, even if you see results in a week. These creams include clotrimazole (Lotrimin, Mycelex), miconazole (Micatin-Derm and Monistat-Derm), tolnaftate (Tinactin, Dr. Scholl's), and undecylenic acid (Desenex).

♦ An antifungal herb is cat's claw, which also enhances the immune system. Take 500 mg of standardized extract three times daily until the condition is completely resolved. (*Note:* Do not use cat's claw if you are pregnant, breast-feeding, or are an organ transplant recipient. Consult with your doctor first if you are taking blood thinners.)

♦ Tea tree oil is a powerful antifungal that speeds up healing and relieves itching. Use tea tree oil as follows: Soak your feet for ten minutes twice a day in 1 quart warm water to which you have added 10 drops of tea tree oil. After each soak, dry your feet and use a cotton swab to apply tea tree oil to the affected areas of your feet. You should soak your feet for ten days, and then continue to use the oil on your feet for another ninety days. If you don't have time to soak your feet, application of the tea tree oil to your feet twice daily is also effective.

Other Options

◆ To relieve itching and redness, use aloe vera gel and calendula (lotion if your skin is damp; ointment if it is dry). Use one of the herbs in the morning and the other at night. Both are soothing and healing for the skin.

◆ The homeopathic remedy thuja can help clear the infection. Rub a few drops of undiluted liquid thuja on the affected areas of your feet twice a day. Continue this treatment for thirty days. If you see an improvement, continue for another month. If you don't see any improvement, try another approach.

When to See a Doctor

Although most cases of athlete's foot can be cleared up at home, you may want to consult with your doctor if the condition is chronic. Also, if the blisters or sores have been opened from scratching or irritation, a bacterial infection can set in. Because an antifungal treatment approach will not take care of a bacterial infection as well, contact your doctor about possibly getting more aggressive treatment for both types of infection.

BOILS

A boil may get its name from the fact that it "boils" up from deep within a hair follicle or a sebaceous (oil-producing) gland and then erupts on the skin's surface. The eruption is a red, tender, pus-filled boil, sometimes referred to as a furuncle, that is about the size of a pea or larger. Boils typically appear on the face, neck, underarms, or buttocks. But why do they boil up in the first place?

Causes of Boils

Most boils are caused by *Staphylococcus aureus* (staph), a very common type of bacteria. In fact, it is estimated that up to 20 percent of people carry the bacteria on their skin. Staph is usually found in the nostrils, cleft of the buttocks, armpits, and between the legs, and is typically transferred under the fingernails to other locations on the body.

A boil is born when the skin in an area inhabited by staph is nicked, rubbed, or irritated in some way, which inoculates the germ into the wall of a hair follicle. Once the follicle is inoculated, the bacteria cause a boil to erupt. Often a single boil appears, but sometimes several will emerge and form a cluster called a carbuncle. Most boils run their course in about ten days.

Naturally, not everyone who experiences a nick or skin irritation develops a boil. People who have diabetes, anemia, or any infection that compromises the immune system are more susceptible to boils. The best way to prevent boils is to keep your skin clean and dry. However, even if you are meticulous, a boil can develop because you have another medical condition, or if you're in a hot, humid environment.

Baby a Boil

While treating a boil, never squeeze or puncture it. If you do, you'll be helping the infection spread. Also do not cover a boil with tape or an adhesive bandage. This may break the boil or increase irritation and possibly cause scarring. The best way to care for a boil is to keep your skin clean and dry, making sure you don't irritate the boil when you wash around it. If a boil breaks, pus will drain out. That's when you want to gently clean the area with a fresh cloth and apply a topical antibiotic, such as bacitracin, to help clear the infection and prevent it from spreading.

Remedies

You've probably heard the expression "lance a boil," which means someone (a doctor; don't do this at home!) uses a scalpel to open up a boil and drain the pus. This, of course, is an option. However, most boils can be treated effectively and safely at home if you can eliminate the infection. Here are some options.

Best Bets

◆ Usnea moss is effective against *Staphylococcus aureus*. The herb is available in an ointment, or can be applied as compress. To make a compress, make a strong usnea tea by adding two tea bags or 3 tablespoons of the whole herb to 8 ounces boiling water. Boil for three minutes and then steep for an additional ten minutes. Allow the tea to cool, then soak a clean white cloth in the tea and apply it to the boil for fifteen minutes. Apply compresses three to four times a day until the boil heals.

◆ The herbs echinacea and goldenseal work together to clear the infection and boost the immune system. These remedies are available in combination formulas. Take 250–500 mg echinacea and 150–300 mg goldenseal three times daily until the boil improves, up to seven days. As an added boost, apply goldenseal topically to the boil for faster healing. Break open a capsule of goldenseal and add enough drops of water to make a thin paste. Using a cotton swab, apply the paste to the boil several times a day until it heals.

◆ Another great combination is ginger tea and green clay. First, prepare a strong ginger tea by steeping two tea bags of the herb in 8 ounces boiling water for fifteen minutes. Allow the tea to cool and then soak a clean white cloth in the tea and apply it to the boil for fifteen minutes at least four times daily. After each application, apply a green clay paste (available in drugstores), which helps dry up the infection. Mix 1 teaspoon clay with just enough water to make a paste. Apply the paste to the boil after you remove the compress. Leave the paste on until it's time to apply the compress again.

Other Options

◆ Help fight infection by taking oregano, which has antibacterial properties. Take 75–160 mg of standardized extract three times daily.

◆ To speed draining of pus, take one dose of silicea 12x or 6c three times a day for two days. This homeopathic remedy can also help bring a boil to a head.

When to See a Doctor

Although at-home treatment is usually sufficient, occasionally a boil will spread beyond the affected area and cause a more serious infection. Indications of an infection include fever, feeling run down, red streaks around the boil, and the presence of swollen lymph glands in your neck, groin, or other areas of the body. If these symptoms occur, call your physician. If a boil grows and does not improve in three to four days with treatment, if you develop a high fever, or if you develop new boils or other members of your family develop boils, contact your doctor.

BUNIONS

There's nothing pretty about bunions. These big, bony knobs that appear at the base of the big-toe joint develop when the joint becomes deformed and the tissue around the joint swells. In medical terminology they are called "hallux vulgus," which certainly doesn't improve their appeal. There are even bunionettes, small bunions that appear on the outside of the little toe. Despite an apparent attempt to make them sound cute, there's nothing attractive about these miniature bunions either.

Causes of Bunions

Bunions are rare in societies where people go barefoot. Why? Because most bunions are caused by wearing "too" shoes: too small, too tight, too high. Look at the shoes that you wear most often. Are the toes pointy? Are the heels an inch or higher? Try on your shoes. Do your feet feel squeezed and pinched?

Although bunions tend to run in families and many people do inherit a weakness of the big-toe joint or flat feet, these ugly bumps would not have a chance to develop in most people if they didn't wear inappropriate, ill-fitting shoes. When we say "they," we are referring primarily to women, because women are the ones most likely to wear "too" shoes, and the ones who typically develop bunions. When such shoes are worn, there is continuous irritation and thus inflammation of the joint. This results in a thickening of the bursa—a fluid-filled sac that serves as a cushion for the big-toe joint. The thicker the bursa, the bigger the bunion.

Some people develop bunions that are so painful they find it difficult to walk. Thus a little bump can become a major problem if the proper steps aren't taken.

Remedies

Once a bunion has developed, the only way to eliminate it completely is to undergo surgery (see "When to See a Doctor" on page 165). However, you can take measures to prevent further growth of a bunion, and to live with one you may have.

Best Bets

◆ Wear appropriate shoes. This is the single most important thing you can do to deal with a bunion. "Appropriate" shoes are those that fit properly: They should be wide enough so your feet and toes are comfortable and not squeezed, with a low heel (no more than $3/4$ of an inch) so your feet are not pushed into the front of your shoes. There should be $1/2$ inch of space between your longest toe and the front of your shoe. Also, get your feet sized. Most women believe they know their shoe size, when in reality they are wearing shoes that are a half or whole size too small. Have both feet sized, as one foot is typically a bit larger than the other, and get the size that matches the larger foot.

◆ A special device that straightens the big toe can be worn to help correct a small, developing bunion.

◆ Foot exercises can strengthen your arches, which can help keep your bones aligned. Use a soft ball, like a Nerf ball, and practice picking up the ball with your toes. Do this for about five to ten minutes a day while watching television or eating dinner.

Other Options

◆ For pain relief, apply Aspercreme to the bunion, or take an over-the-counter painkiller such as ibuprofen (for example, Advil, Motrin) or naproxen (Aleve). An alternative is to crush an aspirin, mix it with a few drops of olive oil, and make a paste. Apply the paste to the swollen joint.

◆ If a foot deformity or abnormality is a contributing factor, you may benefit from orthotics. Orthotics are shoe inserts, which are available either over-the-counter or can be custom made for your feet. They help correct foot problems, such as walking on the sides of your feet. You can try over-the-counter inserts to see if they help. If they do not, see your doctor about getting custom-made orthotics.

When to See a Doctor

See a podiatrist or foot surgeon if you have a bunion that makes it difficult for you to walk, and wearing appropriate shoes does not sufficiently remedy the problem; or if your bunion gets worse despite your attempts to remedy the situation. The solution does not have to be surgery; custom-made orthotics may be what you need. Surgery should be considered as a last resort.

CALLUSES AND CORNS

Shake the hand of a carpenter, and you may feel rough, thickened areas on his hands. Catch a glimpse of the naked feet of a runner and you may see tough yellowish skin on the sides of her toes. These types of skin reactions are calluses and corns, respectively, and they are the body's way of armoring itself against friction and pressure.

The Difference between Calluses and Corns

A callus is a buildup of hard, thick yellowish skin, usually on the bottom of the feet or on the palms of the hands. The buildup is a thickening of the stratum corneum, the outermost layer of skin. It is the body's response to constant friction or pressure, as when you swing a hammer, row a boat, or wear shoes in which there is undue pressure on one part of your foot, such as the heel. The chronic pressure or friction causes an increase in the number of skin cells and the amount of blood flow to the area, both of which work to speed up cell growth. The additional cells form a callus.

A corn is also a thickening of the outer layers of skin prompted by pressure or friction. The difference between calluses and corns is that the latter appear on the feet only, and they develop against bony areas, such as on top of or on the sides of the toes. Corns typically develop when ill-fitting shoes squeeze the foot, resulting in pressure against a bony part of the foot. In some cases, a corn is accompanied by an inflamed bursa (a bubblelike sac that surrounds the toe joint). The bursa becomes inflamed when it fills with fluids in response to pressure and irritation.

How to Prevent Calluses and Corns

The best way to prevent the formation of calluses or corns on your feet is to wear proper-fitting shoes with adequate padding, and low heels. Women who wear high heels much of the time are inviting calluses. Only wear heels that are $\frac{1}{2}$ to 1 inch high. If you feel you must wear higher heels, do so only occasionally, and make sure the shoes have extra cushioning in the forefoot area.

When was the last time you had your feet sized? Many people buy shoes time after time for years and never have their shoe size checked. Feet grow and spread with age, and the size 6A you wore in college may need to be a 6 $\frac{1}{2}$B or 7B by the time you're in your thirties or forties.

Prevention of calluses on the hands can be accomplished by simply wearing gloves. However, calluses on the hands often are not bothersome and are actually a plus for the carpenters, tennis players, rowers, and guitar players who have them.

Remedies

Treatment suggestions for calluses and corns are similar. The number-one remedy for corns and calluses affecting the feet, of course, is getting rid of your tight, high-heeled shoes and wearing shoes that fit. Then there are other options for eliminating these growths and relieving the pain.

Best Bets

♦ To prevent friction in your shoes and the formation of calluses, wear anti-shearing insoles in your shoes. This type of insole is superior to the ordinary foam insoles. Anti-shearing insoles may be made of nitrogen-impregnated foam or a pyrometric material and are available in drugstores and pharmacies.

♦ Steep a chamomile tea bag in 3 to 4 cups of warm water and soak your feet for fifteen minutes. This will soften the calluses. Then, if the calluses are not particularly painful, use a pumice stone to gently remove dead skin. Follow this with application of a moisturizer, such as petroleum jelly. Do this every night or several times a week, depending on the extent of your problem.

♦ Soak your feet in warm water and Epsom salts to soften the thickened skin. Then, if the calluses or corns are not especially painful, use a pumice stone to gently remove the dead skin.

Other Options

♦ Special pads can be worn that protect corns from irritation. The best type has an oval sterile-gauze-covered opening or an oval depression, which allows the corn to bulge into the opening and distributes the pressure onto the surrounding area of the foot. NEVER use pads that contain an acid preparation, because the acid can damage the tissues.

♦ If you have corns that have developed between two adjacent toes, separate them with toe spacers, that is, tiny pieces of foam or lamb's wool that you place between your toes. NEVER use cotton, as it will harden and cause more pressure.

When to See a Doctor

Do not attempt to self-treat calluses or corns on your feet if you have diabetes, poor circulation, a foot infection, or poor vision. Also consult your doctor if your calluses or corns are especially painful and not responding to self-treatment. Sometimes chronic calluses can be relieved by getting custom-made orthotics, shoe inserts that are specially made to address foot abnormalities that may be causing or contributing to excessive pressure on the feet. You must see a podiatrist or foot surgeon for custom-made orthotics.

ECZEMA

Got an itch? Don't scratch it, not if it's eczema. Have you ever taken off your watch and noticed a red, itchy rash where the watchband had touched your skin? Perhaps you washed your clothes in a new detergent and experienced a rash when wearing the newly laundered clothes. Or maybe you got an unexpected surprise when you applied a new facial cream and your face turned red and began to swell and itch.

These situations could represent one of several types of eczema, an inflammatory skin condition characterized by patches of red, dry, itchy skin that may also become swollen, blistered, and oozing. Itching can be so severe that some people scratch until their skin bleeds, which can lead to a bacterial infection.

Eczema can affect people of any age, and it can occur once or twice in a lifetime, or be chronic. It's estimated that 10 million Americans have eczema, and that it's most common among people who have asthma or hay fever. One good thing about eczema is that it is not contagious.

Types of Eczema

Eczema is an allergic reaction that can be the result of either atopic dermatitis (skin inflammation) or contact dermatitis. People with atopic dermatitis, which is believed to be hereditary, are hypersensitive to certain substances in the environment, including pollen, molds, and some foods, that do not harm or affect other individuals. Thus, their immune systems overreact, resulting in irritated, sore, inflamed skin. Unfortunately, atopic dermatitis can be a lifelong problem.

If you have a skin reaction to a watchband, freshly laundered clothes, bubble bath, or cosmetics, you probably have allergic or irritant contact dermatitis. Contact dermatitis is more common than the atopic form. It usually develops over time as the body's immune system reacts to repeated contact with a culprit substance. People who have to wash their hands a lot, like healthcare workers, or who come into contact with detergents and chemicals often suffer with contact dermatitis.

Other types of eczema include adult seborrheic eczema, which usually appears as dandruff (discussed in Chapter 3), and varicose eczema, which affects the lower legs of older individuals.

The one characteristic that binds all the types of eczema together is that it develops in people who have very dry, itchy skin that doesn't hold onto moisture well. Thus, the secret to prevention and treatment is keeping the skin properly moist and thereby more comfortable.

CAN I LIVE WITH ECZEMA?

With a little planning and foresight, you can live with eczema. Here are some tips:

◆ Don't use soap, because it removes natural oils from the body. Instead, use a soap-free cleanser or an emulsifying ointment.

◆ Avoid woolen, fuzzy, or rough clothing. Instead, wear soft cotton clothes.

◆ Avoid cosmetics, lotions, and body products that contain lanolin. Lanolin plugs up oil glands and irritates eczema.

◆ Don't scratch. Sure, that's easy to say, but scratching can make eczema worse by damaging the skin and even causing a bacterial infection.

◆ Use a humidifier in your home or office if the air is dry. It's best to keep your relative humidity higher than 40 percent to protect against dry skin or making dry skin worse.

◆ If you have atopic dermatitis and are sensitive to pollen or other airborne substances, you may need to install high-quality air filters in your home or office. HEPA (high-efficiency particulate arresting) filters can remove nearly 100 percent of molds, pollen, dust, and other particulates from the air in a given space.

◆ Food irritants should be avoided.

Causes of Eczema

Many things can trigger the itching, redness, swelling, and other discomfort associated with eczema. Two very common causes are dust-mite droppings and dander from pets, especially dogs and cats. Many people also have an allergy to nickel, which is found in alloys, including low-carat gold and less expensive silver. Nickel is used in jewelry, zippers, and stainless-steel cutlery. When susceptible people sweat, the moisture releases the nickel from the alloys and results in skin irritation. Stress is a two-pronged factor, as it can trigger eczema and also make an active case worse. And although not believed to be direct triggers, lack of sleep, eating lots of sugar and refined carbohydrates, dry air, temperature extremes, and certain drugs can all lower the immune system defenses and thus increase susceptibility to eczema.

Some people are never able to identify the cause of their eczema. Their skin just starts to itch for no apparent reason. If this sounds like you, the inset "Can I Live with Eczema?" may offer some useful suggestions.

Remedies

Although there is currently no cure for eczema, there are several ways to reduce the itching and other discomfort caused by this skin disorder. The following remedies address eczema caused by both atopic and contact dermatitis.

Best Bets

◆ An antihistamine such as chlorpheniramine (Chlor-Trimeton), diphenhydramine (in Benadryl and other over-the-counter medications), or hydroxyzine (Atarax, Vistaril) can relieve itching. That's because itching is an allergic response associated with the release of histamine.

◆ Vitamin E is the skin vitamin, and it should be taken daily as a preventive measure, and used topically for active cases. Select a product that contains mixed tocopherols or d-alpha-tocopherol. Begin by taking 400 IU every morning for two weeks, then add 400 IU in the evening, and after two weeks add another 400 IU in the middle of the day, for a total of 1,200 IU daily. *Note:* If you have high blood pressure or are taking an anticoagulant (blood thinner), consult with your doctor before you take vitamin E.

◆ Evening primrose oil is rich in omega-6 fatty acids, especially gamma-linolenic acid. This fatty acid has anti-inflammatory properties and provides significant relief of eczema, according to British researchers. You need to take 70–240 mg of gamma-linolenic acid a day; depending on which supplement brand you buy, this translates into two to six standard capsules of evening primrose oil.

Other Options

◆ Take a bath in colloidal (powdered) oatmeal to relieve itching. Pour 2 cups of powdered oatmeal (available in pharmacies and drugstores) into your warm (not hot; hot water can aggravate eczema) bathwater and soak for about fifteen to twenty minutes. If you can't find colloidal oatmeal, buy regular oatmeal and grind it in a blender or food processor until it's finely ground. You can also add 2 tablespoons of baking soda to the bathwater.

◆ After getting out of a bath or shower, apply a lanolin-free emollient, such as calendula ointment or olive oil, to your skin.

When to See a Doctor

If an eczema episode doesn't resolve after two weeks of self-treatment, you may need to ask your doctor for prescription-strength antihistamines or hydrocortisone cream. Also seek help from your doctor if the eczema starts to ooze, has an odor, starts to crust over, or if there are signs and symptoms of infection due to scratching the affected areas (for example, fever, redness and swelling, pus).

HIVES

Imagine a bowl of big, juicy, ripe strawberries. You put the bowl on the table in front of your friends, along with some whipped cream and melted chocolate. They all reach for the plump berries; everyone, that is, except one person. "Chandrea, you don't like strawberries?" you ask. "They don't like me," says Chandrea. "And if I eat one, I'll look like a strawberry in a matter of minutes."

Chandrea, like many people, experiences an allergic response known as hives when she eats strawberries. Hives are a type of itchy rash, also known as urticaria or nettle rash, that usually appears as an allergic reaction to certain foods, medications, insect bites, or plants. Some people get hives from sun exposure, excessive stress, or extreme changes in temperature.

Causes of Hives

About 20 percent of people will develop hives at some time during their lives, with women being more susceptible than men. Hives typically erupt within minutes of eating or coming into contact with an offending food or other substance. They appear when certain skin cells release histamine, a substance that causes the small blood vessels to dilate and the cell walls to become permeable. This action allows a clear fluid called serum to leak into the tissues and cause inflammation and itchy, raised bumps called hives.

Hives can erupt in various sizes and anywhere on the body. Sometimes they even emerge inside the mouth and ears. At first hives are red, but they gradually fade to white at the center with a red outline. An attack can last only a few hours but more typically stays around for a day to a week.

Foods known to cause hives include strawberries, nuts, eggs, milk, and shellfish, although some people do react to other foods and food additives. Medications such as aspirin, penicillin, and other antibiotics are also common culprits. Bites or stings from bees, wasps, beetles, spiders, or other insects, as well as contact with poison ivy, nettle, cactus spines or needles, or other plants may also cause hives.

Remedies

If you've experienced hives and can identify the cause, your best approach is avoidance. That means you may need to pass up the peanuts, find alternative medications if your doctor prescribes antibiotics, or limit your time in the sun. Although hives do go away by themselves, there's no reason you should have to suffer with the intense itching that accompanies them. Here are some ways to relieve the itch.

Best Bets

◆ An over-the-counter antihistamine such as diphenhydramine (Benadryl), hydroxyzine (Atarax), or cyproheptadine (Periactin) can effectively relieve itching and swelling. However, they all can cause side effects, including anxiety, fatigue, drowsiness, dizziness, and dry mouth.

◆ Run a warm bath and add 3–4 tablespoons of baking soda or 5 tablespoons of colloidal oatmeal to the water. Soak for ten to fifteen minutes.

◆ Add 9 cups of white vinegar to a warm bath. Vinegar helps prevent itching by acidifying the skin. If your hives are localized, mix 1 teaspoon of vinegar with a tablespoon of water and apply the mixture with a cotton ball to the affected areas.

Other Options

◆ Take nutrients that have antihistamine and anti-inflammatory properties: 500 mg vitamin C and 300 mg quercetin (a flavonoid) each three to four times daily.

◆ The homeopathic remedy rhus toxicodendron helps reduce redness, swelling, and itching. Take one dose of 30x or 15c three to four times daily for up to two days. If you get minimal or no improvement, take one dose of bovista 6x or 3c three times daily for up to three days.

When to See a Doctor

You should go to an emergency facility immediately if hives affect your mouth or throat, as they may compromise your breathing. Contact your doctor immediately if you get hives after taking medication, or if you experience faintness or rapid pulse.

INSECT BITES AND STINGS

Ants, bees, fleas, flies, gnats, hornets, mosquitoes, scorpions, spiders, ticks, and wasps—collectively there are more of them than there are of us. Sometimes we get in their way, or they get in ours, and the result can be a bite or sting that can be merely annoying and uncomfortable for a short time, or more serious in some people. About 1 in every 250 people is highly allergic to insect bites.

Types of Bites and Stings

The response to a bite or sting is an allergic reaction to the tiny creature's saliva or venom. In most cases that response is pain or itching, redness, and swelling at the site of the attack. If you have been bitten or stung by a venomous spider like the black widow or brown recluse, or you have a severe reaction to a bee sting, you may need immediate medical attention (see "When to See a Doctor" on page 175). Some ticks are also known to transmit disease (see "Going Buggy" on page 174), and mosquitoes can carry various diseases as well. However, in the majority of cases, a bite or sting from a nonpoisonous insect or spider does not cause a serious reaction or disease.

How to Prevent Bites and Stings

You can avoid or significantly reduce your risk of getting insect bites or stings if you take a few precautions.

* Always wear shoes when you're outside. Ants, scorpions, bees, and hornets are usually found on the ground.

* Avoid wearing bright jewelry (including metal earrings) outdoors because insects are attracted to them.

* Keep your skin covered when in areas inhabited by ticks. Gardeners and hikers frequently are the victims of tick bites. Always check your skin and hair carefully.

* Avoid wearing scented soaps, perfumes, hair sprays, and other scented products when you're outdoors. Insects are attracted to them.

♦ You can repel some insects by mixing 5 drops of citronella oil in 8 ounces of water and dabbing the mixture on your skin.

♦ An unlikely insect repellent is permethrin (available in drugstores as Nix, Permanone, or Duranon), a medication used to eliminate head lice. Spray the permethrin on your clothing, not your skin.

GOING BUGGY

A few venomous or disease-carrying insects and spiders are common in some parts of the country. If you are bitten by one of them, seek medical care. Here's how to recognize them or the symptoms they may cause. If possible, capture the creature that has bitten you so the doctor can identify it and better know how to treat you.

♦ *Black widow spider:* This creature has a characteristic red hourglass spot on its underside. Symptoms include sweating, dizziness, stomach cramps, nausea, and headache. An antivenin is available, but healthy adults are usually given medications for the pain and cramps, as well as antianxiety drugs.

♦ *Brown recluse spider:* A bite from this spider causes a bull's eye mark, which looks like a blister surrounded by red and white circles. Symptoms include pain, nausea, chills, and fever. Treatment is critical, as the surrounding tissue may die without it.

♦ *Ticks:* A bite from these creatures can transmit various diseases, including Lyme disease (most Atlantic coast states plus California, Wisconsin, and Minnesota), Rocky Mountain spotted fever (all states except Alaska, Hawaii, and Maine), and babesiosis (California, Connecticut, Massachusetts, Minnesota, New York, and Rhode Island). For Lyme disease, a typical first sign is a bull's eye marking at the bite site: a round, reddish lesion with a pale center. Rocky Mountain spotted fever and babesiosis usually first manifest as fever, chills, headache, nausea, and vomiting.

♦ *Scorpions:* Despite popular opinion, the majority of scorpion bites are not serious unless they happen to infants or the elderly, or if the bite is from an Arizona bark scorpion. Most scorpion bites can be treated according to the "Remedies" section.

- If you know you have serious reactions to insect bites, always carry a prescription epinephrine kit and an antihistamine with you.

Remedies

Everyone reacts to an insect bite or sting differently. Some react immediately; others don't respond for hours or even days. Some break out in hives; others have a few itchy bumps that go away in a day or two. Venom may cause swelling in one person and dizziness and nausea in another. The important thing is to act quickly in order to minimize the reaction, then seek medical help if indicated.

Best Bets

- In the case of a sting, you need to remove the stinger and the attached venom sac to prevent any more poison from entering your body. Never pull the stinger out. Instead, gently scrape the area around the stinger with your fingernail or a knife blade until the stinger and the venom sac have been dislodged. To remove a tick, cover it with petroleum jelly or oil, wait a few minutes, then gently twist it off using tweezers.

- Once the stinger is removed, apply bicarbonate of soda to counteract the acid of the poison. Then apply witch hazel to the area. Apply an ice pack or cold compress for thirty to forty-five minutes to reduce swelling and inflammation.

- Take a twofold homeopathic approach. First, apply liquid natrum muriaticum 6x immediately to the site to relieve burning and itching. Then take apis mellifica 12x, 30x, 6c, or 9c to relieve stinging and swelling. Take one dose as indicated on the package and then subsequent doses one per hour for up to four hours.

Other Options

- If ice is not available, heat is a good alternative. Heat neutralizes a chemical that causes inflammation. A heat pack, hot-water bottle, hot compress, or even aiming a hair dryer on the site will help.

- To relieve inflammation and sting, moisten the area and apply a crushed aspirin to the site.

When to See a Doctor

See a doctor immediately if any of the following occur: you are bitten by a known poisonous spider or scorpion; the bite or sting is on your face or in your

mouth or throat; you develop hives, difficulty breathing, and nausea and vomiting; you had a tick bite and develop a circular rash, joint pain, fever, and flu-
like symptoms.

POISON IVY, OAK, AND SUMAC

It seems to be a childhood initiation rite to get at least one case of poison ivy,
poison oak, or poison sumac. If you were one of the itching victims of these
plants, you probably also remember wearing the calamine lotion on your arms
and legs for days, with the warning from your mother not to scratch lest the
rash spread and cause you even more misery.

Of course, poison ivy, oak, and sumac are not reserved for children. As adults
we are especially susceptible if we're out hiking, working in the garden, or playing with the kids in the park or woods.

Causes of Rash

The rash associated with these plants is an allergic reaction to a resin called
urushiol that is found in their leaves, stems, and roots. The resin is so potent
that you can get the characteristic itchy red rash even if you don't come into
direct contact with the plants. If you brush up against a plant and some of the
urushiol gets on your clothes, you can get the rash if you then touch that part of
your clothing. A serious case of poison ivy/oak/sumac can occur if you breathe
in smoke from the burning leaves of these plants.

Within a few hours, or sometimes even days, of making contact with one of
these poisonous plants, red, itchy pimples can appear on the skin. They usually
develop into small, fluid-filled blisters that can spread the rash even further if
they are broken.

Not everyone is allergic to poison ivy, oak, or sumac, and the extent of the rash
depends on how sensitive you are to the plant. The rash typically lasts one to
four weeks, with the worst itching occurring four to seven days after exposure.

Purging the Poison

Time is of the essence when you've been exposed to urushiol. The quicker you
can eliminate the resin from your body and clothing, the less severe your rash
will be. In fact, it's widely held that if you thoroughly wash away the resin
within thirty minutes of contact, you won't get a rash. Of course, that depends
on how sensitive you are to the urushiol. Why take a chance? As soon as you've

been in contact with urushiol, thoroughly rinse your skin with soap and water or use 70 percent alcohol followed by a water rinse. Rub your skin very gently; do not use a washcloth as it may spread the resin. Clean thoroughly under your fingernails as well, as the resin can hide there and be easily spread to other parts of your body. As a precaution, you should also wash any clothing suspected of having the resin on them. Affected clothing should be washed separately from other clothing.

Remedies

Okay, you've got the rash, so should you reach for the calamine lotion again? Well, mother meant well, but if calamine is used for more than seven days, it can dry the skin and actually create more discomfort. (Calamine can be effective in the short term for mild cases.) Here are some alternative ways to treat the itching and oozing.

Best Bets

♦ Aloe vera gel is very soothing and can be applied three to four times daily.

♦ Soak several times a day in a tub of lukewarm water to which you've added 1 cup of either cornstarch, bicarbonate of soda, or oatmeal. Soak for up to thirty minutes each time.

♦ Apply cold compresses for fifteen to thirty minutes every few hours to reduce swelling and relieve itching. Add 1 tablespoon of sea salt per 16 ounces of water.

Other Options

♦ The homeopathic remedy of rhus toxicodendron, which is homeopathic poison ivy, provides quick relief of itching. Take one dose of 12x or 6c three to four times daily until your symptoms are significantly better.

♦ Calendula gel or liquid extract applied to the skin three to four times a day relieves itching and helps the skin heal more quickly.

When to See a Doctor

You should seek medical help if any of the following occur: if you have difficulty breathing as a result of exposure to these poisonous plants; if the rash is accompanied by pain or swelling on your face or genital area; or if you notice signs of infection such as increased tenderness, swelling, or warmth.

PSORIASIS

Most of us are familiar with a traffic jam. There's a situation—an accident, road construction, a fallen telephone pole in the road—and the cars immediately in front of the situation stop, causing the cars behind them to stop, perhaps suddenly, causing a pileup of vehicles and snarled bumper-to-bumper traffic. The traffic won't resolve until the obstruction is removed.

Psoriasis is something like a traffic jam. Normally, the body sheds old skin cells as the new skin cells move to the surface. This occurs without incident; the traffic flows smoothly. But in psoriasis, the body produces new skin cells about ten times faster than normal, while the old skin cells are still shedding at the normal rate. This causes a traffic jam: the new skin cells can't reach the surface of the skin so they jam up and form thickened patches.

Cause of Psoriasis

While we can identify the cause of a traffic jam, scientists haven't yet been able to uncover the cause of psoriasis. Several of the theories point to diet. Some researchers say that a high-fat diet is the cause, because psoriasis is rare in areas of the world where a low-fat diet is the norm. Others say that the type of fat eaten is more important than the amount: people who do not get enough of the essential fatty acids omega-3 and omega-6 are much more prone to the skin condition.

Another theory is that an accumulation of toxins in the intestinal tract prompts the development of psoriasis; yet another is that a systemic attack of candida (a yeast infection) plays a role. Flare-ups can be triggered by stress, illness, sunburn, alcohol abuse, and use of certain medications such as nonsteroidal anti-inflammatory drugs, lithium, and beta-blockers. And because psoriasis tends to run in families, we can't rule out a genetic link as well. In fact, in 2003 researchers announced that they had identified three genes associated with psoriasis.

Symptoms of Psoriasis

Psoriasis appears as thickened patches of reddened skin covered by white, gray, or silvery scales. The scales are the dead and dying skin that the body has not yet shed. Patches of psoriasis can emerge anywhere on the body, but the most commonly affected sites are the scalp, knuckles, elbows, back, knees, and buttocks. When it affects the nails, it can make them appear discolored and pitted.

An episode of psoriasis may consist of one or two scaly lesions or dozens or somewhere in between. If you have a mild case, the lesions may be barely noticeable, but more severe cases can produce unsightly patches.

Psoriasis usually first appears in people between the ages of fifteen and twenty-five, and overall affects about 2 percent of Americans. It's an unpredictable disorder, because you never know whether your first episode is the last, the first of many, or one of a few during your lifetime. The good news is that it's not contagious, and when the lesions go away they don't leave scars.

Remedies

Although psoriasis isn't a serious condition medically, it can be embarrassing, uncomfortable, and downright annoying. Add to that the fact that no cure has yet been found. But significant relief is possible, especially if you combine several of the suggestions below.

Best Bets

♦ Diet plays a big role in psoriasis, and a shift away from protein-rich foods such as meat and dairy toward cold-water fish can make a significant difference in your symptoms. Some experts recommend getting a daily supply of the essential fatty acids omega-3 and omega-6, which are critical for skin health. These fatty acids are found in cold-water fish, including salmon, herring, and tuna. While you're reeling in the fish, add plenty of plant-based items to your menu, including vegetables, fruits, grains, and legumes, which contain lots of fiber that can help eliminate toxins from the body.

♦ A Swedish study shows that aloe cream produced significant relief in 83 percent of people who used it. Apply the cream according to package directions. In a pinch you can use olive oil; apply twice daily.

♦ Mild psoriasis responds well to over-the-counter hydrocortisone cream. After applying the cream, wrap the treated area in plastic wrap to promote healing.

Other Options

♦ Because chronic stress can both trigger a psoriasis episode and contribute to it, meditation can be of benefit. A study at the University of Massachusetts Medical School in Worcester found that people with psoriasis who used both meditation and light therapy (see next option) healed twice as fast as people who used light therapy alone.

-◆ Exposure to sunlight or to a sun lamp can be very therapeutic for people who have psoriasis. Before you expose yourself to either source, however, ask your doctor how long you can safely use this approach.

When to See a Doctor

If you have a serious episode of psoriasis that is not responding to self-treatment, or if the patches are covering much of your body, your doctor can prescribe various medications, including topical steroids, coal-tar products, calcipotriene (a synthetic derivative of vitamin D3), or etretinate (a synthetic relative of vitamin A). The doctor may also prescribe ultraviolet light therapy along with these prescriptions.

WARTS

The classic picture of a craggy old witch with a large wart on the side of her nose is, fortunately, not the typical case when it comes to warts. For one thing, warts usually appear on the hands or feet, although they can also emerge on the neck, face, and genital area. For another, they can appear in people of any age, but they tend to be more common among younger individuals. Approximately 9 million Americans are affected by warts each year.

Causes and Types of Warts

Warts are skin growths caused by viruses. Scientists have identified about seventy different strains of human papillomavirus, or HPV, that can cause these growths. Warts can be as small as a pinhead or as big as a dime or larger when they appear in clusters. The viruses are contagious, but they need a point of entry on the skin, such as a scratch, puncture, or crack, to get into the body. The virus may then lay dormant for up to six months before it emerges as a wart.

The kinds of warts seen most often are common warts, plantar warts, plane warts, and genital warts. Common warts appear as brown or gray raised skin that is hard, rough, and clearly outlined. They sometimes appear in clusters. Plantar warts are hard, rough areas that develop on the soles of the feet and/or the underside of the toes. Plane warts are small, flesh-colored areas that are flat and tend to grow in clusters. Genital warts are distinguished by their location—the genital or perianal area—and appearance, which is pink or red, rubbery, and clustered like tiny heads of cauliflower.

How to Prevent Warts

While genital warts are transmitted to other people through sexual contact, other types of warts are shared through habits such as walking barefoot on moist floors in locker rooms, pool and spa areas, and communal showers. Always wear shower shoes or flip-flops when walking around in wet areas, and dry your feet well. Don't share towels or washcloths with other people.

With genital warts, use of condoms does not necessarily prevent the spread of the virus, because the warts are often in areas of the pubic region not protected by the condom.

If you have a wart, don't scratch or pick it, even if it itches. Scratching and picking can cause infection and spread the virus.

Remedies

Most warts will disappear by themselves: one-third disappear within six months, while others can take up to five years. But if your warts are painful or in an embarrassing or unsightly location, you probably wanted them gone yesterday. Here are some safe at-home approaches for getting rid of various types of warts.

Best Bets

- For warts on your fingers, wrap the warts with four layers of plain adhesive. Leave the bandage on for six and a half days, remove it for half a day, then put on another bandage. Repeat this cycle for three to four weeks, by which the time the wart should disappear. An alternative is to place a small piece of banana peel against the wart and wrap the finger in adhesive tape. Change the peel once a day and apply it for two weeks or until the wart disappears.

- Over-the-counter acid-impregnated plasters (such as Mediplast) can be used to treat all but genital warts. These plasters are safer than over-the-counter solutions of salicylic acid, which can irritate the skin. Follow package directions for using the plasters. They are typically applied once a day for ten to fourteen days to be effective.

- Crush an aspirin and mix the powder with a few drops of water to make a paste. Apply the paste to the wart and then cover with a bandage for a day or two. The wart should reduce in size and appearance significantly. Don't use this approach, however, if there are any cuts, scratches, or other skin openings near the wart.

Other Options

◆ Although it may be hard to believe, several studies have shown that using visualization to imagine the warts are melting away is effective. It is important that you believe this is possible, and that you practice the technique for about three minutes several times a day until the warts disappear.

◆ Crush several vitamin C tablets, add a few drops of water to make a paste, and apply the mixture to your warts. Cover with a bandage. Reapply the paste and bandage every day for several weeks until the wart disappears. It is believed that the acid in the vitamin C kills the virus.

When to See a Doctor

Although you can treat genital warts at home, they are associated with an increased risk of cervical cancer in women. Therefore, women should be monitored by their doctors during treatment. If you want warts removed because they are unsightly or causing pain, see your doctor, who can use one of several approaches, such as laser surgery, freezing, or burning. Any wart that looks or feels inflamed or infected should be seen by a doctor.

CHAPTER 8

Feeling Down and Out

nlike health conditions that are concentrated in only one part of the body, such as a bunion or a headache or diarrhea, some ailments can make you feel bad all over. For example, if you experience jet lag, insomnia, or chronic fatigue syndrome, you might say that your entire body feels fatigued and generally "worn out." Similarly, if you get a cold, your throat may be sore, your eyes may be tearing, your nose may be runny, you may have trouble breathing, and you probably feel tired all over.

In this chapter we look at health problems that tend to make us feel dragged out, knocked down, and just plain lousy all over. Learn what you can do to kick the symptoms and put the spark back into your life.

ANEMIA

"Iron-poor blood" is often used as a catch-all phrase for anemia, a condition in which the number and/or size of red blood cells is altered, resulting in an insufficient amount of oxygen reaching the tissues. When your cells and muscles are deprived of oxygen, you feel fatigued. You may also feel dizzy or breathless and experience palpitations, headache, insomnia, poor appetite, stomach distress, or chest pains.

Causes and Types of Anemia

Anemia can develop for many reasons, but regardless of the cause, the players include red blood cells, hemoglobin, and oxygen. For red blood cells to stay healthy and function well, they need various nutrients, including iron, folic acid, vitamins B_{12} and C, protein, and copper. One of the functions of red blood cells is to transport oxygen via a pigment found in those cells called hemoglobin. Healthy red blood cells each can carry between 200 and 300 hemoglobin molecules as they circulate throughout the body. But when something causes a reduction in the number of red blood cells or hemoglobin, anemia results. A deficiency of iron is one of those things.

Here's how iron-deficiency anemia works. The formation of hemoglobin requires iron, and thus low levels of iron are a major cause of anemia. About 20 percent of women, 3 percent of men, and 50 percent of pregnant women have iron-deficiency anemia. This form usually results from poor absorption or insufficient consumption of iron, or from blood loss, such as during heavy menstrual periods or surgery. Pregnancy also increases the need for hemoglobin, which many women fail to meet. In addition to the symptoms already mentioned, iron-deficiency anemia can cause a sore tongue, dry, brittle nails, and paleness.

But "iron-poor blood" is actually a misnomer in some cases of anemia. While it's true that most people who have anemia are iron deficient, there are several other causes and types of anemia as well. A deficiency of vitamin B_{12}, for example, results in anemia in about 2 of every 1,000 people. Hemoglobin requires a much smaller amount of B_{12}, so it takes longer for this type of anemia to develop if there is a deficiency of this vitamin. Because B_{12} is found almost exclusively in animal products, people who follow a plant-based diet are susceptible to this type of anemia unless they eat B_{12}-fortified foods or take supplements. Others who may get B_{12}-deficiency anemia include people who have Crohn's disease, celiac disease, or other conditions that interfere with the absorption of nutrients. In addition to the classic symptoms of iron-deficiency anemia mentioned, people with B_{12}-deficiency anemia may have yellowish skin, weight loss, and tingling in the arms and legs.

Another form of anemia is folic acid deficiency. This form is seen most often in pregnant women and the elderly, two populations that have a greater need for folic acid. Poor diet, stress, and absorption problems are the main contributors to folic-acid–deficiency anemia. The classic symptoms typically come on quickly, within weeks of experiencing low levels of the vitamin.

It is also possible to inherit different types of anemia. These include thalassemia, which involves abnormal hemoglobin production, and sickle cell anemia, in which the red blood cells have an abnormal shape. These forms should not be self-treated. Hemolytic anemias are yet another type. These forms involve the premature death of red blood cells. Red blood cells are produced in the bone marrow, and production is steady. Healthy red blood cells live for 120 days, but people with a hemolytic anemia have red blood cells that die prematurely, leaving the body unable to catch up with the deficiency. Hemolytic anemias can be caused by various infectious diseases or in response to certain drugs or toxins. These forms should not be self-treated.

Remedies

If you're feeling run-down and you think you may be anemic, see your doctor for an accurate diagnosis. Then, if you don't have a serious form of anemia, you can treat it yourself. For iron-deficiency anemia, treatment typically includes supplementation with iron. However, taking too much iron can be dangerous, so any iron supplementation should be monitored by your doctor.

Your doctor may also tell you how much folic acid or vitamin B_{12} you need to take to correct your deficiencies. Typical dosages of these nutrients are: 1,000–2,500 micrograms (mcg) twice daily of vitamin B_{12}; and 400 mcg two to three times daily of folic acid. With supplementation and adjustments to eating habits, most anemia corrects in about two months.

In addition to supplementation, here are some remedies you can do yourself for iron-, B_{12}-, and folic-acid–deficiency anemias. (Also see "Eating Anemia Away" on page 186 for more hints.)

Best Bets

♦ Make sure you have lots of iron-rich foods in your diet. These include dried fruits, blackstrap molasses, dark green vegetables, eggs, and fish. To boost iron absorption, consume foods high in vitamin C, such as orange juice, citrus fruits, and broccoli. Also take a vitamin C supplement, 500 mg once or twice daily, depending on the amount of vitamin C–rich foods you eat.

♦ For folic-acid–deficiency anemia, include lots of dark-green leafy vegetables, root vegetables, whole grains, and brewer's yeast in your diet.

♦ Foods rich in vitamin B_{12} include organ meat, egg yolks, and nuts, and to a lesser extent whole grains, legumes, blackstrap molasses, and brewer's yeast. Look for foods that say "B_{12} fortified" such as soy products and whole-grain cereals.

Other Options

♦ Drink a delicious blood-building tonic every evening, composed of 8 ounces of orange juice mixed with 1 teaspoon each of brewer's yeast and thyme. Take this tonic about two hours before bedtime, preferably on an empty stomach. The vitamin C helps with the absorption of iron found in the yeast and thyme.

◆ Foods that contain copper assist iron absorption. Some copper-rich foods include egg yolks, whole grains, green vegetables, apricots, cherries, and dried figs.

◆ The Chinese herb *dong quai* is traditionally used to treat anemia. Take 500 mg twice daily for three weeks.

EATING ANEMIA AWAY

◆ Foods that contain copper assist iron absorption. Some copper-rich foods include egg yolks, whole grains, green vegetables, apricots, cherries, and dried figs.

◆ Avoid coffee, tea, cocoa, soft drinks, and wine when eating, because the tannins in these beverages block absorption of iron from your food. One cup of tea, for example, can block 75 percent of iron from your meal.

◆ Whole grains are healthy foods, but eat them separately from other iron-rich foods, because substances called phytates found in grains can hinder iron absorption.

◆ Cook in cast-iron pots. The iron content of foods increases when cooked in cast-iron cookware. Acidic foods such as tomato sauce, as well as other foods such as oatmeal, soups, and gravies do especially well.

When to See a Doctor

If you have symptoms of anemia, you should see a doctor for a definite diagnosis, especially if you are pregnant or elderly, or if you have a condition that interferes with the absorption of nutrients.

CAFFEINE WITHDRAWAL

For her New Year's resolution, Catherine vowed to give up caffeine, in particular, coffee. She was in the habit of drinking four or five cups a day, but after reading about the impact of caffeine on bone loss and high blood pressure, she decided the health benefits of stopping were very convincing. So she stopped cold turkey.

Catherine had visions of long-term improved health, but what she didn't plan on were the short-term withdrawal effects. Because she quit caffeine suddenly rather than tapering off gradually, she experienced a throbbing headache, bouts of anxiety, and waves of nausea her first two days without coffee. "No one told me I'd feel so bad," she said. Fortunately she switched to a gradual withdrawal plan and was caffeine-free—and nearly symptom-free—in less than a month.

Caffeine is a stimulant that can raise metabolic rate, blood temperature, blood pressure, and blood sugar levels, which is why the International Olympic Committee has banned caffeine use in athletes. In high amounts, generally considered to be five or six cups of brewed coffee daily (or about 525 to 650 mg of caffeine) it can cause anxiety, headache, jitteriness, and insomnia, although these symptoms can occur in people who drink less than this amount.

Stopping caffeine, as Catherine discovered, can cause some very unpleasant symptoms if you do it suddenly. Discomfort usually begins twelve to twenty-four hours after eliminating caffeine, with symptoms peaking about twenty to forty-eight hours after stopping. The symptoms can include severe headache, mood swings, irritability, forgetfulness, muscle stiffness, nausea, alternating waves of hot and cold sensations, slowed reflexes, and an inability to concentrate.

Caffeine: Addictive or Not?

Caffeine is an alkaloid found in coffee, tea, chocolate, kola nuts, and some medications. Most healthcare professionals consider it to be an addictive substance, although the American Psychiatric Association (APA) does not agree. The APA says there is not enough evidence of "clinical indicators of dependence on caffeine" to list it as an addictive substance. This statement is based on the Association's strict criteria in its manual, *Diagnostic and Statistical Manual—Fourth Edition.*

Research, however, supports the view of healthcare professionals that caffeine is addictive. In fact, a Johns Hopkins study published in November 2000 reported that 9 to 30 percent of caffeine users may meet the APA's guidelines for dependency.

Remedies

The following points are not so much remedies as they are tips on how to stop using caffeine with little or no side effects. All of the suggestions refer to coffee, tea, or colas, according to what your "addiction" is. Try them in good health!

Best Bets

◆ Gradually reduce your use of caffeinated products over several weeks. If you normally drink six cups of coffee daily, for example, begin day one of withdrawal by drinking five cups, reduce to four cups by day three, three cups by day five, two cups by day seven, and one cup by day nine. If this program is too fast for you, add another day or two between reducing your intake of caffeine. Substitute decaffeinated coffee (or tea or cola) for the caffeine beverages you are not drinking.

◆ Drink hot caffeine-free herbal teas or herbal coffee substitutes as you gradually withdraw from caffeine. By the time you are rid of caffeine, you'll be enjoying some new beverages.

Other Options

◆ Drink at least eight 8-ounce glasses of pure water daily. This helps flush the caffeine from your body.

◆ Miss that mid-morning kick that a cup of coffee used to give you? Exercise instead. A brisk walk around the block or parking lot is stimulating, too.

When to See a Doctor

If you are still experiencing significant symptoms more than one week after quitting caffeine, or if you have debilitating headaches and/or memory loss that continue past three or four days, you should see your doctor.

CHRONIC FATIGUE SYNDROME

In 1984, in an exclusive resort town in Nevada named Incline Village, about 200 people suddenly became ill with an unknown condition. Most of the affected people were young, white, wealthy, and female, and they complained of severe fatigue and weak, achy muscles. Doctors didn't know what to make of it, but the media found it somewhat amusing and dubbed the malady "yuppie flu" and "yuppie plague," among other names.

Today few people are laughing at what the Centers for Disease Control and Prevention (CDC) has named chronic fatigue syndrome, or, more accurately, chronic fatigue and immune dysfunction syndrome (CFIDS). Much is still unknown about CFIDS, which is one reason why we don't know how many people have it. The CDC has a conservative estimate: 4 to 10 cases per 100,000 adults (translation: up to about 26,000 Americans). However, a study published in the *Archives of Internal Medicine* reports that 422 per 100,000 is more realistic, with 726 per 100,000 among Latinos. Some experts estimate that more than 4 million people in North America have CFIDS.

We do know that women are at least three times more likely to get the disease than men. We also have seen that symptoms typically first appear in people between the ages of twenty-five and forty-five, and that Latinos and African Americans are more likely to get CFIDS than are whites and Asians. And one more thing: we know that it can have a tremendous impact on the life of the person who has it and on the lives of his or her family.

Causes of CFIDS

No one knows exactly what causes CFIDS, but there are several theories. One is that environmental toxins such as mercury, lead, chemicals, and pesticides enter the body and trigger damage to the mitochondria (the energy producers) in cells, causing fatigue and other symptoms of CFIDS. Another is that viruses, such as the Epstein-Barr virus, trigger the disease. Although it's true that many people develop CFIDS after experiencing a lingering viral or bacterial infection, it appears that viruses may play a secondary role instead of a primary one. Stress also seems to play a part.

Diagnosing CFIDS

Adding to the frustration associated with CFIDS is how to diagnose it. The CDC has established a list for this purpose, with the main criterion being debilitating fatigue for six months or longer. Then you must meet at least four of the following criteria:

1. Muscle aches and pains

2. Short-term memory problems

3. Difficulty concentrating

4. Sore throat

5. Swollen or tender lymph nodes

6. Pain in multiple joints without redness or swelling

7. Recurring headaches that differ in severity or pattern than those experienced previously

8. Sleep that does not leave you feeling refreshed

9. Postexercise malaise that lasts more than twenty-four hours

THE "OTHER" SYMPTOMS OF CFIDS

In addition to the symptoms listed by the CDC, many people with CFIDS experience other problems. These symptoms vary in severity, and not everyone has them. They include:

- ◆ Psychological problems (anxiety, depression, mood swings, irritability)
- ◆ Visual disturbances (blurred vision, eye pain, sensitivity to light)
- ◆ Balance problems, dizziness
- ◆ Chills and night sweats
- ◆ Shortness of breath
- ◆ Sensitivity to cold and/or heat
- ◆ Numbness, tingling, or burning sensations
- ◆ Diarrhea, constipation, or intestinal gas
- ◆ Low-grade fever
- ◆ Muscle twitching
- ◆ Irregular heartbeat
- ◆ Rash
- ◆ Dry mouth and eyes
- ◆ Tinnitus (ringing in the ears)
- ◆ Sensitivity to sound, odors, and/or touch
- ◆ Menstrual problems
- ◆ Seizures

Food allergies or sensitivities also are common in people with CFIDS, and can cause many of the symptoms associated with the disease. You should ask your doctor to test you for this possibility. Identifying food problems can make a big difference in your recovery.

Even if you meet all the criteria, doctors must then rule out dozens of other conditions that have symptoms similar to those associated with CFIDS, including anemia, cancer, depression, food allergies, heart problems, hepatitis, hypoglycemia, multiple sclerosis, thyroid problems, and reactions to medications. Establishing CFIDS is not an easy task.

Of course, you may still experience long-term exhaustion and not meet the rest of the CDC's criteria. Just because you don't "officially" have CFIDS doesn't mean you don't want, need, or deserve relief.

So far there is no cure for CFIDS, but many people with the condition eventually recover, although it may take years. The disease is unpredictable: some people have symptoms their entire lives; others experience severe symptoms for months, then go into remission, only to have a flare-up several months later, and eventually recover.

Remedies

The goals of the following suggestions are to relieve symptoms and to help you regain as much control over your life as possible. Because CFIDS has so many facets, it must be approached from many directions as well. Here are a few that have proven effective for people.

Best Bets

- A healthy diet is critical. Focus on organic fruits, vegetables, whole grains, and legumes. Eliminate processed foods, excess sugar, fatty foods, caffeine, and alcohol. If you eat meat or dairy products, choose organic and eat only small portions. Drink six to eight 8-ounce glasses of pure water daily.

- Joint pain can be alleviated with glucosamine sulfate. Take 500 mg three times daily if you weigh less than 200 pounds. If you weigh more, take the same dose four times daily. It takes about two to three months for results, but it's worth the wait. Unlike conventional painkillers, glucosamine sulfate doesn't bother the stomach. It assists in building cartilage in the joints, and it's nontoxic.

- Take a probiotic supplement. Many people with CFIDS have infections and digestion problems, which means the healthy bacteria in their intestinal tracts often don't have a fighting chance. Taking a probiotic such as acidophilus or bifidobacterium, or both in a combination product. Follow package directions. Probiotics are especially critical if you have been taking antibiotics, because these drugs destroy many of the beneficial bacteria in the intestinal tract.

Other Options

◆ Chinese ginseng is a powerful herb that boosts energy, helps the body fight stress, and fights viral infections. Shop carefully for this herb. Choose a standardized extract that contains 7 percent ginsenosides. Begin by taking one-half the dose suggested on the label, then gradually increase until you are taking the recommended amount. (*Note:* Do not take ginseng if you have a heart condition, high blood pressure, hypoglycemia, or if you are sensitive to caffeine.)

◆ St. John's wort can help relieve the depression that accompanies so many cases of CFIDS. Choose a product that contains 0.3 percent hypericin and take 300 mg three times daily. (*Note:* Do not take St. John's wort if you are also taking conventional antidepressants, or if you are pregnant or breast-feeding.)

When to See a Doctor

If fatigue and other symptoms do not improve after a conscientious effort of self-treatment, or if your symptoms are interfering with your work or other aspects of your life, consult your doctor. You should also see your doctor about having food allergy and sensitivity testing performed if you suspect this may be a problem.

COMMON COLD

Feed a cold, starve a fever. Catch a chill, catch a cold. True or false? Both are false. There are lots of myths about the common cold, including a modern-day one that says antibiotics can cure a cold. They can't, and one reason why is that antibiotics attack bacteria, not viruses, which are what cause the common cold. In fact, there are more than 200 different viruses associated with this respiratory condition.

Does that mean there are more than 200 different kinds of the common cold? Technically, and at a cellular level, yes. But regardless of which virus finds itself up your nose, the symptoms it causes are pretty much the same: sneezing, coughing, headache, sore throat, stuffy and/or runny nose, loss of appetite, watery or burning eyes, ear congestion or infection, low-grade fever, and aching muscles and joints. You may suffer one, several, or all of these symptoms when you get your next cold as your body responds to the viral attack.

Causes, Symptoms, and Course of the Common Cold

If you're like most adults, that next cold could be fairly soon. Average, healthy adults can expect to get one or two colds per year, more if they are under lots of stress, have another medical condition, eat a poor diet, or smoke. Children younger than six years tend to have many more, about seven per year, because their immune systems are still developing, while older children average four to five yearly.

Common cold viruses infect the cells that line the nose and throat and are contagious. The viruses are typically passed along to others via droplets put into the air by sneezing and coughing, or via hand-to-hand contact. The viruses can also be transferred from contaminated surfaces to the hands of other people. Cold viruses grow primarily in the nose, but once they enter the body they also travel to the sinuses, bronchial tubes, and ears.

The first symptom is usually a sore throat. As the cold virus multiplies in the body, the mucous membranes along the respiratory tract become inflamed. This swelling, along with an increase in mucus production, blocks the airways and makes breathing difficult. This initial phase of a cold—sinus congestion, runny nose, sore throat, tearing or burning eyes, and sneezing—usually lasts two to five days.

You're usually most contagious during the first three days, when the nasal secretions are watery and composed mainly of viral discharge. When the discharge turns thick and perhaps yellow or green, this means you are healing and also shedding dead viral particles and dead white blood cells.

The average uncomplicated common cold lasts for about five to ten days. According to Elliot Dick, Ph.D., retired chief of the respiratory viruses research laboratory at the University of Wisconsin-Madison, you remain immune to the particular virus that caused your latest cold for three to five years. Of course, you may catch one or more of the other hundreds of cold viruses lurking in the world. This may be the case if you are sick for more than two weeks in a row. If you experience a significant fever (102°F or higher) you probably have the flu and not a cold.

How to Prevent the Common Cold

According to the National Center for Health Statistics, more than 62 million cases of the common cold required medical attention or restricted activity in 1996. Experts estimate that the overall number of cases may be about 1 billion. What can you do to help prevent from being a statistic?

Perhaps the most important thing you can do is wash your hands. The viruses are often carried from the hands to the mouth or nose, where the moist mucous membranes are an ideal environment for them. In fact, cold viruses are transmitted more often from direct contact than from airborne (sneezing, coughing) particles. It's also a good idea to supplement your diet with vitamin C, beta-carotene, and zinc during the cold and flu season (usually October through February or March). Take 10,000 IU beta-carotene and 25 mg zinc once daily, and 500 mg vitamin C twice daily.

While you're taking those supplements, stay positive and chill out. Research results published in May 2001 in *Epidemiology* reported that people who have a negative outlook are at greatest risk of developing a cold, even if they take vitamin C and zinc. Individuals who are under stress are nearly three times as likely to get a cold. Speaking of stress, stay away from tobacco smoke. The nicotine and other pollutants in tobacco smoke stress your body by irritating the nasal membranes and respiratory passages.

Remedies

There's an old saying: "Ignore a cold and it goes away in about a week. Treat a cold and it goes away in seven days." So is it worth treating your cold? Depends on the treatment. Some conventional medications can ease one symptom while causing or aggravating several more. For example, if you take a decongestant to relieve your stuffy, runny nose, you may experience the side effects of restlessness, increased heart rate, and insomnia. Antihistamines dry up your nasal secretions, but they also cause dry mouth and drowsiness. Australian researchers also found that pain relievers (for example, aspirin, acetaminophen, ibuprofen) may lower immune system response or increase nasal symptoms.

We all know there's no cure for the common cold, so once you get a cold all you can do is treat the symptoms and hope for some significant relief. That's what the following remedies are designed to do. Also check out "How to Prevent the Common Cold" on page 193 for more helpful hints.

Best Bets

♦ Drink plenty of fluids, including hot herbal tea, soups (see "Recipe for a Common Cold" on page 195), diluted fruit juices, and pure water. This serves several purposes: it prevents dehydration, which is possible if you have a fever; it helps flush toxins from your body; and it thins nasal secretions, making it easier for your body to eliminate them.

* At the first sign of a cold (usually a sore throat), take 500–1,000 mg vitamin C every hour for up to eight hours. If you develop loose stools, reduce the dose to the level you can tolerate without this side effect. After the first eight hours, take 1,000 mg three times daily for three days.

* Use a cool-mist humidifier in your bedroom and the room you are in most during the day. Humidified air can thin nasal secretions and ease congested sinuses. It's best to use distilled, demineralized water.

Other Options

* The herbal combination of goldenseal and echinacea can help cleanse your system, fight the virus, and strengthen your mucous membranes. Take one dose that supplies 250–500 mg of echinacea and 150–300 mg of goldenseal three times a day for five to seven days.

* To soothe your throat and boost your immune system, take 5–10 mg of zinc in a lozenge form every two to three hours, not to exceed 50 mg daily. Do this for three days.

RECIPE FOR A COMMON COLD

About 800 years ago, an Egyptian doctor named Moses Maimonides recommended chicken soup as a remedy for the common cold. Today we know that it's not the chicken but the hot broth, and the vegetables in the soup that help relieve symptoms. This recipe has added benefits: it contains the herb astragalus, a tonic herb that enhances the immune system and helps detoxify the body; and ginger, which cleanses the body and helps increase perspiration.

1 astragalus root strip

1 inch fresh ginger root

10 cups water

$\frac{1}{2}$ teaspoon each thyme and sage

6 cups vegetables, cut into bite-sized pieces
(choose from carrots, broccoli, cauliflower, turnips, celery,
green peppers, zucchini, string beans, squash, parsley)

1 red onion, chopped

2–4 cloves garlic, minced

1 cup cooked barley

Directions: Place all the ingredients into a stainless steel pot and simmer slowly for one hour. Remove the astragalus and ginger root before serving.

When to See a Doctor

Generally the common cold will go away gradually over about a week's time. However, if you experience a very high fever, shortness of breath, chest pain, or a headache accompanied by a stiff neck, contact your physician immediately. You may have a different type of viral infection.

DEPRESSION

Are you down in the dumps most of the time? Are you feeling so pessimistic, hopeless, or sad that even a crane couldn't lift your spirits? Have you lost interest in things that used to be pleasurable, or do you feel like running away from home (even though you're not thirteen anymore)?

A little depression is common in virtually everyone's life. Stressful situations such as the death of a loved one, a divorce, losing a job, or moving away from people close to you can cause grief and sadness for a while. It's estimated that 10 to 15 percent of all people experience an episode of depression during their lifetime. Most times it is mild and of short duration.

But if sadness and despair overwhelm you for weeks or months on end, and you have other symptoms as well, then you may have major or clinical depression (see "How The Experts Diagnose Major Depression" on page 198). Experts define major depression as that which is significantly more serious than feeling down occasionally. "Clinical" means you need professional help, but that does not mean you need drugs.

Who Experiences Depression

The National Institute of Mental Health says that more than 19 million Americans are clinically depressed, making it America's number-one mental health problem. On top of that number are millions who are mildly and temporarily depressed. These numbers are harder to track, because they often don't seek treatment or treat themselves. More women than men are diagnosed with depression, and one in six seek treatment for it. Only one in nine men get treatment for depression. The gender difference in depression may be related to hormones (see "Causes and Types of Depression" on page 197) or simply that men are less likely to admit they are depressed and to ask for help.

The incidence of depression is higher in the elderly. This increase can be related to a greater number of stress factors in their lives, such as more deaths among friends and loved ones, losing independence because of illness, taking multiple medications (many of which can cause depression), and slowing of mental capacity.

Causes and Types of Depression

Recent studies suggest that depression is linked to suppression of neurogenesis—the growth of new brain cells. It's known that stress can cause depression. Stress can also cause the body to send excessive amounts of certain hormones (glucocorticoids) to the brain, where they suppress neurogenesis. Thus the theory is that in people who are depressed, the brain stops making new nerve cells. When neurogenesis begins again—when depression is relieved because of psychotherapy, drugs, or other means—depression goes away.

One possible reason many of the antidepressant drugs work is that they result in an increase in the level of a specific neurotransmitter (substance that transmits signals between nerve cells) called serotonin. Studies show that people who are clinically depressed often have levels of serotonin that are lower than normal. They also show abnormally high levels of a hormone called cortisol, which is released in high amounts during chronic or excessive stress.

Some types of depression appear to be related to other factors. One of those factors is inadequate nutrition. A deficiency of the B vitamins (especially vitamin B_{12}, folic acid, riboflavin, vitamin B_6, and thiamine) or protein can cause feelings of depression. Even marginally deficient levels of B vitamins can cause or exacerbate depression. While whole grains are rich in B vitamins, most people eat foods made from processed, refined grains, which have been stripped of their nutrients.

Another factor is seasonal affective disorder (SAD), which is related to insufficient exposure to sunlight. This is most common in locations that get little or no sunshine during cold months of the year, such as in northern climates. When the eye doesn't take in enough sunlight, the retina doesn't send the right signals to the hypothalamus in the brain, which in turn transmits signals that regulate the body. The result can be a form of depression.

Yet another form is postpartum depression, which is caused by an imbalance in hormone levels that occurs after a woman has given birth. Postpartum depression fades in the majority of women as their hormones regain equilibrium in the weeks and months after delivery.

Infrequently, people experience drug-induced depression. Several medications can cause or aggravate depression, including diazepam (Valium), oral contraceptives, steroids (prednisone, cortisone), and some cancer chemotherapy drugs.

The bottom line on depression is that, for a variety of reasons not completely understood, a biochemical imbalance occurs. Regaining that balance is the goal of treatment.

HOW THE EXPERTS DIAGNOSE MAJOR DEPRESSION

Experts have devised a list of criteria for a diagnosis of major depression. Five or more of the following nine symptoms must be present during the same two-week period for a diagnosis, and at least one of the five symptoms must be either a depressed mood or loss of interest.

1. Depressed mood for most of the day

2. Loss of interest in things (for example, hobbies, sports, sex) that previously were pleasurable, or an inability to enjoy your usual hobbies or activities

3. Disturbed sleep

4. Disturbed appetite or a change in weight

5. Loss of energy or fatigue

6. Feelings of worthlessness and excessive or inappropriate guilt

7. Difficulty concentrating or thinking clearly

8. Psychomotor agitation or decline

9. Suicidal thoughts or actions

Remedies

Depending on the severity and cause of your depression, you may be able to treat yourself with little or no outside help. However, there are professional outlets available for you to consider, including psychotherapy and various support groups. Here are some ways people have effectively treated mild to moderate depression on their own. A combination of approaches usually works best (but check with your doctor before starting any type of supplement or herbal program).

Best Bets

- Taking a high-potency B-complex supplement every day can help bring the body back into balance, but it won't supply all you need. So also take additional supplements of the following B vitamins: vitamin B_{12}, 300–500 mcg twice daily; folic acid, 800 mcg; vitamin B_6, 50 mg twice daily for two weeks, then 50 mg once daily for three weeks, then continue with just B complex. Always take the B complex at a different time of day than any of the other B vitamin supplements.

- The guru of the relaxation response, Herbert Benson, M.D., reports that people who regularly elicit the relaxation response experience an elevated mood. Choose an approach that is convenient and enjoyable for you, such as deep breathing, yoga, meditation, biofeedback, visualization, self-hypnosis, among others, and practice daily.

- St. John's wort can be very effective for mild to moderate depression. It gradually alters brain chemistry much as conventional antidepressants do. Begin by taking one 300 mg capsule of standardized extract containing 0.3 percent hypericin daily. After two weeks, add another 300 mg capsule; and add a third capsule after an additional two weeks. If you have high blood pressure, consult your doctor before taking this herb. Also, don't take St. John's wort if you are taking amino acid supplements or if you are pregnant or breast-feeding.

Other Options

- The amino acid derivative SAM-e (s-adenosyl-L-methionine) has proven to be as effective as conventional antidepressants, but without the side effects. Begin with 400–500 mg three times daily until you feel results, then take 400 mg daily.

- Here's one more thing exercise is good for. Regular physical activity—at least four to five times a week—has proven to reduce depression, help eliminate insomnia (which often accompanies depression), and ease feelings of anxiety and tension while increasing feelings of well-being. To help keep you motivated, exercise with a friend, and choose something you enjoy.

When to See a Doctor

Generally, it is best to be evaluated by a professional before you begin treating yourself to determine if there are any physical problems that may be causing your depression. Also, if your depression is having a significant negative effect on your work or other aspects of your life, or if you are having suicidal thoughts, see a professional as soon as possible.

HANGOVER

Did you have "one for the road" and now you feel as if you've been run over? Is someone trying to tell you to take the "hair of the dog" to get rid of the headache, dizziness, and nausea plaguing you? Are you paying homage to the "porcelain god"?

Clichés aside, you've got a hangover and you want relief. It may be a bit too late to tell you how to prevent a hangover, or how alcohol works in the body to produce one, but we'll tell you anyhow. And in case you really need some help fast, you can skip to the remedies section. Then come back and find out how you can avoid needing these remedies again.

Causes of a Hangover

When we drink alcohol, several things happen in the body. Alcohol causes the blood vessels to dilate, and too much dilatation can cause headache. The more alcohol we consume, the more our body suppresses the hormones that control fluid balance. Thus, the kidneys are stimulated to excrete more water than usual, which leads to dehydration.

Several factors influence how fast alcohol is absorbed into the bloodstream. If you have food in your stomach before you begin to drink, it will slow absorption of the alcohol. Eating while you drink is also helpful. Some folk customs say that eating cabbage, especially cabbage with an acidic dressing (for example, sauerkraut) is best, but there are no scientific studies to support this.

The more you weigh, the more time it takes for your body to absorb alcohol. However, if a man and a woman of equal weight have drunk the same amount of alcohol, the woman will probably have more alcohol in her blood than the man. Why? It is believed that women produce less of an enzyme that breaks down alcohol, so they are more affected by the same amount of alcohol.

How to Prevent Hangovers

Here are a few tips to help you avoid the dreaded hangover.

◆ Don't drink. Okay, that's obvious. How about, don't drink too much. Simple solutions are always the best.

- Always eat something before you drink, and make sure you snack while you're drinking.

- Alternate nonalcoholic beverages with alcoholic ones.

- Sip slowly.

- Don't mix drinks.

- Watch your consumption of alcoholic beverages high in congeners (see "Champagne, Red Wine, Whisky—Top Offenders?").

- Drink several glasses of water before and after drinking alcohol to help prevent dehydration.

CHAMPAGNE, RED WINE, WHISKY— TOP OFFENDERS?

Are some types of alcohol more likely to cause a hangover than others? It's been found that drinks containing high levels of congeners (impurities such as colorings and preservatives) tend to cause hangovers more than other alcoholic beverages. Drinks high in congeners include brandy, cognac, champagne, sherry, whisky, and red wine. Less impurities are found in "white" alcohol, such as white wine, gin, and vodka.

Have you ever had a glass of champagne and felt that it went "right to your head"? Champagne can cause some of the worst hangovers, because the bubbles speed up absorption of alcohol in the stomach and delivery to the bloodstream . . . and your head.

Remedies

Too late, you're hungover. Avoid the "hair of the dog" (another drink) or coffee (contributes to dehydration and makes you jittery) and try these remedies.

Best Bets

- Drink one cup of milk thistle tea every hour until you feel better. This herb helps detoxify the liver (the organ that processes alcohol) and the blood.

- Drink one cup of rosemary tea every hour until you get relief. Rosemary relieves headache and helps the liver process toxins.

◆ Replace nutrients lost from dehydration by making a Hangover Helper shake: 4 ounces of soy milk, 4 ounces of orange juice, 1 banana, and 2 tablespoons of honey. Process in a blender. This shake gives you needed nutrients and helps raise your blood sugar level, which is lowered by alcohol consumption.

Other Options

◆ The homeopathic remedy *nux vomica* is *the* homeopathic hangover remedy. *Nux vomica* means "no vomit," which tells you what it can do. Take one dose of 30c every thirty minutes for up to six doses.

◆ Eat raw cabbage and/or drink raw cabbage juice. Cabbage is high in the amino acid glutamine, which improves energy and a feeling of well-being, helps concentration, and may curb alcohol cravings.

When to See a Doctor

If hangovers are becoming a habit, it means you're drinking too much and may be addicted. Seek professional help from your doctor, an alcohol abuse center, or Alcoholics Anonymous.

INSOMNIA

According to the National Sleep Research Project, the longest documented period that anyone has stayed awake continuously is eighteen days, twenty-one hours and forty minutes. The record was set during a rocking-chair marathon, and the individual experienced hallucinations, lapses of memory and concentration, blurred vision, slurred speech, and paranoia. We hope the prize was worth it.

Sleepless in America

Insomnia is an inability to sleep, which can involve either difficulty falling asleep or a tendency to wake in the night and be unable to fall back asleep. It is estimated that up to 60 million Americans, mostly women, experience chronic insomnia. Yet only about 10 million people ask their doctors for help with the problem. The rest try to deal with it on their own, or allow it to deal with them.

Experts generally agree that the average adult needs at least eight hours of sound sleep every night, while some need as many as ten hours or more. Yet for most Americans, all this talk about sleep is just a dream. Although Americans were getting about nine hours of sleep each night around 1900, today that number has fallen to seven hours or even less.

Causes and Consequences of Insomnia

Stress and anxiety top the list of causes of insomnia. Although these factors are part of everyone's life, people with insomnia don't let them go. "I can't turn off the day in my head," says one thirty-seven-year-old insomniac, who works as a software engineer. "I'm constantly thinking about problems at work and going over possible solutions in my mind."

Consuming caffeine or alcohol close to bedtime, a deficiency or excess of certain vitamins and minerals (see "Remedies" below), chronic pain, breathing difficulties, jet lag, and undiagnosed illness can also cause insomnia. Infrequent episodes of insomnia usually aren't a problem, but when they are chronic, they can have a significant negative impact on your life.

For example, lack of sufficient sleep does more than put bags under your eyes. Loss of concentration, lack of energy, reduced alertness, foggy memory, and slowed reflexes are some of the common side effects of sleep deprivation. Chronic insomnia stresses the immune system, making you more susceptible to illness and disease, and less productive at your job.

Lack of sleep also makes you dangerous behind the wheel. The National Highway Traffic Safety Administration reports that an estimated 100,000 police-reported crashes related to sleepiness occur each year, and that about 4 percent of all fatal vehicle crashes are caused by sleepy drivers.

Remedies

Remedies for insomnia are not so much about taking something that *makes* you sleep as it is about changing those things that *prevent* you from sleeping, thus *allowing* you to sleep. Take an honest look at your lifestyle and habits and you may discover that you're doing one or more things that are causing or contributing to your inability to sleep.

Best Bets

◆ Manage stress and sleep will come. Rather than medicate against the racing thoughts and whirling problems in your mind, practice five to fifteen minutes of deep breathing and sitting quietly immediately before going to bed. Clear your mind and concentrate on your breath, gently pushing all other thoughts from your mind.

◆ Eliminate caffeine and late-day alcohol consumption. Perhaps your coffee, tea, or cola habit is doing more than keeping you going during the day; it may be keeping you from sleeping at night. Gradually reduce your daily intake of caffeine products (see CAFFEINE WITHDRAWAL on page 186) and replace them with decaffeinated or non-caffeine beverages. Also avoid drinking alcohol within two hours of going to bed. Although drinking may make you drowsy initially, chances are good that you'll wake up in the middle of the night and lose sleep.

◆ Establish a pattern using the Bootzin Technique. Richard Bootzin, Ph.D., developed this successful behavior-therapy program in the 1970s. It may take several nights before you get significant results, because you are creating a new habit. It works by following these five rules:

1. Go to bed only when you feel sleepy, regardless of the time.

2. Do not use your bed for anything except sleeping or sex. Do not read, eat, drink, watch TV, or talk on the phone in bed.

3. If you go to bed and you can't sleep, get up and do something in another room until you feel sleepy again, then return to bed. If you need to repeat this step one or more times during the night, do so.

4. Set an alarm for the same time each morning, regardless of what time you go to bed.

5. Don't take naps during the day.

Other Options

◆ Take a high-potency multivitamin and mineral supplement. Deficiencies in calcium, copper, iron, magnesium, zinc, and the B vitamins can contribute to insomnia. A supplement can help, but you should combine it with a healthy diet that includes lots of vegetables, fruits, whole grains, and legumes, and go easy on fats, meats, and fried foods.

◆ Several supplements can bring on the z's, but choose only one at a time. The herb valerian root can help induce sleep and leave you feeling refreshed in the morning. Take a standardized extract containing 0.5 percent isovalerenic acids and take 200–300 mg thirty minutes before retiring. Valerian is available as a tea, but it doesn't have a pleasant taste. The hormone melatonin, available over-the-counter, is a mild sedative and can facilitate sleep. A typical dose is 3 mg before bedtime. Do not take this supplement if you are pregnant or breast-feeding, or if you suffer with depression. The supplement 5-HTP

(5-hydroxytryptophan, a derivative of the plant *Griffonia simplicifolia*) welcomes sleep at a dose of 100–300 mg taken before bedtime.

When to See a Doctor

If self-treatment methods aren't giving you the z's you need, or if your insomnia is significantly affecting your lifestyle, contact your doctor. Seeing your doctor need not mean you'll get a prescription for sleeping pills. In fact, medications may knock you out, but they also prevent you from getting refreshing sleep and are only good for very short-term use. Your doctor may recommend you go to one of more than 200 accredited sleep clinics in the United States, which have very good success rates.

JET LAG

Roseann loves to travel, so much so that she got a job with a major airline as an airline attendant. Now she travels around the world: London, Berlin, Sydney, New York, San Francisco, Tokyo. She enjoys the adventures, but not the jet lag. "My body clock is constantly confused," she says. "It's hard to get into synch when my body wants to sleep yet I've just arrived in New York from Berlin at 9 A.M. and the sun in shining. I feel out of sorts."

What Roseann and millions of other travelers experience every time they travel across time zones is jet lag, a physical and psychological decline in well-being and performance. The declines are associated with your body clock, the internal clock that controls your body's circadian (daily) rhythms.

Circadian rhythms are orchestrated by areas and portions of the brain that are responsible for such basic bodily functions as sleep, hunger, cardiac activity, energy, alertness, and body temperature. When you cross time zones, the difference between actual time and internal time becomes greater, and the body responds with certain symptoms. Some of those symptoms include headache, tiredness, irritability, problems with memory and concentration, and stomach upset.

Sleep and the Role of the Brain

The hypothalamus, pituitary and pineal glands in the brain maintain your body's circadian rhythms through the production and release of certain hormones. The pineal gland, for example, responds to the level of light in your environment by producing the hormone melatonin. Production of melatonin increases in the evening as light disappears and stops when light reappears. Your body's level of melatonin has an impact on whether you are ready to sleep. Thus, if you left a city when it was light (no melatonin being produced) and then arrived in another city twelve hours later and it was just getting light there (no melatonin), your body would be ready for sleep, but your brain would not be producing melatonin for sleep.

WEST TO EAST, EAST TO WEST, WHICH IS BEST?

When you travel east to west, you lengthen your day. For example, if you take a five-hour nonstop flight from New York to Los Angeles, the local time of your arrival in California is only two hours later, so you actually "gain" three hours. That is, if you leave New York at noon, you arrive in Los Angeles at 2 P.M.

If, however, you fly west to east, you "lose" time. When you make that return trip to New York from Los Angeles on a nonstop flight and leave at noon from California, you will arrive at 8 P.M. New York time. Flying east to west tends to cause more severe jet lag than flying west to east.

How to Prevent Jet Lag

The longer your flight and the more often you fly and cross time zones, the more important it is to try to prevent jet lag. Before you even leave on your trip, you can take some important steps. One recommendation is to get sufficient sleep for each of the several nights before you fly. Don't start your trip already tired. If you will be traveling east, get used to the time change by going to bed one to two hours earlier for several nights. If you will be traveling west, go to bed an hour or two later for several nights before you leave on your trip. If you're taking a very long trip, say, from the United States to Australia, schedule a one- or two-day stopover at an intermediate point so you can better simulate a regular rhythm. Once you're on the plane, avoid dehydration by drinking water or juices rather than alcohol, caffeine, or carbonated drinks.

Remedies

Depending on whether you arrive at your destination during the day or at night, there are several things you can do to reduce or eliminate jet lag.

Best Bets

- If you arrive at your destination during the day, go outdoors immediately and stay there for at least one hour. Exposing yourself to sunlight will help your body clock adjust.

- While outdoors, engage in light exercise—for example, a walk or bicycling—to help you stay awake.

- If you arrive at night, go to bed at the normal hour, even if you aren't sleepy. You can encourage sleep by practicing progressive relaxation or deep-breathing exercises to relax.

RESETTING THE BODY'S CLOCK— TWO INNOVATIVE TECHNIQUES

Light plays a big role in resetting the body's clock. Here are a couple innovative ways scientists have been doing it.

- In 1998, a study showed that shining a bright light on the back of people's knees can reset the brain's sleep-wake clock. Why? No one knows for sure, but if you tape a flashlight onto the back of your knees the next time you fly across several time zones, you may be able to minimize or escape jet lag. You'll probably also attract some attention.

- The British Ministry of Defence has been resetting the body clocks of their soldiers so they can go without sleep for up to thirty-six hours. It requires that the soldiers wear special glasses embedded with tiny optical fibers. The fibers project a ring of bright white light around the edge of the soldiers' retinas, tricking their minds into thinking they have just woken up. This technique was also used on United States pilots during the bombing of Kosovo.

Other Options

- Some people are helped by taking melatonin supplements a few days before and after flying. The suggested dosage varies; some people are helped by 0.3 mg once nightly while others need up to 3 mg. Start low and increase the dosage as needed.

◆ Flying is stressful; flying at 35,000 feet or higher forces the body to work harder at every function, such as digestion and respiration. Therefore, eat lightly before and during your flight (avoid meats, refined starches, and sweets) and avoid smoking and anyone who smokes during the same time period. These approaches can reduce the impact of jet lag.

When to See a Doctor

Jet lag is rarely associated with any serious health problem. However, if you experience severe jet lag for longer than a week, or if you experience a debilitating headache or unexplained internal pain on arrival, see a doctor.

LACTOSE INTOLERANCE

When you hear the "Got milk?" slogan do you say to yourself, "No, but it gets me"? If consuming milk and other dairy products sends your stomach and intestinal tract into a battleground of bloating, gas, cramps, nausea, and diarrhea, then what gets you may be lactose intolerance.

Lactose intolerance is an inability to digest significant amounts of lactose, a milk sugar found in milk and related products such as ice cream, cheese, and yogurt. It occurs in people who have low levels of the enzyme lactase, a substance that helps the body digest lactose. In people who have insufficient lactase, the undigested milk sugar sits in the large intestine and causes the symptoms mentioned, usually within thirty minutes to two hours after consuming the culprit foods.

Lactose intolerance is very common. In fact, 90 percent of Asians, 70 percent of African Americans and American Indians, and 50 percent of Hispanics cannot tolerate lactose. Among whites, it appears in about 25 percent of people of northern European descent and slightly higher or lower percentages among individuals from other areas of Europe.

Symptoms of Lactose Intolerance

If you've experienced the gastrointestinal symptoms mentioned above after you eat dairy products, and then they disappear when you stop eating such foods, you are probably lactose intolerant. However, to find out for certain, your doctor can do a breath hydrogen analysis. This test requires that you fast for eight to twelve hours, then eat a food that contains about 1 ounce of lactose. If your stomach cannot digest the lactose, it will pass into your large intestine, where large amounts of hydrogen will be produced.

One hour after eating the lactose, the doctor will analyze your breath for hydrogen content. If high levels are detected, you are likely lactose intolerant. If your hydrogen levels are normal, you may have another condition that produces similar symptoms, such as irritable bowel syndrome (see IRRITABLE BOWEL SYNDROME on page 149).

Remedies

The severity of lactose intolerance varies from person to person. Some people can tolerate about 1 cup of milk or its equivalent daily without much problem; others get cramps after consuming even an ounce. The ideal remedy is to substitute nondairy foods for the milk products and eliminate your symptoms completely (see "Don't I Need Milk?" on page 210). However, if you want to keep some dairy in your diet, here are some suggestions.

Best Bets

- If you're going to include a dairy food in a meal, eat the nondairy foods on your plate first. This helps prevent symptoms.

- Stick with foods that have a low lactose content ("low" defined as 0–2 grams of lactose per 100 grams, or about 3.6 ounces, of the food). These include certain cheeses (provolone, cheddar, brie, blue, muenster, Camembert, Swiss, and mozzarella), yogurt with active cultures, butter, margarine, and sherbet. Avoid all milk, cream, American cheese, feta cheese, ice cream, cottage cheese, sour cream, and half-and-half.

- Use an over-the-counter lactose supplement, such as Lactaid. Add the suggested number of drops to your milk and then refrigerate it for twenty-four hours. This product and similar ones change the taste of milk by making it sweeter. You can also use Lactaid milk products.

Other Options

- Read labels carefully. Lactose is hidden in many foods, including breads and other baked goods, salad dressings, candy, processed breakfast cereals, instant potatoes, soups, breakfast drinks, and mixes for biscuits, cookies, pancakes, and other similar items. Lactose is also used as a base in many prescription and over-the-counter drugs, and in some nutritional supplements.

- Take the probiotic acidophilus, which restores beneficial bacteria in the intestinal tract and thus aids digestion. Choose a dairy-free brand and take according to package directions daily, or when you eat dairy products.

DON'T I NEED MILK?

Some people worry that if they dramatically reduce or eliminate dairy products from their diet, they will not get enough calcium, putting them at risk for osteoporosis. Milk and milk products, however, are not the only sources of calcium. In fact, the protein in dairy products can actually cause you to lose calcium from your bones. Americans typically eat too much protein; thus, eliminating dairy can be a blessing for many people.

Nondairy sources of calcium typically are lower in fat than dairy products, plus they contain no cholesterol, and provide vitamins and minerals. The following table lists some good nondairy sources of calcium. For comparison, 1 cup of milk contains about 300 mg calcium.

NONDAIRY SOURCES OF CALCIUM

Food	Serving Size	Calcium (mg)
Calcium-fortified orange juice	1 cup	300
Cooked collard greens	1 cup	300
Sardines, canned with bones	3 oz	300
Soybeans, fresh, boiled	1 cup	260
Soy nuts	1 cup	240
Tofu	3.5 oz	204
Almonds	$1/_2$ cup	200
Baked beans, canned	1 cup	200
Kale, cooked	1 cup	180
Figs, dried	$1/_2$ cup	150
Broccoli	1 cup	100
Butternut squash	$1/_2$ cup	45

Also consider taking calcium and magnesium supplements. A dosage of 800–1,000 mg calcium and 400–500 mg magnesium is suggested. If you don't get at least fifteen minutes of exposure to direct sunlight daily, also add 200–400 IU vitamin D to your supplement schedule.

When to See a Doctor

If you eliminate dairy products and you are still experiencing gastrointestinal symptoms, see your doctor. You may have irritable bowel syndrome or other digestive problems.

NICOTINE WITHDRAWAL

Congratulations! If you're reading this, you're probably thinking about stopping smoking, or have already plunged in and need some help. You're doing the right thing, and we hope this section can provide some encouragement and assistance.

Why Quitting Is So Hard to Do

You already know that nicotine is a very addictive drug, but what does it actually do to your body? The "positive" effects include enhancing alertness and relaxing the muscles. Once your body has become accustomed to getting its regular fix of nicotine (not to mention the hundreds of other toxins in cigarettes), it needs to keep getting a steady supply or it will go through physical withdrawal symptoms.

Cons of Smoking Far Outweigh Pros

The negative effects of smoking far outweigh the "positive" ones. The main detrimental impacts of smoking include constriction of your blood vessels (making you more susceptible to stroke and heart attack) and destruction of lung tissue (putting you at high risk for lung cancer, emphysema, and other respiratory diseases). Smoking also puts you at high risk for oral and various other cancers, atherosclerosis, coronary thrombosis, infertility, diabetes, cervical cancer, and high blood pressure. Also, children who are exposed to smoke are twice as likely to develop asthma, asthmatic bronchitis, middle ear infections, or fall victim to sudden infant death syndrome. Infants can even become addicted to nicotine while in the womb of a mother who smokes.

Remedies

Nicotine can be a formidable enemy, so it helps to call in all the reinforcements you need and that work well together. Here are some options.

Best Bets

- Conventional OTC nicotine patches (for example, NicoDerm CQ, Habitrol) and chewing gums (for example, Nicorette) help many people gradually withdraw from nicotine use. They work best when combined with other assistance, such as support groups (for example, SmokEnders), behavior modification, regular exercise, and nutritional supplements. The patches and gum can cause some side effects, such as nausea, increased heart rate, fatigue, and joint pain, but these generally fade over time.

- Behavior modification, such as biofeedback, works very well with any other approach. This does require some assistance from a biofeedback specialist until you learn the technique; however once you learn the method you can do it on your own without the biofeedback device. Self-hypnosis is also successful for some people.

- Join a stop-smoking support group. Emotional and spiritual support from others can be one of the biggest factors in successful quitting.

Other Options

- Vitamin C supplements can not only restore the supply of vitamin C depleted by smoking, but also help you relax and detoxify your body. Take 1,000 mg three times daily.

- To help stop acute cravings, mix 1 tablespoon baking soda in 12 ounces of water and sip the mixture slowly over a twelve-hour period. Also during the day, drink up to three cups of plantain (*Plantago major*) tea to reduce cravings. Sucking on a clove can also do the trick, but not everyone is partial to its taste.

When to See a Doctor

If you've tried many of the remedies and you're still suffering with significant withdrawal symptoms, your doctor may prescribe the antidepressant bupropion (Zyban), which helps some people with withdrawal symptoms. Zyban can be used with a nicotine patch or gum.

CHAPTER 9

Look, Smell, and Feel Good

nitial impressions count, and that's why we like to put our best foot forward when we meet people for the first time. What do you notice when you are introduced to someone new? Although your answers may differ somewhat depending on whether the person is a blind date or the new vice president of your firm, you form an overall impression by what you see (weight, height, condition of the person's skin and nails), smell (perfumes, body odor), and hear (tone of voice, accent).

Various health conditions can have a significant impact on the image you present to others. In particular, the integrity of your skin, hair, nails, and breath can speak volumes when people meet you. This chapter looks at some of the health problems that affect each of these four body factors, as well as weight, and how you can address them so you'll make a good first impression every time.

ACNE

It's the bane of approximately 17 million people in the United States—pimples that erupt on the face, back, neck and shoulders. Nearly 85 percent of young people between the ages of twelve and twenty-four years get acne, yet older individuals are not immune: about 6 percent of men and 8 percent of women older than twenty-four experience outbreaks of acne as well. In fact, many women experience an outbreak of acne right before their menstrual period each month.

Acne is characterized by a collection of skin eruptions that have unappealing names like blackheads, whiteheads, pustules (pus-filled pimples), and papules (inflamed, tender lesions). These skin problems occur when the hair follicles, which are largest and most prevalent on the face, chest, and upper back, become clogged with an oily substance called sebum, which is produced by the oil glands that are connected to the follicles.

Normally, sebum escapes through the hair follicles and reaches the skin, where it can be washed or worn away naturally. But for people who have acne, the lining of the follicles quickly shed their cells. These cells then mix with the sebum and block the passageway to the outer skin surface. When the blocked follicles are filled to capacity, they burst and deposit sebum, bacteria, and cells on the skin, irritating it and causing pimples to develop.

Causes of Acne

Scientists have several theories as to what causes acne. One critical factor appears to be the dramatic rise in hormone (androgens, or male sex hormones) levels that occurs in boys and girls during puberty. These hormones can stimulate the sebaceous glands to produce more sebum. Genetics also appear to be a factor, as do stress, hypothyroidism, and a deficiency of vitamin E, selenium, or zinc.

Some researchers believe that poor digestion is a cause of acne in adults. When the body's main elimination mechanism—the gastrointestinal tract—becomes irritated with toxins that can cause inflammation, such as refined sugar, coffee, alcohol, and hydrogenated and saturated fats, some of this "refuse" may be deposited in the sebaceous glands. Some doctors believe that reducing or eliminating these foods and including foods that have good fats, such as nuts, cold-water fish, and seeds, can rid the body of the inflammatory substances and eliminate acne in affected adults.

Many things can contribute to or make acne outbreaks worse. One is fluctuating hormone levels in girls and women, especially those related to pregnancy, the two-to-seven-day period before menstrual flow begins, or stopping oral contraceptives. Another is stress, especially if it is severe or chronic. The use of some drugs, including barbiturates, lithium, and androgens, can contribute to acne, as can environmental irritants, such as air pollution and high humidity. Things that can make acne outbreaks worse include irritation from clothing, helmets, glasses, or backpacks, and scrubbing the skin too hard. However, three things that are believed *not* to cause acne in young people are greasy foods, chocolate, and dirty skin.

How to Prevent Pimples

You may not be able to completely prevent pimples, but the following tips should help you stop a severe case of acne and turn it into a mild one.

- Use oil-free soap on your face.

- If you use a moisturizer on your face, choose one that is nongreasy.

- Avoid staying in humid environments or getting sweaty. This can make acne worse.

- If you have acne on your forehead and you use mousse or hair gel, stop using these products for a few weeks and see if the acne improves.

- Drink at least eight 8-ounce glasses of pure water daily. Water helps flush toxins from the body.

- Take a high-potency B-complex supplement, which will help promote healthy skin.

Remedies

There are dozens of acne products on the market, both over-the-counter and prescription-only. The major drawback, especially for the prescription drugs, is side effects. For example, long-term use of oral antibiotics to treat acne can largely destroy the beneficial bacteria in the intestinal tract, which can lead to chronic yeast infections. Additionally, the drug isotretinoin (Accutane), usually reserved for severe acne, has a long list of adverse reactions including liver toxicity, cataracts, joint pain, decreased night vision, and inflammatory bowel disease. It should not be taken by women who are or who could become pregnant, as Accutane can cause life-threatening birth defects in infants.

Best Bets

- Over-the-counter benzoyl peroxide cream or gel (at a 5 to 10 percent concentration) helps unblock clogged pores and dry the skin. Another effective over-the-counter treatment is niacinamide gel. Apply 4 percent niacinamide gel twice daily. This should be available at your neighborhood drugstore. It reportedly works better than the antibiotic gel clindamycin.

- Tea tree oil (*Melaleuca alternifolia*), which is obtained from an Australian tree, has potent antibacterial activity. A 5 percent solution is equally effective as 5 percent benzoyl peroxide. Use a cotton ball to dab the oil on any blemishes once or twice daily. This herbal product helps kill bacteria.

- A weekly herbal steam bath for mild acne, or two to three times weekly for more severe acne, can open and drain pores, prevent new outbreaks, and help heal the skin. Add 1 teaspoon of dried yarrow or one tea bag of yarrow tea to 1 cup boiling water and steep for thirty minutes. Pour the tea into a shallow basin of steaming water. Lean your head over the basin (about 12 inches above the water) and place a towel over your head like a hood. Allow the steam to cleanse your face for five to ten minutes.

Other Options

- Zinc supplements have proven very successful, especially in young teenage boys, who are often deficient in zinc. A zinc-sulfate-hydrate supplement (10 ml) taken three times daily for several days, followed by 50–80 mg daily of zinc picolinate for up to twelve weeks is recommended. Because long-term zinc supplementation can deplete copper supplies, also take 2–3 mg copper daily along with the zinc.

- The organic sulfur compound known as MSM (methylsulfonylmethane) can eliminate acne. Take 1,000–2,000 mg daily, either capsules or powder (you can mix the powder, which is flavorless, in juice), divided into two doses. Once the acne has cleared, cut your daily dose in half.

When to See a Doctor

If the skin around your blemishes is red and hot to the touch, you could have cystic acne, which requires professional treatment. Also, if your acne is accompanied by fever and boils, it could be a rare form of acne called *acne fulminans*. See your doctor immediately for treatment.

BODY ODOR

Everyone has his or her own unique body smell—a distinctive, very subtle scent that helps infants identify their mothers and attracts men and women to one another. No amount of soap and water can wash that smell away. Yet there is a big difference between this natural "fragrance," if you will, and smelling funky. Having body odor—and maybe the telltale sweat blotches under your armpits—can be one of life's more embarrassing situations. But just because you may sweat a lot doesn't mean you smell.

That's because sweat itself is odorless; it's what thrives on the sweat that can make you smell. Bacteria are the secret ingredient of body odor, because they live off perspiration and produce bad odors.

Types of Sweat

Humans generate two types of sweat: eccrine and apocrine. Sweat from eccrine glands is produced all over the body and is used to lower body temperature when we exercise or are in a hot environment. Eccrine sweat does not smell.

Apocrine sweat is produced in certain places, like the armpits, hands, feet, and groin. It, too, doesn't smell, but it does contain fat and protein, which seem to appeal to hungry bacteria. After the bacteria feed off apocrine sweat, they break down the chemicals in the "food" and the result is body odor.

Have you ever noticed that young children don't have body odor? That's because they don't secrete apocrine sweat. Apocrine sweat isn't in production until puberty, when levels of the hormone testosterone rise.

Causes of Body Odor

If testosterone is a key factor in the production of body odor, and we know that men have higher levels of the hormone than women do, does that mean men have more body odor?

The potential is certainly there. However, the number-one way to fight body odor is cleanliness, and taking regular baths and showers should know no gender. In fact, women, too, fall victim to the influences of hormones. Hormone fluctuations prior to and during menstruation can cause body odor in some women. Here are some other causes of body odor:

♦ *Zinc deficiency*. The mineral zinc helps regulate detoxification in the body and controls how the body handles waste. Thus a zinc deficiency can worsen body odor.

♦ *Sugar and/or caffeine consumption*. Both of these foods can alter the amount and type of sweat you produce.

♦ *Sexual arousal and nervousness*. Both, whether they occur together or separately, get the sweat glands going.

♦ *Drugs*. Morphine, thyroxine (used for thyroid problems), overdoses of aspirin or acetaminophen, and some antipsychotic drugs can cause excessive sweating, which can lead to body odor.

♦ *Medical conditions*. People who have diabetes, gastrointestinal disorders, liver dysfunction, genetic enzyme deficiencies, or yeast infections may emit certain odors. Individuals with diabetes may smell like nail polish; those with gastrointestinal problems or enzyme deficiencies may have a "fishy" odor; people with liver dysfunction can have an ammonia smell; and those with yeast infections may smell like beer.

Remedies

Good hygiene is certainly the first step you should take to combat body odor. However, keeping clean with an antibacterial soap and water may not always be enough, as there are many other reasons you may be "funky." Here are some things you can do when soap and water don't cut it.

DANGER UNDER YOUR ARMS?

The selling point of many antiperspirants and deodorants is that they contain odor-fighting aluminum compounds including aluminum sulfate, aluminum chloride, aluminum acetate, chlorohydrate, zirconium, and so on, along with alcohol and perhaps a fragrance. These ingredients shrink the pores (alcohol), physically block or clog the pores (aluminum compounds) and mask body odors (fragrance), but do they address the *cause* of the odor? No. There is also evidence--although it is inconclusive--that aluminum causes or contributes to Alzheimer's disease. That's why some healthcare practitioners recommend that people not use products that expose them to aluminum, including antiperspirants and deodorants, which can penetrate the skin day after day, use after use. Aluminum can also cause irritation, stinging, and rash. As an alternative, use products that contain mineral salts, which provide an unfriendly environment for bacteria and so eliminate odor.

Best Bets

♦ Instead of using traditional antiperspirants and deodorants (see "Danger Under Your Arms?" above), try wiping your armpits with a cotton pad damp with white vinegar, apple cider vinegar, or witch hazel. They evaporate quickly and fight bacteria.

♦ Use a crystal stone that contains mineral salts (the primary one is potassium sulfate). Crystal stones do not contain aluminum, are long-lasting, and economical. In fact, one 4-ounce stone typically lasts one year. Several brands are on the market.

◆ Take one or two chlorophyll tablets or take chlorophyll liquid with your meals. This natural green pigment is Mother Nature's deodorizer.

Other Options

◆ If you give off a fishy smell, eliminate foods that are rich in the nutrients lecithin or choline and the amino acids carnitine and lysine, such as chocolate, cereals, eggs, corn, soy products, peanuts, nuts, raisins, and wheat germ.

◆ Herbal deodorants that contain tea tree oil or essential oils of chamomile, sage, walnut, or eucalyptus can eliminate odors without clogging the pores.

When to See a Doctor

Body odor that has one of the smells discussed here—fishy, nail polish, ammonia, beer—is a signal for you to visit your doctor. It could be a sign of something more serious. Because body odor doesn't happen without sweat, another reason to see your doctor may be hyperhidrosis, or excessive sweating. This is not a disease but a symptom of various medical problems, including diabetes, nervous disorders, and hyperthyroidism.

BURNS

You fall asleep on the beach. You grab the lid off a pot of boiling water and get burned by the escaping steam. You spill a cup of hot coffee onto your bare feet. You hold a burning match too long and it singes your finger. Burns happen every day, and fortunately most of them are not serious enough to require medical treatment. Here we will concern ourselves with less serious burns and how you can treat them. However, you should familiarize yourself with the various types of burns so you know how to recognize those that respond to home treatment and those that need immediate professional medical care (see "A Matter of Degrees" on page 220).

Remedies

Do you remember when the first thing people did when they got a minor burn was to put butter on it? If not, you're lucky, because that's one of the things you should *never* do to a burn. You should also never apply oil, grease, lotions, or creams to burns, unless they are specifically designed for burns. Other "never do" items include: covering burns with adhesive bandages, covering a burn too tightly, or applying iodine to raw tissue.

Now here's what you should do. *Remember:* these remedies are for first- and second-degree burns (including sunburn) only.

Best Bets

♦ Immediately immerse the affected area in cool (not cold) running water to help stop the burn and sting and prevent swelling. Keep it there until the pain subsides. If you have serious sunburn, submerse your body in a tub of cool (not cold) water. Gently pat the area dry.

♦ Apply aloe vera pulp, liquid, or gel to the burn. Aloe vera reduces the pain and minimizes scarring. It's a good idea to keep a live aloe vera plant handy especially for this purpose. Break off one of the spongy stalks, split it open, and apply the pulp to your skin.

♦ After the stinging feeling has subsided, apply a topical calendula preparation to help prevent infection. Calendula is available in both homeopathic and herbal formulas.

A MATTER OF DEGREES

There are several types of burns, which are categorized in terms of severity: first-degree burns are the least serious, and fourth-degree burns are the most serious and damaging.

♦ *First-degree burn.* Only the top layer (epidermis) of skin is affected. The burned area is hot, red, and painful, but there is no blistering or swelling. Sunburn is usually a first-degree burn.

♦ *Second-degree burn.* The epidermis and a portion of the layer under it are affected. The skin is red or pink and mottled, and there is usually blistering, along with swelling and seeping. Pain can be severe.

♦ *Third-degree burn.* All layers of the skin are affected, and the blood vessels and nerves in the skin are destroyed. Because the nerves are damaged, there is little or no pain initially. The burned area may be bright red, black, yellow, or white, and the skin may look very dry. This type of burn requires emergency medical attention.

♦ *Fourth-degree burn.* The most serious of all burns, it reaches the muscle and bone. It looks like a third-degree burn but causes much more damage.

Other Options

◆ Take nutrients to speed up healing. They include zinc (15 mg twice a day with food for one to two weeks), vitamin C (1,000 mg three times daily for one to two weeks), and vitamin A (5,000 IU) along with beta-carotene (15,000 IU) twice a day until healing is complete. *Note:* If you are pregnant, intend to get pregnant, or have a liver disorder, do not take vitamin A supplements without first consulting your doctor. Too much vitamin A can be toxic to a developing fetus. Your doctor may recommend beta-carotene instead. This vitamin converts to vitamin A in the body and is not toxic.

◆ Mix 10 drops of healing lavender oil with 1 ounce of jojoba oil and apply the mixture to the burned area several times a day.

When to See a Doctor

Several types of burns require immediate emergency medical attention. These include any third- or fourth-degree burns. You should not attempt to remove any clothing that is burned. Instead, go to the emergency room immediately or contact emergency services. You should also seek medical help for any electrical burn. Although it may look minor, an electrical burn can cause internal damage not visible on the surface of the skin. A chemical burn also should be attended to promptly. Immediately flood the burned area with cool running water and then go to the emergency room.

HANGNAIL

"Ouch! I've got another hangnail!" How often has this happened to you? You know it's a hangnail because it smarts every time you catch it on your clothes, in your hair, or on the fabric of the sofa. How can something so small be so annoying?

Actually, a hangnail isn't a nail at all: it's dead, split skin around your fingernails. Because this area does not get a good supply of oil to keep the skin supple, it dries out easily, and the skin splits.

The people who are most likely to get hangnails are those who have their hands in water a lot, those who bite their nails, and those who handle a lot of paper, such as letter sorters, mail carriers, and people who file most of the day. That's because paper readily absorbs oil from their hands and dries them out quickly.

Remedies

A little tender loving care will keep hangnails away or to a minimum. Here are some tips for prevention and treatment.

Best Bets

- If you get a hangnail, soak it in some water or water and oil (two capfuls of bath oil in 8 ounces of warm water) for ten minutes. Then use small, sterilized scissors to clip off the skin. If you clip the skin when it's hard and dry, you risk ripping the skin.

- To prevent hangnails, moisturize your cuticles daily with hand lotion. If you handle a lot of paper or have your hands in water a lot, keep hand lotion nearby and apply a small amount several times a day as needed. Olive oil or vegetable oil can be used to soften your cuticles as well.

- If hangnails are a chronic problem, apply an emollient cream or ointment on the affected fingers before you go to bed, and wrap a piece of plastic wrap around each one. Secure the plastic with tape and keep your fingers wrapped overnight. Remove the plastic in the morning. Do this nightly or as needed.

When to See a Doctor

Most hangnails can be self-treated and don't cause any problems, but they can become infected if you bite them, pull the skin, or pick at them. See your doctor if you notice signs of infection (hot skin, redness, swelling, or pus formation).

INGROWN NAIL

An ingrown nail: it sounds pretty innocuous, just a minor annoyance. But if you've ever had one and you let it get infected, you know that it can be a big inconvenience and painful. If the ingrown nail is on your big toe, which is where the majority of them develop, it can be difficult to walk or wear shoes until the toe has healed. The problem can be just as inconvenient if the ingrown nail appears on any of the other toes. All this trouble is caused by a little nail that's gone awry.

Causes of Ingrown Nails

An ingrown nail occurs when a portion of the nail curves into the fleshy part of the toe and embeds itself in the soft tissue. Several things can cause the nail to do this, but the most common culprit is wearing tight, ill-fitting shoes with improperly cut nails.

The proper way to cut toenails is straight across without tapering the corners, which should reach out from the sides of the toe. But sometimes you're in a hurry, or you've never known how to properly cut your nails. So you go "snip, snip" and stuff your feet into shoes that are too tight, and off you go to breed an ingrown toenail. In some cases, ingrown toenails are caused by a congenital overcurvature of the nail, a toe injury, or a bunion.

If the nail enters the toe tissue, callused or irritated tissue may grow over the embedded edge. If sweat and dirt become entrapped in this area, an infection can result, causing the toe to become hot, swollen, and red, and to ooze pus.

Remedies

We've already alluded to two ways to prevent ingrown nails from occurring in the first place: avoid tight, improperly fitted shoes and cut your toenails properly. So you didn't do those things, or you did and you got an ingrown nail anyway. Now what?

◆ If your toe is infected, soak it in warm, soapy water three to four times a day.

◆ You can perform your own home procedure to get rid of an ingrown nail by following these steps:

1. Soak your foot in warm, soapy water for ten minutes.

2. Sterilize the tip of a nail file in boiling water for fifteen minutes, let it cool for a moment, then carefully lift the nail away from the affected skin at the outer corners.

3. Soak a tiny piece of cotton in an antiseptic or topical antibiotic and place it under the outer corner of the affected nail.

4. Repeat the above three steps daily until the pressure goes away and the nail begins to grow properly. You must wear sandals or roomy shoes and socks during this healing process or it will not work.

When to See a Doctor

Contact your doctor within a week of self-treatment if the affected toes do not heal, continue to hurt, or if there are signs of infection despite treatment. Also, do not attempt self-treatment if you have diabetes or poor circulation—even for a minor ingrown toenail—as you are more vulnerable to infection.

LIVER SPOTS

"My grandmother and grandfather both had them," says Margaret, as she points to the brown, flat spots on the backs of her hands. "My mother, too. So I knew it was just a matter of time before I got them as well."

Liver spots, which are also known as age spots, senile lentigines, or solar lentigo, look like large freckles. These round or oval areas of increased pigmentation are usually the result of years of exposure to the sun or other forms of ultraviolet light. Like Margaret, many people have a hereditary predisposition for liver spots. They typically begin to appear in people in their forties, and are most often seen on the backs of the hands and on the forearms, shoulders, face, and forehead. Sometimes they appear in clusters.

Liver spots also may result from impaired liver function or a nutritional deficiency. As we age, the liver can become overwhelmed with toxins from our food and the environment. The body's inability to get rid of the toxins, along with a deficiency of antioxidants (for example, vitamins A, C, and E, and other nutrients) may result in liver spots.

Although liver spots can be cosmetically unappealing in some cases, they are harmless and painless. Some people worry that because both liver spots and skin cancer develop from sun exposure, that the former can lead to the latter. However, this is not the case (see "When to See a Doctor" on page 225). Regular use of sunscreen and other sun-shading methods can help prevent new liver spots from forming but cannot help eliminate those that have already appeared.

Remedies

Some experts say that once liver spots appear, there is no way, short of using laser treatments or chemical peels, to remove them. Others say that persistent use of some natural remedies help many people. If you want to try the latter route, here are some suggestions.

Best Bets

◆ Over-the-counter bleaching agents can make liver spots fade. Look for those that contain any of the following ingredients: arbutin (bearberry) glycoside, kojic acid, glycolic acid, hydroquinone, silymarin, and glycyrrhetinic acid (a licorice derivative) and follow package directions.

◆ Some people claim that vitamin E can help make liver spots fade. The recommended daily dose is 400 IU. You can also puncture a vitamin E capsule and apply the oil directly on the liver spots every night before retiring. Vitamin E is an antioxidant and helps with tissue repair. Castor oil, applied twice daily for about four weeks, also is said to make liver spots fade significantly. Vitamin C gel also may make those spots fade. Apply before going to bed.

◆ Help detoxify your liver by taking milk thistle (*Silybum marianum*), a powerful antioxidant that also helps slow down the rate at which the liver absorbs toxins. The suggested dose is one 200–250 mg capsule of a standardized extract (80 to 85 percent silymarin) three times daily.

Other Options

◆ Mix 1 teaspoon onion juice with 2 teaspoons apple cider vinegar and apply to the liver spots twice daily. The spots should fade in several weeks.

◆ Apply fresh lemon juice to the spots twice a day. If you are going to be out in the sun, first allow the juice to dry because it can increase your sensitivity to light. After several months, the acidity in the juice can cause the spots to fade significantly.

When to See a Doctor

Liver spots have smooth, regular borders and are uniform in color. If, however, you notice spots that have irregular borders or shapes and that may have varying shades, contact your doctor. You may have *lentigo maligna,* a noninvasive malignant freckle. Also, if you want to have the liver spots removed medically, there are laser treatments and chemical peels doctors can use.

NAILS (CHIPPED, SOFT, BRITTLE)

They are our miniature coats of armor, composed of a protein substance called keratin, which is also the main component of skin and hair. Fingernails and toenails are designed to shield the tips of our fingers and toes, which are dense with sensitive nerve endings and, thus, very susceptible to pain and injury. Fingernails also allow us to perform certain fine-motor tasks that would be impossible to do with our fingertips alone.

Reading Your Nails

Nails give us hints about various health problems that may be going on in the body. For example:

- White spots in the nails may indicate a zinc deficiency.

- Spoon-shaped nails are associated with low levels of iron.

- Black, splinterlike spots in your nails could indicate a serious heart infection known as bacterial endocarditis.

- Very pale nails suggest anemia.

- Thickened, pitted nails may indicate psoriasis.

- Split, flaky nails may be caused by a lack of linoleic acid (an essential fatty acid).

Most of these nail problems, as well as the most common complaints of soft, chipped, or brittle nails, can be easily remedied by addressing your diet. Nails that break easily may be caused by a deficiency of calcium, silica, and/or other trace minerals, as well as various other nutrients. They may also be caused by poor absorption of nutrients. Discolored nails can result from smoking or regular use of nail polish.

Remedies

The average fingernail takes about six months to grow from its base to tip, and a toenail typically takes twice as long. Yet such growth may be hindered when nails are split, flaky, chipped, brittle, or soft. Here are some home remedies for treating various common nail problems.

Best Bets

- If your nails are brittle or growing poorly, evaluate your protein intake. The average adult needs 0.38 grams of protein per day per pound of body weight (for example, a 150-pound person would need 57 grams daily). If you're not getting enough protein, add a protein supplement to your diet (for example, powdered protein that can be mixed with water or juice) and see if your nails improve after a few weeks.

- For nails that split and break, vitamin A may be the answer. Increase your intake of this vitamin by drinking carrot juice and eating sweet potatoes, parsley, kale, spinach, mangoes, broccoli, squash, and liver. You can also take a supplement, but take beta-carotene (which converts to vitamin A in the body) instead of vitamin A, which can be toxic in high amounts. Take up to 25,000 IU beta-carotene daily. *Note:* If you are pregnant, intend to get pregnant, or have a liver disorder, do not take vitamin A supplements without first consulting your doctor. Too much vitamin A can harm a developing fetus. Your doctor may recommend beta-carotene instead, which is not toxic.

✦ For overall stronger nails, take a sulfur supplement known as MSM (methyl-sulfonylmethane). The recommended dosage is 500 mg three to four times daily with meals.

Other Options

✦ If your nails are brittle and they have white spots under them, try taking zinc (30 mg daily, with food) and vitamin B_6 (pyridoxine; 50 mg daily) for three to six months. Whenever you take individual B vitamins, you also should take a B-complex supplement at a different time of the day, because the B vitamins work together. Also, if you take 30 mg or more of zinc for more than one to two months, also take 1–2 mg copper daily to maintain proper mineral balance.

✦ Nails that split and flake often respond to an increased intake of essential fatty acids, found in oily fish, nuts, seeds, flaxseed oil (1–2 tablespoons daily), and whole grains.

When to See a Doctor

If you believe your nail problems may be related to an iron deficiency, see your doctor for an evaluation before starting an iron supplement program. Also see your doctor if your nail problems don't show improvement after several months of self-treatment; if you suspect you have an underlying condition (especially if you see the black marks related to bacterial endocarditis); or if you experience signs of infection around your nails (inflammation, pain, pus).

OBESITY

Try this the next time you're out and about town or strolling through a shopping mall: notice how many people are overweight. It won't take you long to realize that Americans are fat. According to a Centers for Disease Control and Prevention study published in 2002, the percentages of overweight or obese people twenty years of age or older according to ethnicity look like this:

✦ Non-Hispanic black women: 77.3%   ✦ Non-Hispanic black men: 60.7%

✦ Mexican American women: 71.9%   ✦ Mexican American men: 74.4%

◆ Non-Hispanic white women: 57.3%   ◆ Non-Hispanic white men: 67.4%

Health Problems Linked to Obesity

According to medical experts, you're obese if you weigh 20 percent more than recommended for your height and build, and your body fat accounts for 25 percent of your weight if you're a man and 30 percent if you're a woman. (Women naturally have more body fat, so they are "allowed" the higher percentage.)

Researchers with the ongoing Nurses' Health Study, who have been monitoring more than 100,000 female nurses for thirty years, find that we begin to experience weight-related health problems when we weigh 22 pounds more than we did at age eighteen. Whether or not this claim rings true—and there obviously are exceptions—overweight and obesity are known risk factors for diabetes, gallstones, heart disease, stroke, hypertension, osteoarthritis, sleep apnea and other breathing-related problems, and various forms of cancer (breast, colorectal, gallbladder, kidney, uterine).

Obesity is also associated with high blood cholesterol, menstrual irregularities, depression, excess body and facial hair, pregnancy complications, stress incontinence, and higher surgical risk. The National Institutes of Health (NIH) reports that approximately 280,000 American adults die each year from causes attributable to obesity.

The Importance of Exercise and Diet

We have good intentions: we spend more than $33 billion per year on weight-loss products and services, including low-calorie foods and memberships to weight-loss facilities. Yet most of these foods and services obviously aren't being used effectively or enough, because about 95 percent of people who lose weight gain it all back—and more.

For some Americans, walking to the refrigerator or to the car to get to the drive-through window at a fast-food restaurant is their definition of exercise. About 25 percent of adults say they don't get any physical activity during their leisure time, and only 22 percent say they get the recommended amount (five times a week for at least thirty minutes each time). A mere 15 percent get the recommended amount of vigorous activity (three times a week for at least twenty minutes).

Additionally, we Americans love to eat. The popularity of all-you-can-eat restaurants is a testament to that. So is the fact that the average American eats 756 doughnuts, 60 pounds of cookies and cakes, 7 pounds of potato chips, and 22 pounds of candy per year.

The simple fact is, in the vast majority of cases, obesity is the result of an imbalance in energy exchange. When too many calories are taken in and not enough energy (physical activity) is exerted, the body turns the excess calories into fat and stores it. It takes 3,500 calories to put on 1 pound of fat. Conversely, you need to burn 3,500 calories to lose 1 pound of fat. The healthiest way to lose weight is to moderately reduce the amount of calories you take in, say, eat 500 fewer calories per day; and then add to or increase the vigor of your exercise program. (See Table 9.1 on page 230.) If you were to eat 500 fewer calories per day and exercise away 500 calories three days per week, you could lose about 1½ pounds per week.

Causes of Obesity

Scientists have several theories about why people are fat, and it may well be that the cause is a combination of factors working together. One theory involves heredity. If one or both parents are overweight, then their children have a 40 to 80 percent chance, respectively, to also have a weight problem. When both parents are of normal weight, however, there is only a 7 percent chance that their children will be overweight.

This doesn't mean that fat is "in your genes" if your parents are overweight. They are probably overweight because they eat too many calories and don't get enough exercise. Children follow their parents' lead: if they are raised to eat lots of fried and sugary foods, that's what they usually continue to eat as adults.

Another theory concerns fat cells. This theory says that every fat cell your body produces stays with you for your entire lifetime, unless they are surgically removed. Thus, if you shoveled in high-calorie foods when you were young, you built up a reserve of fat cells that will be around for life.

Recent research indicates, however, that it may be possible to reduce the number of fat cells if there is significant weight loss. Studies also prove that even overweight children of overweight parents can achieve a healthy, slim figure when they eat healthy foods and exercise regularly. Genes—and fat cells—don't have the last say.

Fat Isn't Simple

Being overweight goes a little deeper than simply eating too much and exercising too little. There are cofactors, such as: Why do we overeat? Are we bored, depressed, angry, struggling with low self-esteem, or is it just a habit? Knowing why we overeat is necessary before we can change our eating habits.

TABLE 9.1. MOVE IT TO LOSE IT: CALORIES BURNED PER HOUR

Activity	Calories Burned per Hour*	Activity	Calories Burned per Hour*
Sitting	60–85	Bicycling moderately (8 mph)	300–360
Sleeping	60–85	Tennis (doubles)	300–360
Standing still	120–150	Walking fast (4 mph)	360–420
Walking very slow (1 mph)	120–150	Canoeing (4 mph)	360–420
Walking slow (2 mph on flat surface)	150–240	Walking very fast (5 mph)	420–480
Bicycling slow (5 mph)	150–240	Waterskiing	420–480
Bowling	240–300	Jogging (5 mph)	480–600
Mowing the lawn (power mower)	240–300	Basketball	480–600
		Running (5.5 mph)	600–660
Walking moderately (3 mph)	240–300	Bicycling fast (13 mph)	600–660
		Running (6–10 mph)	> 660

* Based on a 154-pound person. If you weigh more or less, the amount of calories you burn will
  probably be more or less, respectively.

In some cases, factors such as endocrine or metabolic imbalances (for example, hypothyroidism, hypopituitarism), problems with the way the body uses insulin, or use of certain medications may contribute to being overweight.

Remedies

We could make this section really simple: eat less, exercise more. But *how* do you eat less and healthier? How do you resist the cookies and doughnuts and French fries? How do you motivate yourself to exercise? Are there products that can help you achieve these goals more easily? Yes, but there are no magic pills you can take that will make your weight melt away. Anyone who claims to have a product that can do that or anything similar is lying. The tiny print on all of these items tells you to exercise and eat less if you want results. So will any of these products really help you?

When used along with the plan "What's Cookin', What's Shaking" (see the inset on page 231), the following remedies may make your weight-loss efforts easier. And oh yes, you'll need a little patience, too. You didn't gain all the extra weight overnight, so allow some time for it to go away as well.

WHAT'J COOKIN', WHAT'J JHAKIN': A PLAN FOR LOJING WEIGHT

◆ Eat whole foods, preferably organic (fruits, vegetables, grains, legumes), cold-water fish, and, if you eat dairy, make it nonfat.

◆ Avoid processed foods as much as possible. Most contain saturated fats and hydrogenated and partially hydrogenated fats, as well as preservatives, additives, and sugars.

◆ Bake, poach, broil, or steam your food; don't fry, unless it's a quick stir-fry in 1 tablespoon olive oil for vegetables.

◆ Drink at least eight 8-ounce glasses of pure water daily. Water not only makes you feel full, it also helps flush toxins from your body.

◆ Incorporate exercise into your day. Take a brisk walk with a friend during breaks and lunch. Get up thirty minutes earlier in the morning and ride a stationary bike or follow an aerobic video. Walk briskly and with purpose. Park a half mile away from the video store; carrying a video or two back to your car isn't too big of a burden.

◆ Avoid eating a big meal in the evening, and if you snack at night, make it very light (for example, a piece of fresh fruit or air-popped popcorn without butter). The body doesn't burn many calories while you're sleeping.

◆ Eat slowly, chew thoroughly, and be aware of each bite. Eating while watching television can result in unconscious eating: taking bite after bite without being aware of the amount of food you are consuming.

◆ Avoid feeling hungry by eating five or six small, nutritious meals instead of three larger ones. This approach also keeps your energy level steady throughout the day.

Best Bets

◆ Green tea has been shown to enhance the body's ability to burn fat. The recommended dosage is 300 mg of a standardized extract that contains 50 percent catechin and 90 percent total polyphenols. Take one dose thirty minutes before breakfast and another thirty minutes before lunch.

◆ Seek emotional and/or spiritual help. Your emotional well-being is critical if you want to lose weight and keep it off. Why and what we eat is often related to feelings and emotions. Join a support group, share your thoughts with a friend or professional therapist, engage in meditation, yoga, or visualization.

◆ Chromium picolinate can help control blood sugar metabolism, which impacts appetite, and reduce your cravings for sweets. The recommended dosage is 100–200 mcg twice daily.

Other Options

◆ If you crave sugar, take 100 mg of astragalus three times daily (at 9 A.M., 11 A.M., and 1 P.M.). This herb can curb your cravings for the sweet stuff.

◆ If you crave fatty foods, it may be your body's way of telling you that you're not getting the right kinds of fat (for example, essential fatty acids) in your diet. Take 500–1,000 mcg of flaxseed oil, which is an excellent source of essential fatty acids, twice daily.

When to See a Doctor

Consult your doctor before engaging in a weight-loss and exercise program; if your body mass index (BMI) is 30 or greater; if you have experienced a sudden weight gain; or if you have health problems that are caused by or aggravated by excess weight, such as high blood pressure, heart problems, or diabetes.

SKIN TAGS

"For a while I was scared, because I thought it was cancer," says Charlotte, a fifty-nine-year-old teacher in Houston. "Then I remembered that my mother had had the same thing when she got to be sixty years old. She had them checked out and the doctor told her they were harmless. He called them skin tags. I call them ugly."

Skin tags (acrochordons) are small growths of skin that develop on the face, neck, armpits, or groin of some people. They usually first appear among people in their sixties or older. They are harmless and do not become malignant or cancerous, as Charlotte feared at first. And while they tend to be hereditary, no one knows what causes them.

Skin tags first appear as tiny, soft bumps that grow into flesh-colored (or slightly darker) skin attached by a stalk. The tags are easily moved but usually painless. However, if a skin tag is twisted on its stalk, a blood clot may develop within it, and the tag may become painful.

Because skin tags are harmless, they do not need treatment. However, if the tags become sore or red from clothing or jewelry brushing against them, or if they make you uncomfortable, they can be removed surgically. Be warned, however, that even if skin tags are removed, new ones often form.

Remedies

Skin tags are one of those nuisances in life that you can't prevent, and self-treatment is limited to only two approaches.

◆ Avoid wearing clothing or jewelry that will irritate skin tags.

◆ Some people claim that their skin tags disappear after about three months if they take the trace mineral chromium picolinate. The suggested dosage is 200 mcg twice daily. It has also been reported that the skin tags reappear if you stop taking the supplement. However, chromium has been found to be very safe and nontoxic at levels of 1,000 mcg or lower per day, and has the added bonus of helping lower cholesterol and triglyceride levels. Therefore, it seems worth a try.

When to See a Doctor

If you can't live with your skin tags and want them removed, contact a dermatologist, who can remove them by freezing with liquid nitrogen, cutting them off with a scalpel or scissors, or using light electrodesiccation. The procedures can be done in the office or at an outpatient clinic, and healing takes about one week.

SMELLY FEET

Since 1975, Montpelier, Vermont, has been the host of a unique contest: the International Rotten Sneaker Contest, sponsored by Combe, the makers of Odor-Eaters. Dozens of kids from ages five to fifteen bring their sweaty, smelly sneakers to the New England state and have them judged for their "fragrance." In March 2001, Rebeka Fahey, an eleven-year-old from New Mexico, won the honor. In addition to a cash prize and a trip to New York City, her smelly entry has been entombed in the Odor-Eaters Hall of Fumes, a hermetically sealed trophy case, where it can rot in peace along with past winners.

Not many of us would want the dubious honor of having the smelliest sneakers—and thus the smelliest feet. But the truth is, having smelly feet is a common part of life for many people, and not because they don't wash their feet.

Cause of Smelly Feet

Each foot contains about 250,000 sweat glands, which can pump out up to a pint of sweat per day. Because feet have so many sweat glands, it's one of the first places from which heat is released when we are hot. If we are wearing socks and shoes that don't allow our feet to breathe easily, the sweat produced does not evaporate. Moisture is a prime breeding ground for the bacteria (propionic bacteria) on your feet, and the bacterial breakdown of the outer skin layers produces isovaleric acid, resulting in smelly feet.

As an aside, there's actually a connection between smelly feet and your face. The bacteria found on smelly feet are related to the bacteria that cause acne. Thankfully, acne-affected skin doesn't smell, because it's not in an enclosed, moist environment.

Remedies

Having smelly feet is one of the complaints spouses have about their mates. In fact, the inventor of Odor-Eaters, Herbert Lapidus, reported that when he first brought his charcoal-based odor destroyers to market, he was surprised by the number of spouses who contacted him about how their marriages were suffering because of smelly feet. That's when Lapidus knew he had a winning product. His Odor-Eaters and other charcoal-based inserts for shoes are effective ways to treat smelly feet. Here are some other remedies you can adopt to keep on your partner's good side.

Best Bets

- ♦ Wear shoes and socks that breathe. That means wear cotton socks, sandals, or canvas, mesh, or leather shoes.
- ♦ Go barefoot when possible and safe. If you let your feet air out, they won't sweat, thus you eliminate the trigger for the odor.
- ♦ Switch shoes. Don't wear the same pair two or more days in a row. If you wear sneakers a lot, get two pairs and alternate them.

Other Options

- ♦ Change your socks every day, several times a day if your feet sweat a lot.

Bring a few extra pairs with you to the office or to school so you can change them if needed.

◆ Wash your feet every day and dry them completely. Then spray them with a natural antiperspirant foot powder before putting on your socks and shoes.

When to See a Doctor

If your feet continue to reek even after you've tried all these approaches, or if you suspect you have a fungal infection, you should consult a physician.

VARICOSE VEINS

"I can still remember when I was six years old and I pointed to my grandmother's legs and said, 'Grandma, what's wrong with your legs? They're all blue and bumpy,'" says Marilyn, a fifty-two-year-old interior designer. "And now I'm looking at my legs and thinking it could happen to me, too."

Varicose (from the Latin *varix,* meaning "twisted") veins affect approximately 80 million Americans, with four times more women than men having the condition. In most women, varicose veins first appear after age fifty, but if there is a family history of the problem, they can occur sooner. Any vein in the body can become varicose, yet the legs are the most common site. When they develop in the anus, they are called hemorrhoids (see HEMORRHOIDS on page 109).

Varicose Veins—A Closer Look

The legs have two systems of veins: deep veins, which carry about 90 percent of the blood flow; and surface veins, which carry the remaining 10 percent and which are not as well supported as the deep ones. Varicose veins form when there's a dysfunction of the valves in the veins near the surface of the legs.

Normally, when your leg muscles contract, blood is pushed up through the veins in your legs and passes through tiny valves. These valves then shut to prevent blood from flowing back down to your feet. When one or more valves fail to close properly, blood can collect in the veins, causing them to stretch. Over time, the veins expand until bulges are created and push toward the surface of the skin.

Varicose veins appear blue or gray and vary in length and "bumpiness." They cause the legs to ache and swell, and sometimes itch as well. The severity of symptoms does not correspond to how serious the condition looks, however.

Some people who have minimal varicose veins can experience much more pain and discomfort than someone who has large, bulging veins. Unless varicose veins are treated, they usually become worse and can eventually make it difficult to stand or walk without discomfort, or they can lead to other problems (see "When to See a Doctor" on page 237).

Causes of Varicose Veins

The main cause of varicose veins is any condition or activity that hinders blood flow. That includes being overweight, standing or sitting for long periods of time, pregnancy, heavy lifting, and crossing your legs. Hormonal changes at menopause can also cause the veins to bulge, as can chronic constipation and heavy metal toxicity. If you have a family history of varicose veins, a genetic condition that causes overproduction of lysosomal enzymes, or if you've had a vein disease such as thrombophlebitis (vein inflammation), you are more susceptible to varicose veins.

How to Prevent Varicose Veins

Follow these tips to avoid developing varicose veins.

◆ Move. Walking is an excellent exercise to keep your leg muscles contracting and the blood moving through your leg veins. If your job requires that you stand or sit for long periods of time, take walking breaks several times a day.

◆ Stretch your legs often. While sitting, stretch your legs out, extend your toes, and rotate your ankles. If you stand, periodically shift your weight, and rise up on your toes to stretch your calves. You can also stand on one foot while rotating the ankle of the other leg, then alternate.

◆ Keep your weight under control. Excess weight places a great strain on the veins in your legs.

◆ Don't cross your legs. It places a great deal of pressure on your veins.

◆ Elevate your legs when you're watching television or reading. If possible, put your legs up on a stool under your desk at work.

◆ When flying, get up often to stretch your legs. If driving, stop periodically and do the same.

◆ Avoid wearing high heels. They place a lot of pressure on your calves.

Remedies

Treatment and prevention go hand-in-hand for varicose veins, because even if you undergo a medical procedure to get rid of them, new ones can form. So it pays to take several steps when it comes to your legs.

Best Bets

- The herb gotu kola has proven effective for treating insufficient venous blood flow. The suggested dosage is 200 mg twice daily of a standardized extract containing 16 percent triterpenes. Improvement takes about two months to become evident.

- Improve circulation with butcher's broom, an herb from the Mediterranean, and vitamin C. This combination has proven effective in several studies. Take 300–500 mg three times daily of butcher's broom and up to 1,000 mg of vitamin C per day.

- Bilberries contain compounds that strengthen the walls of the veins and reduce production of lysosomal enzymes, which contribute to the development of varicose veins. The recommended dosage is 80–160 mg of bilberry extract three times daily. Another herb that strengthens the blood-vessel walls is horse chestnut. Use a standardized extract and follow the package directions.

Other Options

- Ginkgo biloba improves circulation. Choose a standardized extract containing 24 percent ginkgo heterosides and take 40 mg three times daily.

- Bromelain, an enzyme found in pineapple, helps break down fibrin, a substance that is deposited around varicose veins. Fibrin causes the bumpiness associated with this condition. Take 500 mg of bromelain before meals three times daily. Foods that can help break down fibrin include garlic, onions, and ground red pepper.

When to See a Doctor

Contact your doctor as soon as possible if your veins become red, warm, swollen, or tender to the touch; if you develop a rash or sores near or on the veins; or if your circulation is affected. Varicose veins increase your chance of getting phlebitis, a condition in which veins become inflamed and very painful. Left untreated, phlebitis can progress to thrombophlebitis, in which blood clots form. If a clot becomes dislodged, it can travel to the lungs and become potentially life threatening.

There are procedures that can reduce or remove varicose veins. Mini-phlebectomy involves completely removing the damaged veins. Sclerotherapy involves injecting fatty acids and salt water into the affected veins, which causes them to collapse. However, even if you treat existing varicose veins, new ones can develop unless steps are taken to avoid them.

◆ CHAPTER 10 ◆

Take a Deep Breath

reathing. The average adult breathes in about 6 liters of air per minute at rest and as much as 50 liters per minute immediately after vigorous exercise. We take breathing for granted, and we certainly don't have to think about every breath we take, at least not until something goes wrong. Unfortunately, there are various respiratory and nose and throat conditions that can make us painfully conscious of every breath we take. In this chapter we explore the conditions that have an impact on our ability to breathe, and discuss how we can make each breath an easier one.

ASTHMA

Got asthma? Got cockroaches? What do the two have to do with each other? According to a National Institute of Allergic and Infectious Disease (NIAID) and National Institute of Environmental Health Sciences (NIEHS) Inner City Asthma Study from March 2002, cockroaches are a major cause of asthma throughout the world. In the United States, between 17 and 41 percent of children and adults who have asthma are allergic to these insects.

The NIAID-NIEHS study looked at seven major cities in the United States and measured allergen (allergy-causing factors) levels in urban homes. Seventy-three percent showed evidence of cockroaches. The next culprit on the list was dampness (70 percent), while 47 percent of homes had at least one smoker living there.

Asthma is a chronic respiratory condition in which certain triggers affect the air passages, causing them to become constricted and thus hinder the flow of air in and out of the lungs. The symptoms of asthma, which include chest tightness, wheezing, breathing difficulties, and coughing, are the result of three main forces: inflammation of the air passages, followed by muscle spasms of these air passages, followed by increased production of mucus in the air passages. Symptoms of asthma can last for minutes, hours, or even days, and severely restrict activities.

Asthma Triggers

If you have asthma, you are hypersensitive to one or more triggers, which may include any of the following:

◆ Strenuous exercise, especially when the weather is cold and dry

◆ Allergy-type irritants, such as insects, pollen, mold, dust, and pet dander

◆ Certain foods or food additives, including sulfites (found in red wine, beer, and preserved meats)

◆ Environmental pollutants, such as industrial chemicals, air pollution, tobacco smoke, and irritants found in carpets, wood products, paints, and varnishes

◆ Household products, such as perfumes, air fresheners, hair spray, and cleaners

◆ Respiratory infections, such as the common cold or bronchitis

◆ Stress or strong emotions

◆ Certain foods, including chocolate, milk, eggs, citrus fruits, and nuts (including peanut butter)

◆ Weather changes (for example, an approaching thunderstorm, sudden drop in temperature)

◆ Aspirin or other anti-inflammatory medications

If you have asthma, you're not alone. According to the American Academy of Allergy, Asthma, and Immunology (AAAAI), 20 million Americans have asthma, and this includes about 9 million children. Many famous people, from Beethoven to rock star Alice Cooper, from president John F. Kennedy to Olympic track-and-field star Jackie Joyner-Kersee, have the condition. Obviously it didn't stop them from living full, active lives. And it doesn't have to stop you either.

Conventional Treatment of Asthma

Like it or not, asthma is a complex condition that requires professional medical care. Having said that, we also note that there are many complementary remedies that can be very helpful and reduce the need for some of the conventional approaches. Some of those complementary methods are discussed in "Remedies" on page 242. Here it's important to mention the various medical ways to control different types of asthma.

If you experience symptoms of asthma every day, your doctor will probably prescribe corticosteroids—drugs, usually inhaled, that reduce the chronic inflammation in your lungs and thus help prevent asthma attacks. Along with the corticosteroid you may be given a bronchodilator, a medication you can take when an attack is about to occur in an attempt to prevent it or reduce its severity. Bronchodilators quickly open up the air passages and help you breathe. Oral drugs called mast-cell stabilizers also may be prescribed to help prevent asthma attacks.

If your asthma is caused by an allergic reaction, your doctor may give you cromolyn sodium and nedocromil, drugs that help stop the release of chemicals that make your air passages close up, or constrict. Some people only need to use an inhaler (a handheld device that sprays a dose of medication into the lungs) before exercise or when the lungs are highly upset. Each person's treatment plan is different and depends on individual needs.

THE HARD FACTS

- Despite advances in medical science, the number of asthma deaths continues to rise. Between 1979 and 1998, the number of deaths attributed to asthma increased by 109 percent, according to the American Lung Association.

- Only about 25 percent of children who have asthma outgrow the condition when they reach adulthood. Asthma persists beyond childhood in 72 percent of men and 85 percent of women.

How to Prevent Asthma

Naturally, prevention is the best approach. Once you've identified your trigger(s), do your best to avoid them or minimize their effect on you. For example, if dog or cat dander is a problem, you may need to keep your pets outdoors or find them a more suitable home. Many people who react to dogs or cats find that guinea pigs don't cause asthma attacks. If pollen, mold, or grasses send you wheezing, however, you may find it harder to avoid them. Many people discover that wearing a filtering mask (usually available at neighborhood drugstores) when outdoors is helpful.

If exercise induces an asthma attack, you can try a different exercise or perhaps take your medication before exercise. You should discuss these options with your doctor.

If stress is a trigger for you, learn some techniques for managing stress levels (see "Remedies" below). Speaking of stress: asthma can place great stress on the body, including the adrenal glands, and cause fatigue, among other symptoms. To help prevent stress to the adrenal glands, take a high-potency B-complex supplement daily. Other stressors, such as the common cold, flu, and bronchitis, can be your enemy as well. Avoid people who have these respiratory conditions, and wash your hands frequently. Hands are a major mode of transmission of cold, flu, and bronchitis germs.

Remedies

The following at-home complementary remedies can be used by nearly everyone who has asthma. However, before you try any of these remedies, discuss them with your conventional doctor. Both your conventional doctor and any other healthcare practitioner should be kept up-to-date on your treatment program. Also, never stop using your conventional medication without consulting your doctor.

Best Bets

◆ Get your corticosteroids in candy form—almost. Pure licorice is an anti-inflammatory and can be used to control the inflammation associated with asthma. You want to take the deglycyrrhizinated form of licorice (also known as DGL), which doesn't raise blood pressure like other forms of licorice can. Buy a licorice tincture and put 20 to 40 drops into a cup of hot water, and let it cool slightly before drinking. Do this three times a day, as needed.

◆ If allergies are a part of your asthma picture, try taking the bioflavonoid quercetin. Studies show that quercetin has both antihistamine and antiallergy properties. The suggested dosage is 100 mg three times daily during allergy season.

◆ Yoga combines gentle movements and stretches with breathing exercises. These gentle exercises reduce stress and have proven to be very helpful for asthma sufferers. Yoga breathing exercises relax and strengthen lung muscles, which in turn helps reduce the amount of constriction of the air passages during an attack. Yoga can be learned from local classes, books, and videos. The United States Yoga Association (www.usyoga.org) even has a seven-step program for children with asthma called Yogasthma that provides instructions suitable for adults as well.

Other Options

◆ Good fats—the omega-3s—can help reduce lung inflammation. Omega-3 fatty acids can help stop late-phase inflammation—the inflammation that can occur up to twenty-four hours after an acute asthma attack and last for weeks. Thus, taking omega-3 fatty acids daily, or eating cold-water fish that are rich in omega-3 oils (for example, tuna, salmon, and mackerel) three to four times a week can help keep late-phase inflammation in check. If you choose the supplement route, the suggested dosage is 3 tablespoons daily of flaxseed oil (you can drizzle it over your vegetables or add it to your salad dressing rather than take it straight), or take six to twelve capsules of fish oil (1,000 mg each) daily. If you are allergic to aspirin or if you are at high risk of stroke, fish oil may make your asthma worse or increase your risk of stroke. Talk to your doctor before taking omega-3 fatty acids.

◆ The mineral magnesium is a natural bronchodilator—a substance that relaxes the bronchial passages that lead to the lungs. The suggested dosage is 500 mg of magnesium citrate or magnesium aspartate daily.

When to See a Doctor

If you are having trouble controlling your asthma attacks, if your attacks have increased or otherwise changed in severity or frequency, or if you are having difficulty with your medications, see your doctor as soon as possible. Most asthma medications are inhaled in aerosol form using an inhaler, which must be used properly in order to be effective. Some doctors recommend patients use a peak flow meter, a handheld device that measures the force with which you exhale. Because exhalation levels usually decline hours or days before an asthma attack, you can learn to predict an attack. Instructions on how to use both of these devices are typically provided by your doctor or other medical professional in the office.

BRONCHITIS

It begins like the common cold—stuffy nose, sore throat—but then you get that sinking feeling that it's going to develop into something more. That's when the other symptoms start: a wet or dry cough, chest pain, wheezing, burning in your chest, and a rattle in your throat. You feel worn out and you've got a low-grade fever. Yep, you've got bronchitis.

Bronchitis is a contagious viral infection that attacks the tubes (bronchial tree) that transport air to your lungs. When these tubes become infected, they swell and fill up with mucus, which makes it difficult to breathe. People who have a weakened bronchial tree, such as those who smoke cigarettes or those who have asthma, are more susceptible to bronchitis.

In most cases, bronchitis is caused by viruses, the same viruses that cause colds. Bacterial bronchitis is much less common than the viral type.

Bronchitis is spread through airborne particles from a cough or sneeze, or when handling utensils, plates, cups, or other items that have been used by someone with the virus. The disease comes in two forms. *Acute bronchitis* typically follows a bout with the common cold or flu and then goes away in seven to ten days. *Chronic bronchitis,* which is found most often among smokers, involves persistent inflammation and blockage of the bronchial tubes and increased production of mucus that develop over time. According to the American Lung Association, more than 9.1 million Americans were diagnosed with chronic bronchitis in 2002. Females are more than two times as likely than men to be diagnosed with chronic bronchitis.

Risk Factors for Bronchitis

In addition to smoking, there are other risk factors for bronchitis. They include allergies, exposure to air pollutants (smog or smoke), alcohol abuse, and poor nutrition. Chronic illnesses, such as lung disease, diabetes, chronic sinus infections, kidney problems, as well as a compromised immune system (AIDS), or use of immunosuppressive drugs are also risk factors for bronchitis.

If you suspect you might have bronchitis, a visit to your healthcare provider can confirm a diagnosis through the use of x-rays to identify any infected airways. Blood tests can be used to identify the cause and severity of the infection. A bacterial culture of mucus may be taken, and if you have bacterial bronchitis, antibiotics can be prescribed. Antibiotics are not effective against viral bronchitis.

Remedies

Rest. Lots of fluids. Cough. These are the tried-and-true approaches to cure bronchitis. A rested body heals faster. Fluids help liquefy the mucus, and coughing gets rid of the mucus. Throw in a cool-mist humidifier in your bedroom, steer clear of cough suppressants (remember, you *want* to cough) and dairy products (they produce mucus), and you'll be well on your way to recovery.

Of course, some extra help would be nice, so we've included the following home remedies to make your recovery even smoother.

Best Bets

✦ Help get rid of mucus with the herb astragalus. Look for astragalus root tincture or capsules of the pure root. If using the tincture, add 6 to 8 drops into a few ounces of water and take it three times daily. If you choose the capsules, one 500 or 600 mg supplement three times daily will do the trick.

✦ Another mucus mover is n-acetylcysteine (also known as NAC), a nutrient that causes mucus to turn watery and thus makes it easier to cough up. The suggested dosage is two 600 mg capsules daily: one when you get up and another when you go to bed. Continue taking NAC until your symptoms clear.

✦ Drink your symptoms away with herbal teas. A combination of hyssop (*Hyssopus officinalis*) and thyme (*Thymus vulgaris*) can clear mucus and relieve your cough. Use 3 parts hyssop and 1 part thyme. Place 1 teaspoon of the mixture into 8 ounces of boiled water and steep for several minutes. Drink three to four cups of this tea daily until your symptoms clear. Another helpful herbal tea is grindelia (*Grindelia camporum*). Place 1 teaspoon of the dried herb into 8 ounces of boiled water and steep for several minutes. Drink three to six cups daily until you get relief.

Other Options

✦ Let your fingers do the walking with a massage. Self-massage of your chest—and upper back massage by a willing partner—can break up lung congestion. Lie down or sit in a comfortable chair. Apply massage oil or vegetable oil to your hands. Then, with your fingertips or palms, use long strokes to gently massage your chest. Begin at your lower rib cage and move up toward your neck. Continue these strokes for several minutes, then switch to making small circles, slowly moving over your entire chest. If you have a partner, ask him or her to massage your upper back using the same circular strokes.

◆ Essential oils in a steam treatment are a great addition to any other therapy. Boil several cups of water, pour the water into a bowl, and add 30 drops of eucalyptus essential oil, or 5 drops each of peppermint, pine, sage, and fir oils to the water. Drape a towel over your head and lean over the bowl of water (as close as is comfortable). Breathe in the steam for five to ten minutes two to three times daily to help thin out mucus.

When to See a Doctor

If your symptoms last for more than seven to ten days and you have a fever, you may have pneumonia. Contact your doctor immediately. Other indications that you should place a call to your physician include development of shortness of breath, coughing up larger and larger quantities of mucus, or a change in the color of your mucus. Also, if you have emphysema, asthma, or heart disease and you develop acute bronchitis, you should be under a doctor's care.

HAY FEVER

When they were eleven and twelve years old, Linda and her cousin Bonnie used to have sneezing contests to see which girl would have the most consecutive sneezes. They played this game every spring, when the pollen from the blossoming flowers and trees filled the air. Today Linda and Bonnie are in their thirties, and the sneezing contests are behind them. But they are still living with the symptoms of hay fever.

Hay fever is actually a misnomer in today's world, as it has nothing to do with hay or fever. The term originated centuries ago in England when some people who were pitching hay developed allergic reactions, with some of them experiencing fever as well. Today hay fever refers to an allergic response to pollen or other airborne substances, such as mold or pet dander. This response results in inflammation of the mucous membranes that line the nasal passages. It is also known as seasonal allergic rhinitis, because it tends to occur during the season in which the offending plant is in bloom.

Every year, hay fever affects about 26.1 million Americans who suffer with varying degrees of symptoms. One of the most common symptoms is prolonged and repeated sneezing, along with a stuffy and runny nose, eyes that are red, swollen, and itchy, an itchy throat, mouth, and ears, and breathing difficulties.

Repeated attacks of hay fever can make some people susceptible to nasal polyps (growths in the nose), asthma, chronic sinusitis, or other respiratory tract conditions.

How to Prevent Hay Fever Symptoms

Depending on the type of airborne allergens that affect you, the following suggestions can help prevent or reduce hay fever symptoms.

◆ Change the air filters in your air-conditioning and heating systems once a month.

◆ Consider installing an air purifier in your heating or air-conditioning system, or buy a stand-alone unit for your bedroom or office.

◆ Wear a pollen mask when you are outside in the garden, taking a walk, mowing the grass, or when cleaning the house.

◆ Keep your windows and doors closed during days when there is much pollen in the air.

◆ Do not keep dander-producing pets in the home. Cats and dogs are the biggest culprits. Some people with hay fever find that guinea pigs don't bother them.

◆ If you are allergic to feathers or wool, use cotton or synthetic materials for your pillows, blankets, and clothing.

◆ Get rid of indoor plants and other sources of mildew.

◆ Use plastic barrier wraps around your mattress, box spring, and pillows.

◆ Avoid use of over-the-counter nasal sprays, as they can make symptoms worse.

Remedies

There are many over-the-counter and prescription remedies for hay fever, but all of them cause undesirable side effects, especially dry mouth, drowsiness, dry nose and throat, and dizziness. The natural remedies below are free of side effects.

Best Bets

◆ An Ayurvedic herb called *tylophora* has been used for centuries to treat hay fever symptoms. The recommended daily dose is 200–400 mg of the dried herb (in capsule) or 1–2 ml of the tincture for up to fourteen days.

◆ Stinging nettle (*Urtica dioica*) is an herb that has a long history of effectiveness against hay fever. Look for a product that is standardized to 1 percent silicic acid and take one or two 600 mg capsules every two to four hours or as needed.

◆ Quercetin is a flavonoid that acts like an antihistamine, but without the side effects of over-the-counter or prescription brands. Begin taking quercetin one to two weeks before the start of pollen season and continue until the season ends. The suggested daily dose is one 400 mg tablet twice daily between meals.

Other Options

◆ Bee pollen is helpful for many people, although a very small percentage of people are sensitive to it. Before taking the full suggested dose, break open a capsule and take about half of it in some applesauce or juice. If you develop allergic symptoms, do not take it. If you have no reaction, begin by taking one capsule (450 mg each) daily and gradually increase it to three capsules per day. You should begin this program three to four months before your allergy season begins. If during the allergy season the three capsules per day do not provide sufficient relief, you can increase the dose up to six capsules daily. You can wait until the beginning of allergy season to start taking bee pollen: gradually build up to six capsules daily. Beginning sooner, however, better prepares your body for the onslaught of allergens.

◆ There are several homeopathic remedies that can be helpful, depending on which symptoms are more bothersome for you. If your hay fever produces cold symptoms and runny eyes, take *allium cepa*. If you have typical cold symptoms along with inflamed eyes and a cough, take *euphrasia*. If you have typical cold symptoms and inflamed eyes but no cough, try sulfur. All of these remedies should be taken in a 6c or 12c potency every four to eight hours as needed. Once you begin to experience improvement in your symptoms, you can stop taking the remedy.

When to See a Doctor

Hay fever usually doesn't require a doctor's care. However, if you try various remedies and you do not get significant relief, or if you develop a painful or hacking cough or other symptoms, contact your doctor. Because recurrent bouts of hay fever can reduce your resistance to respiratory conditions, it is possible to develop sinusitis, for example, while experiencing hay fever symptoms.

SINUSITIS

Behind, between, and over your eyes, behind your nose, and inside your cheeks lie four pairs of cavities called sinuses. These tiny caves serve to filter, moisten, and warm the air that you breathe. But sometimes it feels as if the walls of these cavities have caved in. You can't breathe. Your cheeks hurt, your jaw and teeth ache, your head is throbbing, and you have a cough. There's mucus running down the back of your throat, and you wish you knew a good plumber who could clear out your pipes.

You have sinusitis, a bacterial (infrequently a viral or fungal) infection of the sinus cavities that can cause weeks or even months of discomfort and pain.

Types of Sinusitis

Sinusitis can be acute, which means that the infection stays around for less than three weeks and then goes away without treatment. Most cases of acute sinusitis are triggered by the common cold virus. Although the virus itself does not cause symptoms of sinusitis, it does inflame the sinus cavities. Sometimes this inflammation causes mucus and air to become trapped behind the sinuses, which prevents the mucus from draining out. Accumulated mucus is a prime breeding ground for bacteria. All healthy people have bacteria living in their respiratory passages, but when the bacteria become trapped along with the mucus, the stage is set for sinusitis to develop.

People who have hay fever or allergic rhinitis are prime candidates for sinusitis because these respiratory conditions cause chronic inflammation of their nasal passages, which makes them susceptible to sinusitis. Fungal infections can induce sinusitis in some people, usually those who are allergic to fungi.

The other type of sinusitis is chronic sinusitis, which typically lasts three to eight weeks or longer. People who have asthma, who experience severe asthmatic responses to aspirin or aspirinlike medications (for example, ibuprofen), or who are allergic to airborne allergens, such as pollen, dust, and mold, are most likely to get chronic sinusitis.

Alternative health practitioners claim that sensitivity or allergy to foods or environmental substances is believed to be the main cause of chronic sinusitis. If you experience recurring bouts of chronic sinusitis, it may be worthwhile for you to be tested for food and airborne allergens. If sensitivity or allergy is behind your attacks, addressing the root cause should clear up your sinuses.

A SINUS MAP

Four pairs of sinus cavities lie hidden behind your face. Your symptoms depend on which of these cavity pairs are inflamed; in most cases more than one pair is affected. The pairs are as follows:

◆ Frontal, which lie over the eyes

◆ Maxillary, which are inside the cheekbones

◆ Ethmoid, which lie behind the bridge of the nose and between the eyes

◆ Sphenoid, which lie in the upper area of the nose and behind the eyes

Remedies

Because sinusitis is usually caused by a bacterial infection, the standard medical treatment is antibiotics. These drugs are not without side effects, and they also reduce your body's ability to fight off future bouts of sinusitis and other infections. That's why using proven home remedies, like those listed here, can be a safe and effective choice.

Best Bets

◆ Load up on vitamin C and garlic. The immune-system-boosting power of vitamin C and the antibiotic abilities of garlic will help you fight the infection. The suggested dose of vitamin C is 500 mg every two hours that you're awake for the duration of the infection. If this amount causes you to experience loose stools or gas, reduce your intake to 300 mg every two hours. For garlic, take 500–1,000 mg of deodorized garlic capsules once daily.

◆ For acute sinusitis, try the liquefied form of silver known as colloidal silver. This potent natural antibiotic should be used twice daily until two to three days after your infection has cleared. Pour some full-strength colloidal silver into a small nasal spray bottle and use one or two squirts into each nostril twice daily.

◆ Relief of facial pain can be a wet compress away. Place a warm, wet washcloth over the painful area and leave it for about one minute, then replace it with a cold, wet washcloth over the same area for thirty seconds. Keep alternating warm and cold compresses three or four times. The change in temperature helps eliminate congestion and stirs up the mucus. This approach can be used several times throughout the day.

Other Options

◆ Acupressure is a simple procedure that can promote drainage and relieve painful sinusitis. The acupressure point that can provide the best relief is Large Intestine 20, which is located on either cheek in the indentation beside each nostril. Apply steady, firm pressure to both points at the same time for about three minutes.

◆ Eucalyptus essential oil, when dissolved in a steaming bowl of water, provides an aromatic way to open up your sinus cavities. Boil some water, pour it into a bowl, and add several drops of eucalyptus essential oil. Drape a towel over your head, lean over the water (about 12 inches above the bowl), and breathe deeply for about five minutes. Repeat this remedy several times a day.

A LITTLE "POT" FOR YOUR SINUSES

The introduction of salt water into your sinus cavities can kill bacteria and provide relief from pain and discomfort. You'll need a nasal douche (called a neti pot), which looks like a small glass pipe with a hole. Dissolve $1/2$ teaspoon of sea salt in 8 ounces of distilled water. Pour the mixture into the douche and hold a finger over the hole. Take one snort of the mixture and then move your finger from the hole. The saltwater will enter your sinus cavity. Do this twice daily. Alternate nostrils each time.

When to See a Doctor

If you don't get relief when using the remedies suggested here, or if your symptoms worsen, contact your doctor. Also, if you have chronic, recurring sinusitis, you should be tested for allergies and sensitivities as the cause of your attacks.

SNORING

It may not be a shot heard around the world, but you can surely hear it halfway down the block. According to the *Guinness Book of World Records*, a man in England holds the record for the loudest snore. He clocked in at 92 decibels, which is 2 decibels louder than a loud shout and 10 decibels greater than the sounds of heavy traffic.

Fortunately, not everyone who snores creates such a roar. According to a National Family poll taken in 1997, about 100 million Americans snore at least occasionally, with about 37 million of them being habitual noise makers. Men out-snore women. An estimated 33 percent of men and 20 percent of women snore, and these figures rise to about 60 percent and 40 percent, respectively, after people reach age sixty.

Causes of Snoring

Snoring is the result of the vibration of the soft tissue of the throat (the uvula, the small piece of flesh that hands downward from the soft palate) as air passes over it with each inhalation and exhalation during sleep. The result is a buzzing, rattling, snorting, and/or wheezing sound. Most people who snore sleep with their mouths open, usually because there is an obstruction in the throat or nasal passages. The blockage could be caused by nasal congestion from a cold or aller-gies, nasal polyps, loose dentures, swollen tonsils or adenoids, or a deviated septum. Some people snore simply as a result of lying on their backs, which causes the jaw to open and the tongue to fall backward and partially close off the windpipe.

Obesity is an important risk factor in snoring. Being significantly overweight increases the chance of snoring by threefold. Also, obese people who snore are prone to having sleep apnea, a potentially dangerous condition in which breath-ing stops for as long as two minutes during sleep (see "Snoring and Sleep Apnea" on page 253).

Remedies

Your long-suffering sleep partner has rolled you over and elbowed your rib cage until it's sore. She or he has tried earplugs and banished you to another room, but these are not long-term solutions. A Mayo Clinic study reports that non-snoring bedmates lose an average of one hour of sleep per night because of their thunderous partners. For the sake of your own health—and that of your mate—try the following remedies to reduce or eliminate the roar.

Best Bets

- Drop a few pounds. Most people who snore are overweight, and losing weight can significantly reduce, or even stop, your snoring.

- Sleep on your side. Most people who snore do so, or more loudly, on their backs. Changing position can take some getting used to. Turn on your side and place firm pillows behind your back to prevent yourself from rolling onto your back. One home remedy is to sew a tennis ball into the back of your pajamas so when you roll over, you'll be jolted awake or back to your side.

◆ Breathe through your nose. Mouth breathing is a cause of snoring. If your snoring seems to be caused by nasal congestion that is causing you to breathe through your mouth, one of the products on the market may help you. Two of them are Breathe Right and Chin-Up strips. The strips work by holding congested nasal passages open, and the Chin-Up strip holds the bottom lip and chin up. When used together, these products may reduce or eliminate snoring.

SNORING AND SLEEP APNEA

Sleep apnea is a condition in which an individual has chronic cessation of breathing, often several hundred times a night, during which the blood levels of oxygen can drop to dangerously low levels. It's estimated that 18 million Americans have sleep apnea and that it affects 4 percent of middle-aged men and 2 percent of middle-aged women.

Individuals most likely to have or develop sleep apnea are those who are overweight and snore loudly, have a physical abnormality in the nose or other part of the upper airway, or have high blood pressure. It appears that sleep apnea runs in some families and so may have a genetic basis.

Snoring is a symptom of sleep apnea. You may snore and not have sleep apnea, but if you have sleep apnea, chances are pretty good that you snore. Sleep apnea can have long-term health consequences, such as heart attack, stroke, and high blood pressure. It's recommended that if you snore or you live with someone who does, you should be evaluated at a sleep center with a sleep test to determine if you suffer from sleep apnea so your doctor will know how to treat you.

Other Options

◆ Use homeopathic remedies. These may reduce mucus congestion and swelling in the throat, which may be contributing to your snoring problem. Several different products are on the market, in pill, spray, and nasal-drop form, including SnoreStop (pills), Snore Control (spray), and Ysnore (drops and spray)

◆ Spray your throat. People who snore usually have dry, sore throats. This can occur because the constant vibration of the soft palate can bruise and dry out your throat tissues. Special throat sprays, which typically contain natural oils and are formulated to last about eight hours, can reduce the volume of your snoring.

When to See a Doctor

If you suspect you have sleep apnea, or your partner has observed regular breathing cessation while you sleep, see your doctor for a sleep test. Also, if you have tried the home approaches mentioned above and snoring is still a problem, contact your physician. You may have sleep apnea or physical abnormalities that are causing your problem.

CHAPTER 11

The Body Internal

The inner workings of the human body are truly fascinating and complex. All components, from individual cells to the entire organ system, work together in often mysterious ways. Sometimes those inner workings go awry, causing discomfort, pain, or emotional distress, or limiting activities and lifestyle. In this chapter we focus on health conditions that affect various organs or organ systems, such as the circulatory system, the gallbladder, the liver, the bones and joints, and others, all of which make up the body internal.

COLD HANDS

"My hands are so cold they hurt," said Colette, a thirty-eight-year-old graphic designer. That's not such an unusual statement, except that Colette made it in the middle of June in Florida. "My husband says my cold feet eliminate the need for air-conditioning at night," she added wryly. "But I have to live with the pain."

Millions of people like Colette have hands and feet that become cold, painful, and numb in response to slight changes in temperature. Simply turning on the air-conditioning in the car can make their hands so frigid they can't hold the steering wheel.

Most people expect their hands or feet to get cold when the temperature dips around freezing. But for individuals like Colette, frigid fingers and toes are a year-round problem and a sign of Raynaud's disease, a condition that affects an estimated 5 to 10 percent of the United States population.

Raynaud's Disease

For people with Raynaud's disease, cold hands and feet are just the tip of the iceberg. Although cold normally causes the muscles in the arteries to contract (grow smaller), people with Raynaud's disease have arteries that overreact. The small arteries in the hands and feet go into spasms when they are exposed to cold temperatures, and blood flow is severely restricted. This causes the hands and feet to turn white or bluish and to sting, tingle, or go numb as they get progressively colder.

Initially, only the tips of the toes and fingers are affected. In some people, the disease progresses, and over time the attacks extend to the entire digit and ultimately all the digits. When the hands and feet begin to get warm again, they become red and throb with pain, often for hours. Anxiety and emotional distress can make symptoms worse.

Raynaud's disease can be either primary or secondary, and each type occurs about equally. The primary form is usually milder, while secondary Raynaud's disease has more severe symptoms and is more likely to progress. Medical conditions that may predispose you to secondary Raynaud's disease include rheumatoid arthritis, lupus, scleroderma, atherosclerosis, some blood diseases, and carpal tunnel syndrome, among others. Women are five times more likely than men to get Raynaud's disease, and it is usually diagnosed between the ages of twenty and forty. In about 1 percent of people with Raynaud's disease, the condition progresses until the digits become gangrenous.

Remedies

Even though we don't know exactly *why* people get Raynaud's disease, we do know that treatment should focus on helping keep the extremities warm. Here are some natural ways to achieve that goal.

Best Bets

◆ Sometimes the simplest solutions are the best, and so here goes: cover up. Donning mittens and woolen socks, two pairs if necessary, can offer much relief. Always keep a few pairs of mittens (these tend to keep your hands warmer than do gloves) and socks handy—at home, in your car, at work—so you'll be prepared when the cold encroaches. Wear mittens and socks to bed, especially in the winter months. Tuck a battery-powered warming device into your pocket, mittens, or boots when you're outside in the cold weather.

◆ The heat-producing herb cayenne should be on your kitchen shelf. Add a teaspoon of cayenne or chili powder into a glass of water, stir well, and drink it down once daily when symptoms strike. Or, you can take capsules: 40,000–80,000 heat units daily. And don't worry about cayenne bothering your stomach: although this herb produces heat, it is actually good for your stomach.

◆ Exercise to help stimulate blood circulation. While traditional physical activity—jogging, dancing, bicycling—can be helpful, you may get faster relief by standing with your feet comfortably apart and twirling your arms like you are pitching a softball. Twirl your arms at a rate of sixty to eighty rotations per minute until you get relief, and repeat as necessary.

Other Options

◆ A technique called thermal biofeedback, which does require some professional guidance before you go out on your own, can be very effective. During a few lessons with a biofeedback instructor, you will learn how to voluntarily control the temperature of your fingers and toes, using the power of your mind. During those lessons, you'll have painless lead wires attached to your hands and/or feet. As an instructor helps you mentally warm your hands or feet, you will get feedback on a device that is connected to the wires. After a few sessions, you'll be able to get the same results without using the machine, which means you will be able to warm your extremities anytime, anywhere.

◆ Some substances can improve blood flow; others can hinder it. Helpful supplements include vitamin E (400 IU daily), magnesium (200 mg three times daily), coenzyme Q_{10} (60 mg daily), and fish oils (1,000 mg three times daily). Avoid caffeine and nicotine, as both can restrict blood flow.

When to See a Doctor

If your attacks are severe and debilitating, contact your doctor. He or she may prescribe a mild sedative or a vasodilating drug (one that helps open up the blood vessels) to help prevent the spasms. Also, contact your doctor if the attacks occur on one side of the body only (one foot or one hand), or if the attacks result in sores or ulcers that develop on the fingers or toes.

DIABETES (TYPE II)

Americans have a love affair with sugar. We develop that relationship at a very early age, and it often begins with the jarred baby food we were fed, is nurtured by grandma's cookies and years of soda and ice cream, and the urge stays with most of us. In fact, the average American consumes about 140 pounds of sugar in various forms each year.

Thank goodness for the pancreas, an organ whose main job is to produce a hormone called insulin. Insulin transports the sugar you eat from your bloodstream and into your cells, where it is used for energy or stored.

At least, that's what's supposed to happen. But for some people—at least 6 percent of the population—the insulin receptors in the cells don't recognize the insulin, or they don't accept the insulin that comes to them. The result is that too much sugar remains in the bloodstream, and you have a condition known as type II diabetes, or high blood sugar.

Type II diabetes accounts for 90 to 95 percent of all cases of diabetes. The other form, type I diabetes, develops in childhood and is characterized by a complete lack of insulin production. The American Diabetes Association estimates that 6 percent of the United States general population older than forty has been diagnosed with type II diabetes, and that an equal number have the disease but have not yet been diagnosed.

HOW SWEET IT'S NOT

Having high levels of sugar in the blood can lead to a variety of health problems, including kidney disease, eye problems, serious nerve damage to various parts of the body, damage to the blood vessels, heart attack, and stroke. People who have type II diabetes are two to four times more likely to have heart disease or stroke than people without diabetes. Loss of kidney function occurs in about 100,000 people with diabetes every year. Blood circulation to the lower legs and feet can be so poor in some people that they develop gangrene and must have their toes, feet, or lower legs amputated. In fact, more than half of all lower-limb amputations performed in the United States each year are done on people who have diabetes.

Risk Factors and Symptoms of Type II Diabetes

Type II diabetes usually develops after age forty, although doctors are seeing it in younger and younger patients every day. One reason for the increasing prevalence of type II diabetes is that obesity, a risk factor for the disease, is a growing problem among individuals younger than forty as well as older folks. Another risk factor for type II diabetes relates to ethnicity: African Americans and Hispanics are twice as likely, and Native Americans are many times more likely, to develop type II diabetes than are whites. A family history of diabetes is yet another risk factor to consider.

Signs that you may have type II diabetes include the following:

- Frequent urination
- Extreme hunger
- Extreme thirst
- Blurred vision
- Unexplained weight loss
- Itchy skin
- Frequent vaginal or urinary tract infections
- Slow healing of sores and cuts
- Numb extremities
- Extreme fatigue

Remedies

While people who have type I diabetes must take insulin for the rest of their lives, individuals who have type II diabetes can usually control their disease by making some lifestyle changes, namely, maintaining a healthy diet and regular exercise. We'll throw in a few herbs along the way, and you'll have the ingredients you need to deal with type II diabetes.

Best Bets

- Increase the amount of whole foods (fruits, vegetables, legumes, grains, beans, seeds, nuts) that you eat and dramatically reduce sugars and refined foods, like those that contain white flour and other processed grains. Sugars and refined foods send too much sugar into your bloodstream. Whole foods are rich in fiber and they help maintain balanced blood sugar levels.

- Regular exercise is critical for effective diabetes management. Walking, jogging, dancing, handball, tennis, bicycling, swimming, or other fun aerobic activities need to be done daily. Exercise not only helps prevent type II diabetes from occurring in the first place, it also helps transport sugar out of the bloodstream and into the cells. Regular daily exercise helps control weight as well. Plan on at least twenty to thirty minutes of exercise per day.

- The herb bilberry is recommended for individuals who want to help stop damage to their capillaries (the smallest blood vessels) and the resulting medical problems. When purchasing bilberry, look for a brand that is standardized to 24 percent anthocyanosides, which means it has high concentrations of the substances that help heal the blood vessels.

Other Options

◆ Supplements of chromium, a trace element that plays a major role in the proper functioning of insulin, can help make sure your cells accept sugar. Although chromium supplements don't help everyone who has type II diabetes, many people report better control of their blood sugar levels once they begin supplementation. The average dose is 200–600 micrograms (mcg) daily, available in tablets, capsules, and liquid. Look for chromium picolinate, which is easily absorbed by the body. Another form, chromium polynicotinate, contains both chromium and niacin, which causes flushing and itching in some individuals.

◆ Magnesium deficiency is common among people who have type II diabetes. This finding lead scientists to study the relationship between the nutrient and the disease. They believe that abnormally low levels of magnesium may worsen blood sugar control and interrupt insulin secretion in the pancreas in people with the disease. Evidence also suggests that a magnesium deficiency may contribute to some complications of diabetes. Thus, a diet rich in magnesium (whole grains, leafy green vegetables, legumes) and a magnesium supplement (300–500 mg daily) is suggested.

When to See a Doctor

If you have type II diabetes, you should have regular checkups (at least once a year) with your doctor. Also contact your doctor if you experience any change in the signs or symptoms of the disease, or if you develop any new ones. Because of the risk of diabetic retinopathy (leakage of blood into the retina of the eye, which can lead to blindness), everyone who has type II diabetes should have an eye examination once a year.

FIBROCYSTIC BREASTS

"It was the same thing every month," says Nancy, a fortysomething account executive. "About two weeks before my period, my breasts would become so tender I could hardly bear to put on my bra. When the pain subsided and I did my self-breast exams, I'd feel these cottage-cheese-like lumps in my breasts. I was worried that I might have breast cancer until my doctor examined me and told me it was just fibrocystic breast changes. Boy, was I relieved!"

About 50 percent of women experience fibrocystic breast changes. Symptoms include breast lumpiness, breast cysts, breast tenderness, and pain. These symptoms, while uncomfortable, are harmless and do not increase your risk of breast cancer. They typically appear about two weeks before your period should begin, and then subside.

Causes of Fibrocystic Breast Changes

During the two weeks before your menstrual period begins, extra blood and bodily fluids begin to flow to the breasts and accumulate there. The result is pain and tenderness in your breasts. Some women experience more lumps, tenderness, or pain than others, and the reason is related to hormone levels. In menstruating women, levels of estrogen and progesterone fluctuate throughout the month. The amount of discomfort any one woman feels depends on how sensitive her breast tissue is to hormone changes, her age (women in their thirties often have more tenderness and pain than do younger women), and the actual levels of their hormones.

The good news is that after menopause, which typically occurs when a woman is in her late forties or early fifties, these symptoms stop because estrogen and progesterone levels have declined dramatically. Women who elect to take hormone therapy after menopause, however, may experience symptoms of fibrocystic breast changes because the therapy reintroduces the hormones to their bodies.

Remedies

When it comes to relieving symptoms of fibrocystic breast changes, you need to practice a little patience. You may not notice a significant change the first month you try a remedy, so stick to it through several menstrual cycles.

Best Bets

◆ Although experts disagree about the effectiveness of this suggestion, so many women swear it works that we must mention it: cut out caffeine. That includes coffee, tea, colas, chocolate (sorry!), and medications that contain caffeine, such as NoDoz, Exedrin, Anacin, and some prescription drugs (for example, Darvon). In one study, 83 percent of women who eliminated caffeine from their diets also eliminated fibrocystic breast discomfort, while 98 percent experienced significant relief.

◆ If fluid retention is a cause of your breast tenderness and discomfort, try an herbal diuretic. Here are three to consider.

1. Black cohosh (*Cimicifuga racemosa*): Add ½ teaspoon powdered root to 8 ounces water. Boil for thirty minutes. Drink up to one cup daily, 2 tablespoons at a time. Black cohosh should not be used if you have a heart condition.

2. Dandelion (*Taraxacum officinale*): Place 1 heaping teaspoon of finely cut root into 16 ounces of boiling water and simmer for fifteen minutes. Drink up to two cups daily. Avoid dandelion if you are pregnant or breastfeeding.

3. Parsley (*Petroselinum crispum*): Steep 1–2 teaspoons dried leaves in 8 ounces of boiling water for ten minutes. Drink up to three cups daily. Parsley has no known adverse side effects.

◆ To help eliminate breast lumps, try essential fatty acids. Take your choice of either evening primrose oil or flaxseed oil. If you choose primrose oil, take two 500 mg capsules three times daily for six weeks. If flaxseed oil is your preference, take 1 tablespoon three times daily for six weeks. Flaxseed oil is easy to add to your diet: drizzle it over your vegetables or pasta, or mix it with your favorite salad dressing to get your daily dose in a delicious way.

Other Options

◆ Vitamin E reportedly can soften breast lumps. Some women even claim that their lumps disappeared completely after they took vitamin E for several months. For best results, take 400–800 IU of vitamin E daily, and add vitamin B_6 as well: 150 mg daily for ten to fourteen days before your period begins.

◆ Chaste berry (*Vitex agnus castus*) provides relief from breast symptoms for many women. Add 30 drops of the tincture to water twice daily during your menstrual cycle. You should notice significant improvement after two to three periods.

When to See a Doctor

If these at-home remedies do not offer you significant relief, or if your symptoms do not respond to over-the-counter pain relievers or anti-inflammatory drugs such as acetaminophen and ibuprofen, contact your doctor. Also, if you notice unusual changes in your breast lumps, if you detect a lump that does not feel like your "normal" cottage-cheese lumps, or if a lump becomes painful, contact your physician for a professional examination. Sometimes a painful breast lump or cyst (a type of lump that is filled with fluid) needs to be aspirated (drained of its fluid using a needle). Aspiration is an in-office procedure that can eliminate your discomfort and pain.

GALLSTONES

They can be as tiny as fine grains of sand or as large as a golf balls. But if you've ever had one lodged in your bile duct, it probably felt as big as a basketball. Gallstones are solid lumps composed of cholesterol, by-products of bile (a digestive juice made by the liver), and minerals such as calcium. About 10 percent of people in the United States have gallstones, but only one in five of those people ever experience symptoms that let them know they're there. The other four out of five have silent, or dormant, stones.

Bile, a substance produced by the liver, is stored in a pear-shaped organ called the gallbladder. Bile is necessary to break down fats so the body can use them. Fatty foods, such as meat, whole milk, egg yolks, and other animal foods, as well as hydrogenated oils, make bile more concentrated. If the bile stored in the gallbladder becomes too concentrated, stones can begin to form. Individuals can have one or hundreds of stones. Sometimes the stones irritate the gallbladder and cause the ducts (the tubes that connect the gallbladder and the small intestine) to become inflamed. In some cases, stones become lodged in the ducts, causing intense pain.

Although about 500,000 people a year who have gallstones have their gallbladders removed, many alternative physicians believe that up to 85 percent of these surgeries are not necessary. That's because only about 15 percent of people who undergo surgery have large gallstones, while the remaining patients have smaller stones, which often can be managed with diet, nutritional supplements, and herbs (see "Remedies" on page 265).

Risk Factors for Gallstones

In addition to a fatty diet, other factors may cause gallstones to develop. One is obesity, especially among women. Results of a large study show that even women who are moderately overweight are at increased risk of developing gallstones. Also, women between the ages of twenty and sixty are twice as likely to have gallstones as men. However, both men and women over the age of sixty are more likely to develop gallstones than younger individuals. Diabetes, which is common among people who are obese, also increases the risk of developing gallstones. If we look at ethnicity, Native Americans have the highest rate of gallstones in the United States. This is because they have a genetic predisposition to release a large amount of cholesterol into the bile. Most Native American men can expect to have gallstones by age sixty.

Many people take medications to reduce their cholesterol, but these drugs can also increase cholesterol levels in the bile, which then increases the risk of gallstones. Another factor that can raise cholesterol levels in bile is high levels of estrogen, which are often associated with pregnancy, use of birth control pills, or hormone replacement therapy. And if you practice fasting or experience rapid weight loss, beware: these activities cause gallbladder activity to decline, which causes bile to become overconcentrated.

How to Prevent Gallstones

Because diet is a key factor in the formation of gallstones, it's no surprise that taking some precautions with your diet can help prevent these potentially painful lumps. Here are a few ways to help prevent gallstones:

◆ Limit or eliminate your consumption of foods that contain animal fat (meat, cheese, whole milk, butter, baked goods, egg yolks). They cause bile to become more concentrated.

◆ Reduce your intake of sugar. Sugar and sugary foods can irritate the gallbladder ducts.

◆ Lecithin is a substance derived from soybeans and sunflowers that dissolves fat and thus helps increase elimination of fatty compounds from the body. Lecithin granules can be taken as a supplement, sprinkled on cereal or other foods, to help prevent gallstones.

◆ Thirty to sixty minutes before breakfast each morning, drink a cup of hot water to which you've added the juice of half a lemon.

◆ Eat lots of foods rich in vitamins C and E, such as vegetables and fruits.

◆ Consume brown rice and whole-grain cereals, breads, and pastas.

◆ Avoid coffee.

- Drink lots of water. Bile can become highly concentrated if you are not properly hydrated. As a general rule, drink $\frac{1}{2}$ ounce of water for each pound you weigh.

- Drop a few pounds. Being overweight is a common risk factor for gallstones. That's because fat stresses the gallbladder, which makes it work harder and increases the likelihood of gallstones.

Remedies

Surgery is still the primary way doctors deal with gallstones, and sometimes an operation is necessary. In many cases, however, people who have small gallstones can flush them out using various home treatments.

Best Bets

- Take 1 tablespoon cold-pressed olive oil and the juice of one lemon daily. You can mix them together in some tomato juice to help it go down more easily.

- Make the recommendations included in "How to Prevent Gallstones" part of your lifestyle. Not only do they prevent gallstones, but they also help keep stones from becoming larger and keep the gallbladder ducts from becoming inflamed.

- Perform a gallbladder flush (see the inset below).

GALLBLADDER FLUSH

Under the supervision of a healthcare professional, follow these steps to perform a gallbladder flush:

1. Thirty minutes before you retire for the night, blend $\frac{1}{4}$ cup olive oil and $\frac{1}{4}$ cup fresh lemon juice and drink the mixture.

2. Then take the herbal laxative cascara sagrada according to package directions.

3. Lie on your right side for thirty minutes, then go to bed.

4. In the morning, see if your stools contain stones.

5. Repeat the flush for two to three more days.

Other Options

- Chinese herbs such as pyrrosia leaf and rhubarb can dissolve very small gallstones. However, you need to consult a skilled practitioner who can blend these herbs for you.

- The herb milk thistle protects the liver and also stimulates the flow of bile. The suggested dose is 600 mg of extract daily, standardized to 70 to 80 percent silymarin, which is the active ingredient in the herb.

When to See a Doctor

If you are experiencing severe pain in the upper right area of your abdomen, or you have pain accompanied by nausea, vomiting, or fever, see a doctor immediately. Also seek medical help if your skin or eyes turn yellow, as this is a sign of jaundice, which means your liver is not functioning properly.

HEPATITIS C

An estimated 4 million Americans are harboring a virus that can cause irreparable, life-threatening damage when it attacks the liver. That virus is HVC—hepatitis virus C—and the disease it causes is hepatitis C. Hepatitis C is one of the more common types of hepatitis, a disease in which the liver becomes infected and inflamed. The other types of hepatitis—A, B, D, and E—like hepatitis C, are named for the specific virus that causes the disease.

Hepatitis C is a blood-borne disease, which means it is transmitted via exposure to contaminated blood. About 50 percent of all cases are associated with injection drug use, with remaining cases being attributed to blood transfusions, sexual contact (especially among people who have multiple partners), health-care workers who are stuck by an infected needle, tattoos, household contact with an infected individual, and mother-to-infant transmission. In up to 30 percent of cases, doctors cannot identify the source of the disease.

Hepatitis C—Life Threatening Disease

You can't live without a liver. One of this organ's most important functions is to filter your blood to remove toxins that have entered your body from your environment, food, and water. Nearly 2 quarts of blood pass through the liver every minute, where up to 99 percent of bacteria and other harmful substances are removed from the blood before it is allowed to flow through the rest of your body. If your liver is damaged, an untold number of dangerous elements can be released into your body. The hepatitis C virus can cause that kind of damage.

Types and Symptoms of Hepatitis C

Hepatitis C can be either acute (short-term) or chronic (long-term). Extreme fatigue is one of the most common symptoms of acute hepatitis C, along with dark urine, pain in the lower right abdomen, loss of appetite, nausea, fever, vomiting, jaundice (yellowing of the skin or whites of the eyes), headache, itching, diarrhea, and muscle and joint pain. Most people recover completely within sixteen weeks, but up to 40 percent can go on to develop the chronic form of the disease.

Symptoms of chronic hepatitis C are the same as those of the acute form, although some people don't have any symptoms or only have mild ones. Their prognosis is generally good. At the other end of the spectrum are those who have severe symptoms and serious liver damage. These individuals eventually develop cirrhosis (scarring of the liver; often fatal) or liver cancer.

Patients who are in the middle of the spectrum typically have mild to moderate symptoms and an uncertain prognosis. Overall, at least 20 percent of patients who have chronic hepatitis C go on to develop cirrhosis over a ten- to twenty-year period.

Conventional Medical Treatment

Because hepatitis C is a potentially life-threatening disease, it's critical that you consult a conventional medical doctor to help with your treatment and care. Along with that care, however, there are several complementary remedies that can easily be incorporated into your treatment program. It is your responsibility to make sure both your conventional doctor and qualified alternative health practitioners are fully informed of all the remedies and treatments you are using.

In the world of conventional medical treatment, an antiviral drug called interferon is the standard approach. When it is used alone, the response rate is only 15 to 35 percent. When combined with other antiviral drugs, such as ribavirin, response can be as high as 47 percent.

Unfortunately, along with the less-than-desirable response rates there is an even higher rate of side effects from these drugs. About 60 percent of patients experience adverse reactions, including depression, muscle and joint aches, fatigue, weight loss, hair loss, and fever. In addition, anyone who is taking these drugs (treatment lasts up to one year) must be monitored very closely by his or her doctor.

These facts have made many people who have hepatitis C seek alternative, complementary remedies. Along with these remedies, you can follow a liver-friendly diet (see "A Be-Kind-to-Your-Liver Diet" below).

A BE-KIND-TO-YOUR-LIVER DIET

Because your liver's job is to filter your blood and remove potentially damaging substances, it makes sense to eliminate or reduce the number and amount of those dangerous factors as much as possible. One way you can do that is to avoid foods that stress the liver. Here are some dietary tips you will find useful if you have hepatitis C:

◆ Meat is difficult for your liver to digest. In addition, animal products (including dairy products) are loaded with growth hormones, steroids, antibiotics, and other substances that can severely stress your liver. Limit your consumption of these foods, and choose organic varieties when you do eat them.

◆ Alcohol has known liver-damaging effects. Avoid it.

◆ Caffeine, found in colas, coffee, tea, chocolate, and some medications, stimulates the liver. Avoid it.

◆ Artificial sweeteners, such as aspartame, are very difficult for the liver to process. If you're looking for a low-calorie sweetener, use liquid stevia, which is an herb, available in most health food stores.

◆ Sugary foods, including fruit juices, stress the liver and the digestive system. Enjoy fresh fruit, but no more than three servings daily.

◆ Protein sources that are easy for your liver to process include fish, soy products, lentils, chickpeas, beans, and organic turkey and chicken.

◆ Enjoy lots of steamed green vegetables.

Remedies

If you have hepatitis C, the goal of treatment is to prevent further damage to your liver. This means you need to boost and support your immune system and protect your liver. As a complement to conventional treatment, the following remedies have proven helpful for many people.

Best Bets

◆ Of all the herbs, milk thistle (*Silybum marianum*) is best known for its ability to protect the liver. Milk thistle contains silymarin, a combination of flavonoids that have powerful antioxidant abilities. Silymarin is effective in treating both acute and chronic hepatitis. Because the dose of milk thistle is based on its silymarin content, you should look for standardized extracts that contain 70 to 80 percent silymarin. Take two 150 mg capsules or tablets of the extract, three to four times daily.

◆ Garlic is one of Mother Nature's most potent antiviral substances, and a good enhancer of the immune system as well. If you like the taste of fresh or cooked garlic, include a few cloves in your daily diet. If you choose the supplement route, look for those that contain 3,000–4,000 mcg of allicin (an active ingredient in garlic) per capsule.

◆ The shiitake mushroom (*Lentinus edodes*) has been called the Elixir of Life, and for good reason. Both the National Cancer Institute (U.S.) and the Japanese National Cancer Institute have found that shiitake mushrooms enhance the immune system and have powerful antiviral abilities. Include these magic fungi in your diet by eating two to six per week, or take a daily supplement: 1,500–2,000 mg in tablet or capsule form twice daily with meals.

Other Options

◆ Help protect your liver while enjoying a cup of herbal tea. Add 1 teaspoon of dried or fresh lemon balm to 8 ounces of boiling water. Steep for fifteen minutes, strain, and drink two to three cups daily.

◆ An ingredient called glycyrrhizin, found in licorice, is effective against both acute and chronic hepatitis. Glycyrrhizin has been used in Japan for several decades as a treatment for hepatitis. Suggested doses are 1–2 grams of the powdered root taken three times daily; 2–4 ml of the fluid extract, taken three times daily; or 250–500 mg of the dry powdered extract (5% glycyrrhetinic acid content) taken three times daily.

When to See a Doctor

You should see your doctor when you first notice symptoms of hepatitis C, and then continue follow-up visits as needed. If at any time during your treatment, whether conventional or complementary, you experience a worsening of symptoms or develop new ones, contact your doctor immediately.

HIGH BLOOD PRESSURE

When Eric's doctor told his forty-four-year-old patient that he had high blood pressure, the slightly overweight attorney was not surprised. After all, he typically put in an eighty-hour work week, ate too much fast food, and enjoyed an occasional cigar. But he was surprised when his doctor presented him with two treatment options: diet and exercise, or medication. He had thought drugs would be his only solution.

"I was real tempted to choose the drugs and just be done with it," confessed Eric. "But I knew there were side effects, so I figured, why not try a natural approach? So I choose diet and exercise. And after a few months, it really worked!"

High blood pressure, or hypertension, is a very common chronic condition that can lead to life-threatening medical problems, including heart attack, heart failure, stroke, and kidney damage. It is estimated that more than 50 million Americans have high blood pressure, including 25 percent of whites and 33 percent of blacks.

The number of affected Americans is estimated because, in most cases, high blood pressure is a symptomless condition. Too often, people discover they have hypertension only after they have suffered a stroke or heart attack. If hypertension is detected before such life-threatening events, they can often be prevented.

If your doctor takes your blood pressure once and it is high, that does not mean you have hypertension. You need to have your pressure checked several times, over a period of weeks or months, before a diagnosis of high blood pressure can be made. That diagnosis is made by looking at two numbers: systolic and diastolic levels.

Measuring Blood Pressure

When the blood pressure cuff is placed around your arm, the medical professional is looking for two numbers on a gauge or meter. The systolic reading, which is the larger of the two, is a measure of the force of the wave created when your heart contracts. The smaller number, or diastolic reading, is a measure of the constant force inside your arteries when your heart relaxes. Although you need to maintain a certain blood pressure to keep your blood vessels open and your blood circulating throughout your body, too high of a pressure damages the lining of your vessels.

Both systolic and diastolic levels are measured by recording the height in millimeters (mm) that a column of mercury (Hg) rises. If your blood pressure is between 120/80 mmHg and 139/89 mmHg, you have what is called *prehypertension*. This means although you don't have high blood pressure now, you could develop it in the future. A blood pressure level of 140/90 mmHg or above is considered high. About two-thirds of people older than sixty-five have high blood pressure.

About 90 percent of cases of high blood pressure are essential hypertension, which means the cause is unknown. Essential hypertension is a lifelong condition that has no cure, but it can be controlled. The other 10 percent of cases are associated with a specific medical condition, such as kidney disorders, which can cause blood pressure to rise. If the underlying condition can be treated successfully, blood pressure will likely be reduced.

Risk Factors for High Blood Pressure

Even though the specific causes of high blood pressure have not been clearly defined, experts have identified some of the risk factors. They include:

- ✦ African or Hispanic ancestry
- ✦ Older age
- ✦ Excessive intake of salt or salty foods
- ✦ Excessive intake of alcohol
- ✦ Family history of high blood pressure
- ✦ Obesity
- ✦ Sedentary lifestyle
- ✦ Use of oral contraceptives

Do two or more of these risk factors identify your life? Then it's time to roll up your sleeve and get your blood pressure checked.

Remedies

For many people, positive changes in their lifestyle can help keep their blood pressure under control. They pay attention to diet (maintaining a low-fat, low-salt, high-fiber diet high in fresh fruits and vegetables), exercise, lose weight, and stop smoking. For these people, drugs and their accompanying side effects are not needed. Others achieve some control with lifestyle changes, but need a little help from medications. Here are some specific lifestyle remedies, including nutritional supplements, that may help you steer clear of high-blood-pressure medications.

Best Bets

♦ Potassium-rich foods can lower your body's level of sodium, or salt. Include four to five servings of these foods daily. Potassium-rich foods include bananas, oranges, avocados, raisins, papayas, honeydew mellons, dates, apricots, Swiss chard, celery, spinach, endive, broccoli, tomato juice, cucumbers, asparagus, potatoes, and winter squash. Before you embark on this approach, however, check with your doctor to make sure you don't have kidney disease. High intake of potassium can be harmful if you do.

♦ Garlic—either fresh, cooked, or in supplement form—can help lower blood pressure. Two or three cloves of raw or cooked garlic, added to your favorite dishes, is sufficient. If this is too much for you, or if you want to eat garlic only occasionally, find a garlic supplement (now available in odor-free varieties) that provides you with the equivalent of 4,000 mg of fresh garlic daily.

♦ Coenzyme Q_{10} deficiency has been found in more than a third of people who have high blood pressure. That finding led experts to investigate a possible connection between the substance and blood pressure. The result of their research: coenzyme Q_{10} lowers blood pressure, but it takes about four to twelve weeks of therapy to see results. Suggested dosing is 50 mg two to three times daily if you have moderate to severe hypertension (minimum of 140 systolic and 105 diastolic).

Other Options

♦ The mineral magnesium relaxes blood vessels, which in turn helps lower blood pressure. A total of 500–1,000 mg daily of magnesium gluconate, taken in two to three divided doses, is suggested. If you have heart problems, talk with your doctor before taking this supplement, as it can cause problems.

♦ Sometimes referred to as the heart herb, hawthorn is good for both your heart and your blood vessels. One 250 mg capsule of a standardized extract of the herb, taken daily, relaxes your arteries and can help get your blood pressure under control. Keep taking the herb until you reach your goal, then you can stop.

When to See a Doctor

Because high blood pressure is symptomless, you should have your blood pressure checked regularly, either at your doctor's office, a clinic, or by qualified professionals at a health fair. If you show a pattern of high blood pressure, see your doctor about a treatment plan. Also, if you have two or more of the risk factors for high blood pressure, a visit to your doctor is recommended.

HIGH CHOLESTEROL

Every day, your body synthesizes up to 1,500 mg of cholesterol, or roughly the equivalent found in ten eggs. Wait, you say. You mean to say that even if I never eat another egg or another steak or another piece of cheese, that my body will continue to manufacture large amounts of cholesterol? Why does it do that?

Cholesterol: Misunderstood

Cholesterol has been given a bad rap over the years, when, in reality, it performs some very essential functions in the body. For example, it plays a role in membrane structure, and it is a precursor for the synthesis of bile acids and steroid hormones, substances that are critical for our health.

It is true that a high level of low-density lipoprotein (LDL) cholesterol, the "bad" cholesterol, is a risk factor for heart attack and stroke. It is not, however, the only risk factor. In fact, more than 50 percent of people who have a heart attack have cholesterol levels in the normal range. This information is not a license for you to forget about your intake of dietary cholesterol, but it does highlight the fact that many factors are involved in maintaining your health. (See "High, Low, Total Cholesterol: What Does It Mean?" on page 274.)

Remedies

Winning the war against high cholesterol involves bringing down high levels of LDL cholesterol and raising levels of high-density lipoprotein (HDL) cholesterol. If it sounds like a balancing act, it is. Fortunately, there are some effective natural approaches you can use to achieve that balance.

Best Bets

◆ Antioxidants can help prevent the damaging oxidation process initiated by LDL cholesterol. The antioxidants that work well together to prevent this process are vitamin C, vitamin E, and glutathione. And here's how to take them: 1,000–4,000 mg daily of vitamin C in divided doses; 800 IU natural vitamin E that contains mixed tocopherols (alpha-, beta-, and gamma-tocopherol); and 3,000 mg n-acetylcysteine (NAC), a form of amino acid that allows your body to create glutathione. NAC is recommended because the body does not adequately absorb most glutathione supplements.

♦ The mineral selenium carries a powerful punch against high cholesterol. Not only does it help reduce LDL and boost levels of HDL, it also raises the body's glutathione levels. The suggested daily dose of selenium is 200 mcg, which can be found in many high-quality multivitamin and mineral supplements.

HIGH, LOW, TOTAL CHOLESTEROL: WHAT DOES IT MEAN?

If you've ever had your cholesterol level checked, you may have been wondering about all the different readings you were given. Here's a brief overview of what the terms and figures mean.

Low-density lipoprotein (LDL) cholesterol is the "bad" cholesterol because it increases the risk of heart disease. It is manufactured and secreted by the liver, and then enters the bloodstream and travels through the arteries to the heart. Once it reaches the heart, it can be oxidized, which means it causes inflammation. The immune system then responds to eliminate the inflammation. Unfortunately, the anti-inflammatory process causes damage to the arteries, which in turn allows plaque to build up in the arteries. One way to fight the oxidation process is with antioxidants (see "Remedies"). Desirable levels of LDL are 60–130 mg/dL (milligrams per deciliter of blood).

High-density lipoprotein (HDL) cholesterol helps remove the LDL from your arteries and bring it back to the liver, where it can be processed. Naturally, higher levels of HDL are necessary to perform this function. Desirable levels of HDL are 40–70 mg/dL or higher.

Very-low-density lipoproteins (VLDL) is like LDL, because it carries cholesterol to your heart and thus raises your risk of heart disease. Desirable levels are less than 30 mg/dL.

Total cholesterol is the sum of the three types of cholesterol. Desirable levels are less than 200 mg/dL.

♦ Don't let the name inositol hexanicotinate scare you; it's just a form of niacin that doesn't cause the itchy, tingling hot flashes that are associated with other forms of the nutrient. The other good news is that inositol hexanicotinate brings down LDL levels and raises HDL levels. It's also less expensive than prescription cholesterol-lowering drugs. The suggested starting dose is 500 mg, increasing the dose by 500 mg per week until you reach 1,500 mg daily. The only caveat is that in high doses, niacin may cause liver problems. Although 1,500 mg daily is safe for most people, you should consult with your doctor before taking inositol hexanicotinate.

EAT YOUR WAY TO LOWER CHOLESTEROL

Here's the scoop on cholesterol: your liver manufacturers all the cholesterol your body needs. So whenever you eat foods that contain cholesterol, you're at risk of getting too much. Modification of your eating habits can help keep your cholesterol levels in a healthy range. Foods that are high in fiber, such as whole grains, seeds, nuts, beans, vegetable, and fruits, help remove cholesterol from the body. For example, oat bran contains high amounts of soluble fiber, a substance that attaches to cholesterol in the intestinal tract and helps eliminate it from the body. The best source is cooked oat bran cereal: a mere $3/4$ cup daily can reduce your cholesterol by up to 10 percent. If you prefer oat bran muffins, you can enjoy them as well.

Not only are grains, nuts, seeds, fruits, vegetables, and beans high in fiber; they also contain zero cholesterol. The same cannot be said for foods like butter, beef, lamb, pork, chicken, eggs, and ice cream, which contain high levels of cholesterol and no fiber.

Other Options

♦ Red yeast rice is another supplement proven to lower total and LDL cholesterol levels and to raise HDL levels. The suggested daily dose is two 600 mg tablets; you can take one in the morning and one at night. Along with red yeast rice you should also take the powerful antioxidant coenzyme Q_{10}; take two 50 mg tablets daily. The coenzyme Q_{10} is needed because the red yeast rice lowers the level of this antioxidant.

♦ An Ayurvedic remedy called guggul, derived from the Indian mukul myrrh tree, contains an ingredient called guggulsterone, which stimulates the liver to metabolize LDL cholesterol and thus reduces cholesterol levels. Take 500 mg three times daily of guggul that contains 25 mg of guggulsterone per pill.

When to See a Doctor

High cholesterol is a life-threatening condition, yet it is without symptoms—that is, until you're rushed to the hospital with a stroke or heart attack. If you don't know what your cholesterol levels are, the time to see a doctor is now. If your total cholesterol is 200 mg/dL or higher, it's also time to work on bringing it down.

HYPOGLYCEMIA

In 1978, San Francisco Supervisor Dan White shot and killed San Francisco Mayor George Moscone and Supervisor Harvey Milk. White's defense attorney, Dr. Martin Blinder, got his client convicted of manslaughter rather than murder partly because of his "Twinkie" defense. Basically, Blinder testified that White's diet of Twinkies and soda contributed to his erratic behavior.

This defense could also be called the "hypoglycemia" defense. Hypoglycemia, a condition in which an individual has an abnormally low level of sugar in the blood, is characterized by irrational behavior, irritability, confusion, mental disturbances, and nervous habits. Apparently, on the day Moscone and Milk were murdered, White hadn't had his Twinkie and soda fix.

Hypoglycemia Explained

The amount of glucose (sugar) in your bloodstream is controlled by several mechanisms. The hormones insulin and glucagon, which are produced by the pancreas, are key players in this control. Less influential hormones include cortisol, growth hormone, and catecholamines (epinephrine and norepinephrine).

When you eat, your blood sugar levels rise, prompting release of insulin by the pancreas. The insulin helps sugar enter cells, which in turn reduces the level of sugar in the bloodstream. If the level of sugar in the blood drops too low, the pancreas releases glucagon. This hormone triggers the liver to release stored supplies of glycogen, which is changed back into glucose, which in turn raises blood sugar levels again.

Hypoglycemia can be an early sign of a problem with insulin secretion (dysinsulinemia) or diabetes. In fact, hypoglycemia most often occurs as a complication of diabetes, a condition in which people either don't produce insulin (type I diabetes) or their bodies do not properly process or utilize the insulin they produce (type II diabetes). Low blood sugar levels occur in diabetics for various reasons, including taking too much medication, consuming too little food compared with the amount of medication taken, overexercise, drinking too much alcohol, missing a meal, emotional stress, or a combination of these factors.

Although it occurs far less often, people who do not have diabetes can experience hypoglycemia. Chronic alcohol consumption, binge drinking, early pregnancy, prolonged fasting, prolonged strenuous exercise (for example, marathon running), and use of beta-blocker drugs may induce hypoglycemia in some people.

How to Prevent Hypoglycemia

If you have diabetes, you can reduce or prevent bouts of hypoglycemia if you learn to recognize the symptoms of an oncoming attack and any circumstances that may trigger it. You also need to monitor your blood sugar levels often to head off an incident.

Most people who have diabetes are aware when symptoms of hypoglycemia occur, and they can take preventive measures, such as eating a piece of candy or fruit to get sugar into their system quickly. Occasionally, however, individuals who have had diabetes for many years develop what is called "hypoglycemia unawareness," which means they have difficulty recognizing the symptoms of low blood sugar. On rare occasions, people with type I diabetes may lose consciousness when hypoglycemia occurs. For these individuals, when hypoglycemia sets in, it may be necessary for another person to give them an injection of the hormone glucagon. That's why it's important for family and coworkers to know how to recognize hypoglycemic symptoms and how to treat them if they occur and individuals are unable to treat themselves.

Remedies

Natural remedies are geared toward keeping your blood sugar levels in balance and strengthening your pancreas. Especially if you have diabetes, you need to talk to your doctor before taking any supplements or changing your eating plan.

Best Bets

◆ Center your diet around foods that are natural, low in fat, and high in fiber. These include whole grains, fresh fruits and vegetables, legumes, seeds, nuts, and fish. Generally, these foods are more slowly digested, which prevents the sudden spikes and valleys of energy associated with simple carbohydrates, such as sugars and white flour.

◆ A well-rounded vitamin and mineral program can help normalize your blood sugar levels. Look for a high-potency multivitamin and mineral supplement that contains at least 400 mg magnesium, 100 mcg selenium, 20 mg zinc, 500 mg vitamin C, 200 mcg chromium, and 400 IU vitamin E. Because no multivitamin and mineral supplement could possibly contain all the nutrients you need in the optimal amounts, you will need to take some individual supplements as well. They include: 1,000 mg vitamin C, 1,000 mg bioflavonoids, 400 IU vitamin E, 200 mcg chromium, 100–200 mg coenzyme Q_{10}, and 250–500 mg milk thistle extract standardized to contain 70 to 80 percent silymarin.

◆ According to traditional Chinese medicine, *chi* is the energy flow that circulates throughout the entire body along paths called meridians. If you apply pressure to certain points on the body, the flow of chi can be balanced and redirected to organs that require healing. When it comes to hypoglycemia, the pancreas and spleen are the organs in need of healing power. The following points can be treated if you want to restore energy to your pancreas and spleen. (See Chapter 2 for an acupressure point chart and an explanation of how to do acupressure on yourself.) Treat each of the following points for two minutes at each session.

  • ST36—four finger widths below the lower edge of the kneecap, located in the indentation at the front of the shinbone

  • BL20—located two finger widths from the spine, midway between the waist and the middle of the shoulder blades (You may need a partner to treat this point.)

  • CV6—located two finger widths below the navel

  • SP4—located on the inside of the foot at the beginning of the arch, behind the bone of the big toe

Other Options

◆ Chinese or Korean ginseng may help the liver convert glycogen to sugar. (American and Siberian ginseng do not have this quality.) It also promotes energy in the pancreas and spleen, which makes it a good complement to acupressure. Take it according to package directions. Allow at least two to four weeks to see results. Consult your doctor before taking ginseng if you have high blood pressure.

♦ Another herb that acts similarly to ginseng but works more slowly is *Codonopsis pilosula*. It is also known as bellflower or dang shen. The suggested dose is five 300 mg capsules three times daily. One major advantage of codonopsis is that it is much less expensive than Chinese or Korean ginseng.

When to See a Doctor

If you have diabetes, you need to see your doctor regularly as recommended. Also contact your doctor if you are experiencing frequent episodes of hypoglycemia, you are having difficulty regulating your blood sugar levels, or you develop new symptoms.

HYPOTHYROIDISM

"I kept telling my doctor that I was always tired, my hands and feet were cold even during the summer, and that I was depressed and constipated," said Cynthia, a forty-six-year-old marketing analyst. "I asked him if it could be a thyroid problem, so he took a blood test and said I was fine. But I knew better. I certainly didn't *feel* fine."

What Cynthia's doctor, and many others do, is rely on conventional blood tests to rule out thyroid problems, such as the type affecting Cynthia. She eventually went to another doctor, who ran the necessary battery of tests to uncover thyroid problems. What he found was hypothyroidism—an underactive, sluggish thyroid gland, which was making Cynthia feel fatigued, moody, bloated, and sore, among other complaints. Detecting this condition requires a range of medical tests that detect levels of specific substances, a detection process that is more sensitive than conventional blood tests.

Here's how hypothyroidism works: The thyroid gland secretes hormones that, among other things, regulate your body temperature. If the level of the hormones is low, then your body temperature is abnormally low. A lower-than-normal body temperature causes many of the body's functions to perform less than optimally.

That's why Cynthia, along with millions of other people with hypothyroidism, experience a wide range of symptoms. In addition to the ones already mentioned, hypothyroidism is characterized by confusion, slow heart rate, aching muscles, weight gain, dry skin, coarse hair and hair loss, puffy face, hoarseness, decreased sexual drive, apathy, and changes in the menstrual period in women who are still menstruating.

More Reasons Why Hypothyroidism Is Not Diagnosed

Many people who have hypothyroidism are misdiagnosed or undiagnosed because the symptoms can easily be mistaken for other conditions. Some doctors, especially when blood tests come back normal, declare their patients are depressed and prescribe antidepressants. Others tell patients their symptoms are a normal part of aging, that they are experiencing symptoms of perimenopause or premenstrual syndrome, or that they are overworked.

If you suspect you have a thyroid problem, find a doctor who is willing to go beyond conventional blood tests in the search for the truth. In the meantime, you can also conduct your own at-home test. Although not foolproof, if you have the symptoms we've already described and the results of the at-home test are positive, then chances are good that you have an underactive thyroid gland (see "Your At-Home Test for Hypothyroidism" below).

Remedies

Hypothyroidism requires professional care, but there are remedies you can take that will facilitate your healing. Find a doctor who is willing to work along with you in applying the complementary remedies you wish to include in your treatment plan. Complementary approaches often can reduce the dosage of medication you will need.

YOUR AT-HOME TEST FOR HYPOTHYROIDISM

All you need for this simple test is a glass mercury thermometer. Before you go to sleep, shake down the thermometer and place it within easy reach of your bed, like on a nightstand. When you wake up in the morning, reach over, pick up the thermometer, and tuck it under your armpit for ten minutes. Do not make any other movements either before placing the thermometer or once it is in place. After ten minutes, take the reading and note it on a piece of paper. Repeat this process every morning for five to six days. If your temperature is consistently in the low 97 or 96 degrees Fahrenheit range, this is a good indication that your thyroid is underactive. Take this information to a knowledgeable physician.

Best Bets

◆ One of the thyroid hormones, thyroxine, is produced in the body when the amino acid tyrosine and iodine combine. A tyrosine supplement, 500–1,000 mg daily, along with a balanced diet, can help keep your thyroid in balance. Take the supplement for three months and then be reevaluated by your doctor.

◆ Among other things, thyroid hormones are composed of fatty acids. Thus, daily supplementation with either flaxseed oil or fish oil can help maintain thyroid health. The suggested daily intake is 3,000–6,000 mg. Flaxseed oil has the added advantage of being a wonderful ingredient to add to salad dressing. To get the amount of flaxseed oil you need, add 2–3 tablespoons of the oil to your favorite salad dressing, or drizzle the oil over vegetables, potatoes, pasta, or bread.

◆ Many of the foods Americans eat contain synthetic hormones, which can have a significant effect on the functioning and balance of the thyroid gland. The foods that typically contain these hormones are meat, eggs, and dairy products. If you continue to eat these foods, choose organic products.

Other Options

◆ We know that exposure to the sun is necessary for the body to manufacture vitamin D, but did you know that sunlight also stimulates the pineal gland? Stimulation of this gland, which lies in the center of the brain, in turn positively affects the thyroid gland. Early morning sunlight (within one hour of sunrise) is the most beneficial. Don't look directly at the sun, but gaze toward it to allow the sunlight to enter your eyes and thus reach the pineal gland.

◆ Several vitamins and minerals are involved in the manufacture of thyroid hormones, including zinc, vitamins A, C, and E, and the B vitamins riboflavin (B_2), niacin (B_3), and pyridoxine (B_6). A high-potency multivitamin and mineral supplement can help your thyroid function properly.

When to See a Doctor

If you have the symptoms discussed in this chapter and/or you tested positive on the at-home test, contact your doctor. Tell him or her if anyone in your family has had a thyroid problem.

KIDNEY STONES

"It's a pain you'll never forget, and one you don't want to repeat," said Glenda, a thirty-nine-year-old middle-school teacher in Chicago. "Giving birth is a piece of cake compared with passing a kidney stone."

That doesn't mean that every kidney stone, when it passes out of the body, causes excruciating pain. Most stones are so tiny—like grains of sand—they exit the body without you ever knowing they were there. Others let their presence be known but can be "delivered" with the help of natural remedies. Occasionally, stones must be removed surgically, as they can grow to the size of a golf ball.

Kidney Stones Defined

A kidney stone is a hard mass composed of crystals that have separated from urine and have accumulated on the inside of the kidney. Although urine contains substances that prevent the formation of crystals, these chemicals fail to do their job in some people, and stones form.

Not all kidney stones are alike. The most common type contains calcium along with phosphate or oxalate, all chemicals that are found in a normal diet. A less common type is called a struvite, or infection stone, because it is caused by an infection in the urinary tract. Even less common are stones composed of uric acid or cystine. It's important to know the type of stone you have because preventive treatment can be tailored to it. Your doctor can make this determination for you (see "Know Thy Stones" below).

KNOW THY STONES

If you have passed a kidney stone, you should take it to your doctor to have it analyzed. To capture your stone, urinate into a strainer once your pain has subsided. If you're unable to get a specimen, take a urine sample to your doctor for analysis to see whether it contains traces of crystals.

Risk Factors for Kidney Stones

For reasons unknown, more and more people in the United States are developing kidney stones. More than 1 million cases of kidney stones are diagnosed in the United States each year. Whites are more likely to get stones than blacks, and men are more likely to develop stones than women. Most kidney stones are diagnosed in people between the ages of twenty and forty. Once you develop more than one stone, you're very likely to develop more.

Exactly why kidney stones form is unknown. Some experts believe that certain foods, such as those high in fat and low in fiber, promote the formation of stones in people who are susceptible, yet they don't believe those same foods cause stones to form in people who are not susceptible. You may be more likely to develop kidney stones if you have a family history of the disease, or if you have cystic kidney disease, a rare hereditary disease called renal tubular acidosis, urinary tract infections, or a metabolic condition such as hyperparathyroidism.

Remedies

The following suggestions are not as much remedies as they are preventive measures. If you have had a kidney stone, you'll need little incentive beyond the memory of the pain to convince you that prevention *is* the best medicine.

Best Bets

◆ Drink lots of water. An insufficient amount of fluid intake is a major contributor to the formation of crystals in the urine. Drink six to eight 8-ounce glasses of purified water daily.

◆ The traditional American diet (high-fat, low-fiber, lots of red meat and dairy products) contributes to the formation of calcium oxalate crystals in the urine. Thus, the opposite dietary approach—low-fat, high-fiber, and little or no red meat—helps prevent kidney stones. Although leafy green vegetables are usually highly recommended, there are a few you should avoid because they are high in oxalates, acids that the body cannot process properly. Thus, if you have had calcium stones, avoid spinach, beet greens, and Swiss chard.

◆ Believe it or not, to help prevent calcium stones from forming, you should take calcium supplements. Calcium binds to the oxalate in your body, which helps prevent stone formation. Take 600 mg daily. Along with the calcium also take 300 mg of magnesium and 400 IU of vitamin D, both of which help your body absorb calcium. For added protection, add 100 mg of vitamin B_6, which reduces the production of oxalates.

Other Options

◆ If your problem is uric acid stones, help prevent them by drinking two to three glasses of orange, grapefruit, or tomato juice every day. These beverages keep the chemistry, or pH, of your urine in balance.

♦ People who have uric acid stones should avoid substances called purines, which are found in certain foods. Those foods include anchovies, liver, kidney, sweetbreads, meat extracts, gravies, and fried foods. Also limit your consumption of any one of the following foods to no more than one serving daily: asparagus, cauliflower, crabs, tuna, ham, lima beans, mushrooms, peas, spinach, oatmeal, oysters, or 3 ounces of lean meat.

♦ If you are passing a kidney stone and are looking for some natural pain relief, try one of the following. (You may need some help with the first one.)

1. Heat some water in a large pot and soak a washcloth in the water. Remove the washcloth and wring it out so that it's wet but not dripping. Place the hot washcloth on your lower back over the painful area and cover the cloth with a piece of plastic, and then a dry towel. Keep the hot towel on your back for five to ten minutes, then replace it with another one. Repeat this cycle for forty-five minutes.

2. Take the herb corn silk. This herb reduces the friction caused by the stone as it moves through the urinary tract. Corn silk is available in capsules and liquid. Take according to package directions.

When to See a Doctor

You should call your doctor if you begin to experience the symptoms of a kidney stone attack, especially if you are unable to relieve the pain using one of the above methods or by drinking lots of water. Also contact your doctor if you have blood in your urine, you have difficulty urinating, or you develop a fever.

OSTEOPOROSIS

Candace hopes other women don't find out about osteoporosis the hard way, like she did. At fifty-three years of age, she got her diagnosis literally by accident. "I was getting out of my car and I tripped over the curb," she says. "I instinctively tried to brace myself by putting out my hand, and I broke my wrist. I wasn't too concerned until my doctor told me that the bone density test they ran showed I had osteoporosis."

Osteoporosis, which means "porous bones," is a disease characterized by loss of bone density or mass. An estimated 44 million Americans have the disease or are at risk: 10 million have been diagnosed with osteoporosis (8 million of them are women), and the remaining 34 million have low bone mass, which places them at an increased risk for the disease. And when it comes to broken bones,

Candace is not alone: osteoporosis is responsible for approximately 1.5 million fractures per year.

Until people reach their mid-thirties, their bones are either building up bone density (about 98 percent of bone density is achieved by age twenty) or staying stable. Then begins a decline in bone density, a loss that can be accelerated by many factors.

Risk Factors for Osteoporosis

Despite what many people think, osteoporosis is *not* an inevitable part of aging. Bone loss is a natural part of the aging process, but that doesn't mean you can't do anything to significantly slow that loss, enough so that your bones stay healthy. That said, there are some risk factors for the disease you should know about, so you'll know which ones you can change, and which ones you can't.

- *Sex.* Eighty percent of people who get osteoporosis are women. One reason for this high percentage is that women lose most of their estrogen during menopause, and estrogen is essential for maintaining bone health.

- *Age.* As we age, our ability to absorb and use calcium and other nutrients necessary for bone health declines. Also, the longer women live, the longer their bodies have low levels of estrogen and calcium.

- *Menopause.* Menopause increases the risk of developing osteoporosis as it causes a dramatic decline in estrogen levels. Women experiencing early menopause (before age forty-five) should be particularly aware of this risk factor.

- *Calcium and vitamin D deficiency.* Although there are many important nutrients required for bone health, calcium and vitamin D are regarded as the most essential. Calcium makes up a major portion of bone structure, and vitamin D is needed by calcium in order to be absorbed adequately. Unfortunately, many women are deficient in one or both of these critical vitamins: they don't consume enough in their diet, nor do they supplement enough to make up the difference. Premenopausal women need 1,000 mg of calcium daily, while postmenopausal women need 1,500 mg. All women need at least 400 IU of vitamin D daily.

- *Exercise.* Weight-bearing exercise, such as walking, jogging, dancing, skiing, and tennis, helps maintain bone mass.

- *Personal and family history.* You're at an increased risk of osteoporosis if you've had a fracture earlier in your lifetime, or if your mother had the disease or vertebral (spinal) fractures.

◆ *Use of medication.* Medications that are often taken by women, including those for thyroid, gastrointestinal, and arthritic conditions, can contribute to bone loss. Women should talk to their doctors about any drugs they are taking and, if they have bone loss as a side effect, discuss other drug options.

◆ *Caffeine.* The caffeine in coffee, tea, colas, chocolate, and some medications may cause you to lose calcium through your urine. While some studies have shown caffeine to have a negative effect, a few other studies have not. This is still an area of controversy.

◆ *High-protein diets.* Eating too much protein (the average adult needs 0.38 grams per pound of body weight; thus a 125-pound women needs 48 grams daily) can actually increase your requirement of calcium to maintain adequate bone density.

◆ *Smoking.* Smoking affects the production of bone cells and also interferes with bone healing.

◆ *Excess alcohol.* Alcohol consumption interferes with the absorption and use of calcium.

Screening for Bone Loss

A broken bone is often the first symptom of osteoporosis; others include severe back pain; a stooped, round-shouldered posture; and loss of height. But there's no reason to wait and see if you develop symptoms. You can undergo a painless and quick screening procedure for osteoporosis and, if you show signs of significant bone loss, you can then take aggressive steps to protect your bone health.

One of the screening procedures is a heel ultrasound, an inexpensive procedure that scans the heel. This approach is generally suggested for younger women who have not yet gone through menopause, unless they have a prior history of fracture or family history of the disease. Heel ultrasound is less accurate than a DEXA (dual-energy x-ray absorptiometry) scan, an ultrasound of the spine and hip areas, which are the areas most susceptible to fracture and bone loss. All women of menopause age and older are encouraged to get a DEXA-scan every two years.

Remedies

The good news about osteoporosis is that it can be prevented. If you already have osteoporosis, there are steps you can take to minimize your bone loss.

TABLE 11.1. DIETARY SOURCES OF CALCIUM

Food		Serving Size	Calcium (mg)
Beverages	Orange juice (fortified)	1 cup	300
	Grapefruit juice (fortified)	1 cup	280
	Cow's milk (whole)	1 cup	290
	Soymilk (fortified)	1 cup	160
	Rice milk (fortified)	1 cup	240
Dairy Foods	Cottage cheese (low-fat)	1 cup	150
	Yogurt, plain (low- or nonfat)	1 cup	480
	Yogurt, flavored (low- or nonfat)	1 cup	330
	American cheese	1 oz	195
	Cheddar cheese	1 oz	200
	Swiss cheese	1 oz	250
Soy	Tofu (processed with calcium sulfate or calcium chloride; firm has more calcium than soft)	4 oz	400
	Tempeh	4 oz	170
	Soybeans (cooked)	1 cup	200
	Soy nuts (dry roasted soybeans)	$\frac{1}{2}$ cup	185
Vegetables (cooked)	Bok choy or turnip greens	1 cup	230
	Collard greens	1 cup	350
	Kale	1 cup	180
	Broccoli	1 cup	160
Beans, Grains, and Legumes (cooked)	Amaranth	1 cup	275
	Black beans	1 cup	135
	Black-eyed peas	1 cup	210
	Lima or white beans	1 cup	160
	Navy beans	1 cup	120
	Pinto beans	1 cup	130
Nuts and Seeds	Almonds (shelled)	$\frac{1}{2}$ cup	190
	Brazil nuts (shelled)	$\frac{1}{2}$ cup	130
	Walnuts	$\frac{1}{2}$ cup	140
	Sesame seeds	1 oz	280

Best Bets

- Calcium, calcium, calcium. You know how much you need, now where will you get it? See Table 11.1 for ideas. And because you may not get all you need from your food, take a supplement to make up the difference. Calcium carbonate and citrate are the two most common supplements. Calcium carbonate should be taken with meals; citrate can be taken with or without food.

- Get your vitamin D. Ten to fifteen minutes of sun exposure per day on your face (without sunscreen) is enough for your body to produce the vitamin D it needs. Food sources include fatty saltwater fish such as halibut, tuna, and herring, and low-fat dairy foods. If you take a supplement, look for 400 IU daily. Some calcium supplements contain vitamin D as well.

- Bone up on minerals. Along with calcium and vitamin D, bones also need other nutrients, including magnesium (400–500 mg; helps move calcium into the bones), boron (3 mg; helps convert estrogen and vitamin D to their active forms and thus helps maintain bone health), manganese (6 mg; helps bones absorb calcium); and vitamin K (80 mcg; helps hold calcium in the bones). Because vitamin K thins the blood, check with your doctor before taking this supplement.

Other Options

- Move it! Although exercise is especially critical during the bone-building years, regular weight-bearing exercise later in life can help slow the rate of bone loss. What is the best exercise? Walking, because it's easy to do, doesn't cost anything except the price of a good pair of shoes, and can be done just about anywhere.

- Manage stress. When you're under a lot of stress, your levels of cortisol, epinephrine, and other hormones rise, which can deplete the body of magnesium and other minerals that are necessary for bone health. A daily routine of yoga, meditation, deep breathing, tai chi, visualization, or other relaxation techniques can help keep your stress levels down.

When to See a Doctor

If you have symptoms such as hip or back pain or loss of height, see your doctor immediately. But don't wait until it's too late! Women are encouraged to get an ultrasound screening for bone density premenopause if they have risk factors for osteoporosis, and at menopause if they do not (see "Screening for Bone Loss" on page 286).

Resources and Further Reading

ORGANIZATIONS

American Association of Oriental Medicine
P.O. Box 162340
Sacramento, CA 95816
866-455-7999 (toll-free)
www.aaom.org

American Botanical Council
6200 Manor Road
Austin, TX 78714-4345
512-926-4900
www.herbalgram.org

American College for Advancement in Medicine
24411 Ridge Route, Suite 115
Laguna Hills, CA 92653
949-309-3520
800-532-3688 (toll-free)
www.acam.org

American Herbalists Guild
141 Nob Hill Road
Cheshire, CT 06410
203-272-6731
www.americanherbalistsguild.com

American Holistic Health Association
P.O. Box 17400
Anaheim, CA 92817-7400
714-779-6152
www.ahha.org

American Holistic Medical Association
P.O. Box 2016
Edmonds, WA 98020
425-967-0737
www.holisticmedicine.org

American Naturopathic Medical Association
P.O. Box 96273
Las Vegas, NV 89193
702-897-7053
www.anma.org

Association for Integrative Medicine
Box 1
Mont Clare, PA 19453
610-933-8145
www.integrativemedicine.org

The Center for Mind-Body Medicine
5225 Connecticut Avenue, NW,
  Suite 414
Washington, D.C. 20015
202-966-7338
www.cmbm.org

**Complementary and Alternative
  Medicine Program at Stanford**
Stanford University School of
  Medicine
Stanford Prevention Research Center
Hoover Pavilion
211 Quarry Road, N229
Stanford, CA 94305-5705
650-723-8628
http://camps.stanford.edu/

**Foundation for the Advancement
  of Innovative Medicine**
2 Executive Boulevard, Suite 206
Suffern, NY 10901
877-634-3246
www.faim.org

Herb Research Foundation
4140 15th Street
Boulder, CO 80304
303-449-2265
www.herbs.org

**The Institute for Functional
  Medicine**
4411 Pt. Fosdick Drive, NW,
  Suite 305
P.O. Box 1697
Gig Harbor, WA 98335
800-228-0622 (toll-free)
www.functionalmedicine.org

**National Center for
  Homeopathy**
801 North Fairfax Street,
  Suite 306
Alexandria, VA 22314
703-548-7790
www.homeopathic.org

**The National Health Association
  (formerly American Natural
  Hygiene Society)**
P.O. Box 30630
Tampa, FL 33630
813-855-6607
www.anhs.org

**The National Institute of
  Ayurvedic Medicine**
584 Milltown Road
Brewster, NY 10509
845-278-8700
http://niam.com

**North American Society of
  Homeopaths**
P.O. Box 450039
Sunrise, FL 33345-0039
206-720-7000
www.homeopathy.org

**Physicians Committee for
  Responsible Medicine**
5100 Wisconsin Avenue, NW,
  Suite 400
Washington, D.C. 20016-4131
202-686-2210
www.pcrm.org

**The Richard and Hinda Rosenthal Center for
  Complementary and Alternative Medicine**
Columbia University, College of Physicians
  and Surgeons
630 W. 168th Street, Box 75
New York, NY 10032
212-342-0101
www.rosenthal.hs.columbia.edu

FURTHER READING

Books

Adderly, Brenda D. *The Complete Guide to Nutritional Supplements.* Los Angeles: New Star, 1998.

Craig, Selene, and editors of *Prevention. The Complete Book of Alternative Nutrition.* New York: Berkley Books, 1997.

Duke, James A. *The Green Pharmacy.* Emmaus, PA: Rodale Press, 1997.

Gach, Michael Reed. *Acupressure's Potent Points: A Guide to Self-Care for Common Ailments.* New York: Bantam Books, 1990.

Gillanders, Ann. *The Family Guide to Reflexology.* Boston: Little, Brown, 1998.

Graedon, Joe, and Teresa Graedon. *The People's Pharmacy Guide to Home and Herbal Remedies.* New York: St. Martin's 1999.

———. *Dangerous Drug Interactions: How to Protect Yourself from Harmful Drug/Drug, Drug/Food, and Drug/Vitamin Combinations.* New York: St. Martin's Press, 1999.

Hayfield, Robin. *Homeopathy for Common Ailments.* Berkeley, CA: Frog, 1993.

Lockie, Andrew, and Nicola Giddes. *Homeopathy: The Principles and Practice of Treatment.* London and New York: Dorling Kindersley Ltd., 1995.

Mindell, Earl. *Earl Mindell's New Herb Bible.* New York: Simon & Schuster, 2000.

North American Vegetarian Society. *The Vegetarian Voice.* Magazine, available through the North American Vegetarian Society, P.O. Box 72, Dodgerville, NY 13329; 518-568-7970.

Null, Gary, and Barbara Seaman. *For Women Only!* New York: Seven Stories Press, 1999.

Peirce, Andrea. *The American Pharmaceutical Association Practical Guide to Natural Medicine.* New York: William Morrow, 1999.

Weil, Andrew. *Natural Health, Natural Medicine.* Boston: Houghton Mifflin, 1995.

Weil, Andrew. *Spontaneous Healing: How to Discover and Enhance Your Body's Natural Ability to Maintain and Heal Itself.* New York: Knopf, 1995.

Online Reading

Dr. Andrew Weil's Self-Healing Newsletter
www.drweilselfhealing.com

Good Medicine, magazine of the Physician's Committee for Responsible Medicine
www.pcrm.org

Let's Live Magazine
www.letsliveonline.com

Life Extension Magazine
www.lef.org

McDougall Newsletter
www.drmcdougall.com

Natural Health
www.naturalhealthmag.com

Center for Science in the Public Interest
www.cspinet.org/nah

Index

Abreva, 48

Abscesses, 157–159

Accutane (isotretinoin), 215

ACE inhibitors, 104

Acetaminophen, 33, 34, 35, 80

Aches, 76–102

Acid reflux, 143

Acidophilus, 119, 123, 126, 131, 134, 138, 155, 158, 191, 209

Acne, 213–216, 234

Acrochordons. *See* Skin tags.

Acupressure, 21, 28, 78, 80–81, 99, 152, 251, 278
    point charts, 28, 29

Acupuncture, 21, 28, 80, 100

Addiction, 187, 211

Adrenal glands, 242

Adrenaline, 15

Aerophagia, 128

Aging, 40, 45, 67, 85, 89, 103, 138, 184, 196–197, 271, 285

Air and air pollution, 11–13

Air purifiers, 247

Alcohol, 6, 9–10, 41, 55, 67, 93, 105, 115, 118, 121, 122, 128, 142, 144, 148, 155, 200, 204, 268, 270, 286

Alcoholics Anonymous, 10, 202

Allergies and food sensitivities, 45, 58, 82, 92, 150, 168, 171–173, 173, 176, 239, 240, 246, 248, 249

Allium cepa, 248

Aloe vera, 36, 95, 126, 145, 155, 161, 177, 179, 220

Alopecia areata, 63

Alpha-lipoic acid (ALA), 46

Alprostadil, 106

Aluminum, 218

Alzheimer's disease, 218

Amerge (naratriptan), 84

American Academy of Allergy, Asthma, and Immunology (AAAAI), 240

American Hair Loss Council, 63

American Psychiatric Association, 187

American Tinnitus Association, 70

Amino acids, 199

Amoxil (amoxicillin), 133

Amputations, 258

Amylase, 138

Anacin, 261

Androgenetic alopecia, 61, 63

Anemia, 183–186, 226

Anthocyanosides, 60

Antiacids, 33, 130, 133, 144

Antibacterials and antifungals, 33, 160

Antibiotics, 45, 50, 119, 133, 137, 148, 155, 192, 215, 250

Anticoagulants, 158, 160, 170

Antidepressants, 40, 55, 104, 130, 192, 199

Antihistamines, 33, 40, 55, 130, 170, 172, 175
Antihypertensive drugs, 34, 55, 130, 133
Antioxidants, 6, 46, 68, 85, 224, 273–274
Antipsychotics, 34, 130, 217
Anxiety and nervousness, 54, 55, 128, 199, 203, 217
Apis mellifica, 50, 175
Appendicitis, 149
Apples, 144
Arava (leflunomide), 92
Arbutin, 224
Argentum nitricum, 50
Arginine, 48, 105
Arnica, 36
Aromatherapy, 25–26
Arsenicum album, 142
Arthritis
    osteo, 84–86
    rheumatoid, 90–93
Aspartame, 268
Aspirin, 60, 80, 101, 155, 172, 175, 181, 217, 240, 249
Asthma, 239–243, 249
Astragalus, 195, 232, 245
Atarax (hydroxyzine), 170, 172
Athlete's foot, 111, 159–161
Attitude, 17–19
Auras, 82, 84
Automobile Association of America (AAA), 152

Babesiosis, 174
Back, 76–79
Bacteria, 39, 45, 73, 121–122, 123, 140, 161, 216, 234
Bacterial endocarditis, 226, 227
Baking soda, 212
Baldness, 60–64

Bananas, 181, 202
Bath oils and salts, 123, 125, 222
Baths, 90, 220, 222, 223
    cornstarch, 177
    baking soda, 170, 172
    bubble, 123, 125
    oatmeal, 170, 172, 177
    sitz, 29, 109
    steam, 215–216, 246, 251
    vinegar, 172
Beans, 137, 139, 151
Bee pollen, 248
Belching, 127–129
Bellflower. See Codonopsis pilosula.
Benadryl (diphenhydramine), 170, 172
Benign prostatic hyperplasia, 117
Benign prostatic hypertrophy (BPH).
        See Benign prostatic hyperplasia.
Benson, Herbert, 199
Benzoyl peroxide, 215
Beta-carotene, 45, 46, 194, 221, 226
Beverages
    carbonated, 55, 121, 128, 142, 148, 186, 261
    iced, 148
    sports, 134
Bicarbonate of soda, 175, 177
Bicycling, 104
Bifidobacteria, 119, 123, 138, 155, 158, 191
Bilberries, 60, 68, 237, 259–260
Bile, 263
Biofeedback, 72, 83–84, 90, 99, 199, 212, 257
Bioflavonoids, 43, 46, 70, 108, 278
Bisacodyl, 133
Black cohosh, 113, 262
Bladder, 119–120, 121
Bleach, chlorine, 125, 160
Bleaching agents, 224

Blisters, 94, 95
Blood
    type A, 154
    type O, 154
Blood pressure, 270–271
    high. *See* Hypertension.
Blood thinners, 60
Blueberries, 123
Body
    balance within, 15, 28, 31
    clock, 205, 207
    odor, 216–219, 233–235
    temperature, 279, 280
Body mass index, 232
Boils, 161–163
Bone density. *See* Bones and bone
    density.
Bones and bone density, 284–285
Bootzin, Richard, 204
Bootzin Technique, 204
Boric acid, 126
Boron, 288
Botulism, 141, 142–143
Bovista, 172
Bowel movements, 129, 130, 131
Brandy, 201
Bread, 147
Breastfeeding, 96–98, 158, 160, 192,
    199, 204
Breasts, 96–98, 115
    fibrocystic, 260–263
Breath, bad, 39–41
Breath hydrogen analysis, 208–209
Breathe Right strips, 253
Breathing, 32, 33, 147, 239–254,
    252–254
    deep, 17, 55, 62, 99, 128, 130,
        149, 150, 155, 199, 203, 207,
        288
Brewer's yeast, 185
Bromelain, 102, 138, 237

Bromocriptine, 90
Bronchitis, 242, 244–246
Bronchodilator, 241
Broth, 134
Bunions, 163–165
Burns, 219–221
Burrow's solution, 95
Bursa, 100, 101, 102, 164, 166
Bursitis, 100–102
Butcher's broom, 237

Cabbage, 151, 200, 202
Caffeine and coffee, 6, 25, 55, 73, 93,
        118, 121, 122, 142, 144, 155,
        192, 201, 204, 217, 257,
        261–262, 264, 268, 286
    withdrawal, 186–188, 204
Calamine lotion, 95, 177
Calcipotriene, 180
Calcium, 210, 226, 283, 285, 286,
        287, 288
Calcium channel blockers, 55, 104
Calendula, 126, 161, 171, 177, 220
California Dry Beans Advisory Board,
    139
Calluses, 165–167
Calories, 229
Cancer
    breast, 10
    cervical, 13, 182
    colorectal, 130
    lung, 13
    mouth and throat, 14
    prostate, 119
    skin, 14
Candida. *See* Vaginitis.
Canker sores, 43–45
Cantharis, 124
Capsaicin, 86, 95
Carbohydrates, 4–5, 115–116,
        136–137

Carbuncles, 162
Carnitine, 219
Carob, 134
Carpal tunnel syndrome, 87
Cartilage, 84, 85
Cascara sagrada, 265
Cat's claw, 158, 160
Cataracts, 14, 45–47
Catecholamines, 9
Catnip, 142
Cavities, 73
Cayenne, 256
Celecoxib, 92
Cells
  fat, 229
  red blood, 183–184
  white blood, 157
Cellulose, 138
Cernilton, 119
Chamomile, 36, 50, 58
Champagne, 201
Chaparral, 34
Charcoal, 41, 44, 138, 151, 152, 234
Chaste berry, 116, 262
Cheese, 209
Chemical peels, 225
Chi, 28, 278
Chicken pox, 94
Chin-Up strips, 253
Chlorophyll, 40, 219
Chlor-Trimeton (chlorpheniramine), 170
Chocolate, 121, 151, 214, 261
Cholesterol, 6, 9, 104, 233, 264, 273–276
  high-density lipoprotein (DHL), 274
  low-density lipoprotein (LDL), 274
  very-low-density lipoprotein (VLDL), 274

Choline, 219
Chondroitin sulfate, 85
Chromium picolinate, 233, 260, 278
Chronic fatigue and immune dysfunction syndrome (CFIDS). See Chronic fatigue syndrome.
Chronic fatigue syndrome, 188–192
Cialis (tadalafil), 106
Cinnamon, 42
Circadian rhythms, 205
Circulation, 89, 258
Cirrhosis, 267
Clay, green, 163
Cleaning supplies, 12
Clothing, 122, 125, 160, 169, 233, 234
Clotrimazole, 111
Clove, 212
Cockroaches, 239
Cocoa, 186
Codonopsis pilosula, 279
Coenzyme Q10, 42, 56, 257, 272, 275, 278
Coffee. See Caffeine and coffee.
Cognac, 201
Cold sores, 43–44, 47–49
Colds, 192–196, 242, 244
Colitis
  spastic. See Irritable bowel syndrome (IBS)
  ulcerative, 147, 148
Colostrum, 98
Comfrey, 34
Compresses
  cold, 29, 60, 81, 88, 95, 101, 110, 175, 177, 250
  hot, 29, 98, 99, 101, 159, 162, 175, 250, 284
Compression, 88
Congeners, 201
Conjunctivitis, 49–50

Constipation, 129–132, 149
Consumer Lab, 28
Copper, 46, 108, 183, 186, 216, 227
Corn silk, 284
Corns, 165–167
Correctol, 133
Corticosteroids, 34, 45, 241, 242
Cortisol, 15, 197, 288
Cotton, 125, 160, 169, 234, 247
Coughing, 245
COX-2 inhibitors, 92
Craddock, Sandie, 114, 115
Cranberries, 123
Cranial manipulation, 100
Cream of Rice, 135
Crohn, Burrill, 147
Crohn's disease, 147, 148
Cromolyn sodium, 241
Crystal stones, 218
Cuticles, 222
Cystitis. *See* Urinary tract infections.

Daily value (DV), 26–27
Dairy products, 6, 58, 115, 155, 245, 281
Dandelion, 262
Dander, pet, 169, 241, 246, 247
Dandruff, 51–52, 63, 168
Dang shen. *See Codonopsis pilosula.*
Darvon, 261
Davis, R. Carter, 154
Decongestants, 40
Dehydration, 133, 142, 194, 200, 206
Deodorants and antiperspirants, 218, 219, 235
Depression, 130, 196–200, 204
Dermatitis, 51, 168
Desenex (undecylenic acid), 160
Detergents, 125

Diabetes, 40, 60, 104, 130, 217, 264, 276–277
  type II, 257–260
Diaphragm, 146
Diaphragm (birth control), 122
Diarrhea, 132–135, 142, 147, 149
  traveler's, 135
Dick, Elliott, 193
Diet. *See* Foods.
Dietary Supplement Health and Education Act (DSHEA), 27
Digestion, 136, 144, 214
Dihydrotestosterone (DHT), 61, 63, 116, 118
Dill, 144
Disks, ruptured, 77, 79
Diuretics, 55, 130, 262
Diverticulitis, 132
Dong quai, 186
Douches, herbal, 126
Dr. Scholl's (tolnaftate), 160
Driving, 9
Drugs, recreational, 73, 105
Drusen, 67
Dry eye syndrome. *See* Dry eyes.
Dry eyes, 52–54
Dry mouth, 54–56
Duranon, 174
Dust, 12
Dust-mites, 169
DV. *See* Daily value (DV).

Ears, 56–58, 70–72, 99
  infections of, 56–58
Echinacea, 36, 42, 58, 126, 158, 162–163, 195
Eczema, 168–171
Electrolytes, 133
Elevation, 88
Engorgement, 97, 98
Enzymes, 217

digestive, 41, 138
lysosomal, 236, 237
Epinephrine, 175, 288
Epsom salts, 167
Erectile dysfunction (ED), 103–106
Erections. See Erectile dysfunction (ED).
Eructation. See Belching.
Essential fatty acids, 227, 232, 243, 262
Essential oils. See Oils, essential.
Estrogen, 112, 113, 261, 264, 285
Etretinate, 180
Eucalyptus, 42
Euphrasia, 248
Eustachian tube, 57
Exedrin, 261
Exercise, 7–8, 18, 77–78, 80, 86, 90, 93, 113–114, 116, 120, 130, 144, 155, 188, 199, 207, 228, 229, 230, 231, 236, 240, 241, 242, 257, 259, 271, 285, 288
Ex-Lax, 133
Eyebright, 50
Eyes, 45–47, 49–50, 52–54, 58–60, 66–69, 83, 260
Eyewash, 50

Fahey, Rebeka, 233
Famvir (famciclovir), 95, 108
Fare You, 155
Fasting, 93, 264
Fatigue, 82
Fats, 4, 5, 93, 232
Fecal impaction, 132
Feet, 30–31, 159–161, 163–165, 166, 233–235
Feminine hygiene products, 123, 125
Femstat, 126
Fennel seeds, 138

Fetal alcohol syndrome, 10
Fever blisters. See Cold sores.
Feverfew, 35, 83
Fiber, 6, 129, 130, 132, 149, 179, 259, 275
Fibrin, 237
Fillers, 27
Fillings, dental, 73
Filters, 247
     HEPA (high-efficiency, particulate arresting), 169
Finasteride, 104
First aid kits, 35
Fish, 115, 140–141, 179, 227, 243, 288
5-alpha-reductase, 61, 62, 63, 118
5-hydroxytryptophan (5-HTP), 83, 204–205
Flatulence, 131, 136–139, 151
Flaxseed Dressing, 86
Flexibility, 77, 78
Flu, 193, 242, 244
Fluoride, 73
Folic acid, 44, 183, 184, 185, 197, 199
Food poisoning, 139–143
Food sensitivities. See Allergies and food sensitivities.
Foods, 4–7, 42, 48, 54, 85, 92–93, 99, 110, 113, 114, 115, 117, 121, 128, 129–130, 132, 134, 137, 142, 143, 148–149, 150, 153, 154, 155, 179, 185–186, 191, 200, 201, 204, 208, 209, 210, 214, 226, 228, 230, 231, 240, 259, 264, 268, 271, 277–278, 283, 284, 287
     canned, 141, 142
     contamination of, 140–141
     raw, 141
     temperature of, 140, 141

Free radicals, 6, 12, 67
Fruits, 6, 48, 121, 122, 135, 155,
    264, 268

Gallbladder, 152, 152, 263
    flush, 265
Gallstones, 153, 263–266
Gamma-linolenic acid (GLA), 114, 170
Gargling, 147
Garlic, 35, 35, 40, 57, 126, 134, 237,
    250, 269, 272
Gas, intestinal. See Flatulence.
Gastritis, 146, 153
Gastroenteritis, 140
Gastroesophageal reflux disease
    (GERD), 145
Gastroesophageal reflux. See
    Heartburn.
Gas-X Extra Strength, 144
Genetics and heredity, 45–46, 82
Ginger, 36, 128, 135, 142, 144, 152,
    153, 195
Ginger ale, 142
Gingivitis, 42
Ginkgo biloba, 34, 59, 69, 72, 88,
    105–106, 237
Ginseng, 34, 106, 192, 278–279
Ginsenosides, 106, 192
Glaucoma, 58–60
Glucagon, 276, 277
Glucosamine sulfate, 85, 191
Glucose, 276, 277
Glutamine, 156, 202
Glutathione, 46, 274
Glycolic acid, 224
Glycoside, 224
Glycyrrhetinic acid, 224
Glycyrrhizin, 269
Goldenseal, 34, 56, 58, 126, 155,
    158, 162–163, 195
Golfer's shoulder, 100

Gotu kola, 237
Gout, 101
Grains, whole, 186, 197, 227, 264
Guggul, 275–276
Guided imagery. See Visualization.
Gum, 41, 128
Gums and gum disease, 39, 42, 56, 74
    bleeding, 41–43
Gyne-Lotrimin, 126

Habitrol, 212
Hair, 51–52, 60–64
    brushing of, 63
    loss of, 60–64
    myths, 63
    washing of, 52, 63
Hair follicles, 162, 213–214
Hair sprays and products, 173, 215
HairClean 1–2–3, 66
Halitosis. See Breath, bad.
Hallux vulgus. See Bunions.
Hands, 30
    cold, 255–257
    washing of, 194, 242
Hand lotion, 222
Hangnails, 221–222
Hangover, 200–202
Hangover Helper shake, 202
Hats, 63
Hawthorn, 34, 272
Hay fever, 246–248, 249
Head and Shoulders, 51
Headaches, 79–84, 99, 187, 200
    migraine, 81–84
    rebound, 79–80
    tension, 79
Headstands, 63
Health, 3–19
    children's, 57, 65–66, 151, 193,
        241
    holistic, 3

men's, 61, 103–106, 116–119, 217,
  252, 283
women's, 61–62, 96–98, 112–116,
  119–126, 151–153, 164, 184,
  189, 197, 200, 235, 244, 256,
  264, 285, 286, 288
Heart, 9
  attacks, 145, 270, 273
  disease, 113, 192, 226, 258, 272,
  274
Heartburn, 143–145
Helicobacter pylori, 153
Hemoglobin, 183–184
Hemorrhoids, 109–110, 235
Hepatitis C, 266–269
Hepatitis virus C (HVC), 266
Herbs, 22–24
Herpes, genital, 105, 106–109
Herpes simplex virus (HSV), 47, 106
Herpes zoster. *See* Varicella zoster.
Hiccups, 145–147
Histamines, 82
Hives, 171–173
Home safety, 10–11
Homeopathy, 24–25
Honey, 36, 64, 202
Hops, 34
Hormone replacement therapy (HRT),
  114, 261
Hormones, 115, 116, 196, 214, 217,
  261
Horse chestnut, 237
Hot flashes, 112
Huang Lian Yang Gan Wan, 60
Huff, John D., 46
Human papillomavirus (HPV), 180
Humidifiers, 64, 169, 195, 245
Humidity, 70
Hydrocortisone, 179
Hydrogen, 208, 209
Hydrogen peroxide, 74, 97

Hydrogen sulfate, 137
Hydroquinone, 224
Hydrotherapy, 21, 29, 60, 93
Hyperhidrosis, 219
Hypertension, 60, 104, 145, 170, 192,
  199, 270–273, 279
Hypnosis, 99, 199, 212
Hypoglycemia, 192, 276–279
Hypothyroidism, 214, 279–281

Ibuprofen, 35, 80, 101, 155, 249
Ice, 147
Imitrex (sumatripan), 84
Immune system, 15, 16, 48, 57, 94,
  118, 158–159
Impotence. *See* Erectile dysfunction
  (ED).
Incontinence, stress, 119–121
Indocin (indomethacin), 133
Inflammatory bowel disease (IBD),
  147–149
Inositol hexanicotinate, 275
Insect bites and stings, 172, 173–176
Insoles, 167
Insomnia, 199, 202–205
Insulin, 258, 259, 276
Interactions, herb-drug, 23, 33,
  34–35, 60
Interferon, 267
International Headache Society, 79
International Olympic Committee,
  187
International Rotten Sneaker Contest,
  233
Intraocular pressure (IOP), 58, 59, 60
Ipecac, 35
Iron, 183, 184, 185, 226, 227
Irrigators, oral, 42
Irritable bowel syndrome (IBS), 130,
  149, 209
Isovaleric acid, 234

Jacob, Stanley W., 78, 101
Jaundice, 266
Jaw, 98–100
Jet lag, 205–208
Jewelry, 173, 233
Jock itch, 110–112
Jock straps, 110, 111
Jogging, 99
Joints, 84, 91, 92, 98, 163, 164
Journaling, 99
Juices
    apple, 121
    beet, 152
    cabbage, 155, 202
    fruit, 134, 194
    grapefruit, 283
    onion, 225
    orange, 185, 202, 283
    potato, 145
    sauerkraut, 134
    tomato, 134, 265, 283
    vegetable, 152

Kava, 34
Kegel exercises, 120
Keratin, 225
Keratoconjunctivitis sicca. *See* Dry
    eyes.
Ketoconazole, 51
Kidney stones, 282–284
Kidneys, 40, 258, 272, 282–284
Knees, 207
Kojic acid, 224

Lacrimal glands, 52, 53
Lactaid, 209
Lactase, 136–137, 138, 208
Lactose intolerance, 208–211
Lanolin, 97, 169
Lapidus, Herbert, 234
Larson, David, 19

Laryngitis, 64–65
Larynx, 64
Laser treatments, 225
Latch on, 96–97
Laughter, 18
Laxatives, 33–34, 265
Lecithin, 219, 264
Legs, 89–90, 235–238
Lemon balm, 48, 108, 269
Lemons, 36, 64, 108, 225, 264, 265
Lentigo maligna, 225
Levitra (vardenafil), 106
Levodopa/carbidopa, 90
Lice, 65–66
Licorice, 34, 108, 144–145, 242
Lifestyle, 7–14, 18, 67, 93, 113, 129,
    143–144, 154
Lifting and twisting, 77
Light electrodesiccation, 233
Light therapy, 179, 180
Lighthouse International, 68
Linoleic acid, 226
Lipase, 138
Liver, 152, 218, 224, 266–267, 274,
    275
    disease, 40, 266–269
Liver spots, 224–225
Lotrimin (clotrimazole), 160
Lower esophagal sphincter (LES),
    127
Lungs, 241
Lutein, 46, 68
Lycii-Rehmannia, 54
Lycopene, 117
Lyme disease, 174
Lysine, 44, 48, 95, 105, 108, 219

Ma huang, 34
Maalox, 133
Macula, 66
Macular degeneration, 66–69

Magnesium, 72, 83, 90, 116, 133, 210, 243, 257, 260, 272, 283, 288

Makeup, 50

Maltase, 138

Manganese, 288

Marijuana. *See* Drugs, recreational.

Marriage, 19

Masks, 242, 247

Massage, 21, 28, 62, 88, 89, 245

Mast-cell stabilizers, 241

Meadowsweet, 142

Meals, 231

Meat, 116, 281, 268

Medications, 40, 55, 64, 133
  over-the-counter (OTC), 33–34, 79–80, 126, 133

Medicine, 21–36
  allopathic, 3, 21–22
  alternative, 21–22
  Ayurveda, 21, 40, 55, 247, 275
  herbal, 21, 22–24
  self-care, 22
  traditional Chinese, 21, 28, 31, 54, 134, 278

Mediplast, 181

Meditation, 16–17, 32, 62, 90, 99, 128, 149, 150, 155, 179, 199, 232, 288

Melatonin, 204, 205–206, 207

Melissa officinalis. See Lemon balm.

Menopause, 112–114, 120, 122, 261, 285

Menstruation, 82, 112, 114–116, 213, 217, 261

Methane, 137

Methylsulfonylmethane (MSM), 46, 78, 101–102, 145, 216, 227

Micatin-Derm (miconazole), 160

Miconazole, 111

Microcides, 107–108

Milk thistle, 224, 225, 266, 269, 278

Milk. *See* Dairy products.

Mineral salts, 218

Minerals, 27, 133–134, 226

Mini-phlebectomy, 238

Mints, 128

Mittens, 256

Moisturizers, 215

Mold and mildew, 246, 247

Monistat, 126

Monistat-Derm (miconazole), 160

Mononucleosis, 153

Morning sickness, 151, 152, 153

Morphine, 217

Motion sickness, 151, 152

Mouth, 54–56, 98–100

Mouthwashes, 56

Movements
  leg, 89–90
  repetitive, 87–88, 100

Mucus, 244, 245, 249, 250

Multiple sclerosis, 130

Murray, Michael, 108

Muscles, 77, 79, 88, 99–100

Mushrooms, shiitake, 269

Music, 72

Mycelex (clotrimazole), 160

Mylanta, 133

Myrrh, 44

N-acetylcysteine (NAC), 46, 245, 274

Nails, 225–227
  cutting of, 223
  ingrown, 222–223

Naprosyn (naproxen), 80, 133

Nasal sprays, 247

National Clearinghouse for Alcohol and Drug Information, 10

National Sleep Research Project, 202

Natrum muriaticum, 56, 175

Nature, 7, 18, 19

Naturopathy, 21
Nausea and vomiting, 142
Nedocromil, 241
Neo-Synephrine, 69–70
Nervousness. *See* Anxiety and
    nervousness.
Neti pots, 251
Nettle, 63, 247
Neurogenesis, 197
Niacin, 71, 84, 275, 281
Niacinamide, 215
Nickel, 169
NicoDerm CQ, 212
Nicorette, 212
Nicotine gums and patches, 212
Nictotine, 257
    withdrawal, 211–212
Nipples, 96–98
Nitrates, 105
Nitric oxide synthesis, 106
Nitrogen, liquid, 233
Nits, 65–66
Nix, 174
Nizoral, 51
NoDoze, 261
Non-steroidal anti-inflammatory
    drugs (NSAIDs), 34, 35, 60, 92,
    93, 155
Nosebleeds, 69–70
Nurses Health Study, 228
Nuts and seeds, 227
Nux vomica, 36, 142, 202

Oat bran, 275
Obesity, 227–232, 252, 253, 258,
    263–264, 265, 271
Odor-Eaters, 234
Odor-Eaters Hall of Fumes, 233
Oils
    black currant, 54, 86, 114
    borage, 54, 86, 114

castor, 133, 225
chamomile, 58
citronella, 174
essential 25–26, 219, 246
eucalyptus, 251
evening primrose, 54, 86, 114,
    170, 262
fish, 86, 243, 257, 281
flaxseed, 51, 86, 93, 227, 232,
    243, 262, 281
garlic, 57
jojoba, 221
lavender, 36, 42, 58, 221
mineral, 133
mullein, 57
olive, 6, 36, 66, 171, 222, 265
omega-3, 83, 86
sesame, 51–52
tea tree, 36, 51, 66, 108, 111, 126,
    160–161, 215, 219
vegetable, 222
Onions, 128, 151, 237
Opiates, 130
Oregano, 119, 158, 163
Orthotics, 165, 167
Osborne, Charles, 145
Osteoporosis, 113, 210, 284–288
Oxalates, 283
Oxidation, 67
Oxygen, 183, 253

Pain, 76–102
Pancreas, 257–258, 276, 277
Panty hose, 125
Papaya, 138, 144
Parkinson's disease, 130
Parsley, 40, 262
Passionflower, 34
Peak flow meters, 243
Peas, 36
Pectin, 149

Pencillin, 172
Penile implants, 106
Penis, 104
Pepcid (famotidine), 155
Pepper, 135
Peppermint, 42
Peppers, red, 86, 237
Pepsin, 153, 154
Perfumes, 173
Pergolide, 90
Periactin (cyproheptadine), 172
Perimenopause, 112
Perio-aids, 42–43
Periodontitis, 43
Peristalsis, 150
Permanone, 174
Permethrin, 65, 174
Perspiration, 159, 160, 215, 216,
    234, 235
Petroleum jelly, 110
pH, 73
Phlebitis, 237
Phytates, 186
Phytoestrogens, 113
Pimples. *See* Acne.
Pineal gland, 205, 281
Pityrosporum ovale, 51
Pizzorno, Joseph, 68, 108
Plants, indoor, 12
Plaque, 42
Pneumonia, 246
Podophyllum, 142
Poison ivy, 176–177
Poison oak, 176–177
Poison sumac, 176–177
Pollen, 246, 247
Pollutants, 82, 240
Pope Pius XII, 146
Porridge, 135
Postherapetic neuralgia, 94, 95
Posture, 76, 87

Potassium, 218, 272
Pots, cast-iron, 186
Pregnancy, 10, 109, 120, 122, 130,
    151, 158, 160, 184, 192, 197,
    199, 204, 215, 221, 226
Premenstrual syndrome (PMS), 114
Probiotics, 45, 118–119, 123, 137,
    138, 155, 158, 191
Progesterone, 115, 261
Prolactin, 116, 118
Propecia, 62, 63
Propylene glycol, 51
Prostaglandins, 114
Prostate, 116–119
Prostate-specific antigen (PSA), 119
Prostatitis, 117, 118
Protease inhibitors, 35
Protease, 138
Protein, 5, 6, 43, 183, 210, 226, 268,
    286
Psoriasis, 178–180, 226
Psychotherapy, 198
Psyllium, 131
Puberty, 214, 217
Pulsatilla, 50
Pumice stone, 167
Purines, 284
Pus, 157, 161, 162
Pyelonephritis, 121
Pygeum, 62
Pyrethrin, 65
Pyrrosia, 266

Qi. See Chi.
Quercetin, 172, 242, 248

Radon, 13
Raynaud's disease, 255–257
Recipes, 86, 195, 201
Red yeast rice, 275
Reflexology, 21, 30–31, 151

Refrigerators, 140, 141
Relationships, 19
Relaxation, progressive, 32–33, 99,
    150, 207
Repetitive strain injury (RSI), 87–89
Restless leg syndrome, 89–90
Retina, 66, 207
Rhubarb, 266
Rhus toxicodendron, 172, 177
Ribavirin, 267
Riboflavin, 197, 281
Rice, 135, 264
RICE (rest, ice, compression,
    elevation), 88
Rocky Mountain spotted fever, 174
Rogaine (minoxidil), 62
Root canals, 73

Salicin, 80
Salicylic acid, 80
Saliva, 40, 54, 73
Salt, 6, 36, 93, 115, 271
SAM-e (s-adenosyl-L-methionine),
    199
Saunas, 29
Saw palmetto, 34, 62, 118
Sciatica, 78
Sclerotherapy, 238
Scorpions, 174
Scratching, 168, 169
Seasonal affective disorder (SAD), 197
Seasonal allergic rhinitis. See Hay fever.
Sebum, 214
Selenium, 46, 51, 68, 214, 274
Self-care remedy kits, 35–36
Senna, 133
Senokot, 133
Serotonin, 81–82, 197
Sexual arousal, 217
Sexual intercourse, 106, 123
Shampoos, 51, 65–66

Sherry, 201
Shingles, 94–95
Shoes, 164–165, 166, 167, 173, 223,
    234, 236
Shower slippers, 159, 160, 181
Showers, 159,160
Sickle cell anemia, 184
Silicea, 163
Silver, colloidal, 250
Silymarin. See Milk thistle.
Simethione, 139
Similasan, 54
Sinuses, 249, 250
Sinusitis, 40, 248, 249–251
Sitting, 77
Sjögren's syndrome, 53
Skin, 157–182
Skin tags, 232–233
Sleep, 9, 10, 78, 82, 88, 202–205,
    206, 251–254
Sleep apnea, 252, 253, 254
Slippery elm, 142, 145
SmokEnders, 212
Smoking, 12, 13–14, 45, 46, 67, 83,
    93, 104, 122, 144, 154, 155, 194,
    208, 211–212, 244, 271, 286
Snacks, 231
Sneezing, 246
Snore Control, 254
SnoreStop, 254
Snoring, 251–254
Soaps, 111, 123, 125, 169, 173, 215,
    218
Socks, 159, 160, 234–235, 256
Sorbitol, 137
Soups, 194, 195
Soy products, 113, 202
Spiders, 174
Spinal column, 76–77, 100
Spirituality, 19, 232
St. John's wort, 34, 35, 57, 192, 199

Staphylococcus aureus, 161
Stevia, 268
Stingers, 175
Stomach acid, 143, 144, 154
Straws, 128
Strep throat, 153
Stress and stress management, 14–17,
    18, 43, 54, 55, 62, 71, 80, 83, 87,
    90, 94, 99, 118, 128, 130, 133,
    144, 149, 150, 154, 155, 169,
    179, 194, 197, 199, 203, 214,
    240, 242, 288
Stress incontinence. See Incontinence,
    stress.
Stretching, 88, 90, 236
Strokes, 243, 258, 270
Sufites, 240
Sugars, 4–5, 6, 93, 122, 147, 155,
    217, 257, 259, 264
Sulfur, 248
Sun, exposure to, 14, 45, 46, 67, 180,
    197, 207, 210, 224, 281, 288
Sunburn, 220
Sunglasses, 14
Supplements
    high potency, 27
    nutritional, 26–28
    safety of, 27–28
Support groups, 212, 232
Sweat. See Perspiration.
Swimmer's calculus, 73
Swimmers's ear, 56–57
Swimming, 73

Tagamet (cimetidine), 104, 155
Tai chi, 16, 31, 62, 90, 99, 150, 288
Tampons, 122
Tannins, 186
Tardive dyskinesia, 34
Tea, 73, 121, 186, 261
    chamomile, 151, 167

corn silk, 123
garlic, 134–135
ginger, 163
green, 231
grindelia, 245
herbal, 134, 150–151, 188, 194
hyssop, 245
lemon balm, 269
milk thistle, 201
pau d'arco, 151
peppermint, 151
plantain, 212
rosemary, 201
thyme, 245
Tears, 52–53
    artificial, 50, 53–54
Teeth, 72–75
    bonding, 74, 75
    cleaning, 73–74
    grinding, 98
    veneers, 74, 75
    whitening, 74–75
Temporomandibular disorder (TMD),
    98–100
Tendonitis, 100–102
Tendons, 100, 102
Tennis elbow, 100, 101
Tension, 79, 80, 88, 99, 19
Testosterone, 61, 63, 116, 118, 217
Tetracycline, 73
Thalassemia, 184
Thiamine, 71, 197
Throat sprays, 254
Thrombophlebitis, 236, 237
Thrush, 126
Thuja, 161
Thyme, 42, 185
Thyroid gland, 279, 280
Thyroxine, 217, 281
Ticks, 173, 174, 175
Time and time zones, 206

Tinactin (tolnaftale), 160
Tinea cruris, 110–111
Tinea pedis. *See* Athlete's foot.
Tinnitus, 70–72
Tinnitus masker, 72
Toast, 138
Tobacco, 73
Toe spacers, 167
Toes, 163, 165, 166, 222
Tomatoes, 117, 121, 128
Tongue scrapers, 40
Tonsillitis, 40
Toothpastes, 75
Toxins, environmental, 11–13
Triglycerides, 233
Tumeric, 102
Twinkie defense, 276
Tyler, Varro E., 108
Tylophora, 247
Tyrosine, 281

Ulcers, 153–156
Ultrasounds
    DEXA (dual-energy x-ray
        absorptiometry), 286
    heel, 286
Underwear, 111, 122, 125
United States Pharmacopeia (USP),
    27
United States Yoga Association, 243
UPS. *See* United States Pharmacopeia
    (USP).
Urease, 154
Urethra, 117, 121, 122
Urethritis, 121
Urinary tract, 121
Urinary tract infections, 121–124
Urine and urination, 117, 188,
    119–120, 122, 123, 282, 283
Urushiol, 176
Usnea moss, 162

Uva ursi, 123

Vacuum devices, 105
Vagina, 125
Vaginitis, 124–126
    bacterial, 124, 125
    protozoan, 124, 125
    yeast, 124, 125–126, 218
Valerian, 34, 204
Valtrex (valacyclovir), 95, 109
Varicella zoster, 94
Varicose veins. *See* Veins, varicose.
Vasotec (enalapril), 133
Vegetables, 6, 7, 48, 115, 135, 142,
    185, 264, 268, 283
Veins, 235
    varicose, 235–238
Viagra (sildenafil citrate), 105
Vinegar, 126, 172, 218, 225
Vistaril (hydroxyzine), 170
Visualization, 31–32, 62, 90, 99, 128,
    149, 150, 182, 199, 232, 288
Vitamin A, 57, 61, 85, 221, 226, 281
Vitamin B-complex, 15, 57, 71, 80,
    116, 118, 197, 198, 215, 227,
    242
Vitamin B6, 54, 83, 116, 118, 153,
    197, 199, 227, 262, 281, 283
Vitamin B12, 44, 71, 183, 184, 185,
    197, 199
Vitamin C, 15, 36, 43, 45, 46, 54, 57,
    60, 68, 70, 83, 85, 108, 123, 172,
    182, 183, 185, 194, 195, 212,
    221, 225, 237, 249, 264, 274,
    278, 281
Vitamin D, 14, 210, 281, 283, 285,
    288
Vitamin E, 45, 46, 51, 57, 62, 68, 83,
    85, 108, 170, 214, 224–225, 257,
    262, 264, 274, 278, 281
Vitamin K, 288

Vitamins, multi, with minerals, 48, 80,
    116, 204, 278, 281
Viva-Drops, 54
Vomiting. *See* Nausea and vomiting.

Walking, 236, 288
Warts, 180–182
Water, 41, 55–56, 113, 123, 130, 135,
    142, 188, 194, 201, 215, 230,
    264, 265, 283
  salt, 251
Wax treatment, 93
Weather, 82, 240
WED (water, exercise, diet), 113–114
Weight, 121, 200, 227–232, 236, 252,
    253, 258, 263–264, 265, 271
Weil, Andrew, 134
Wheat, 58
Whirlpools, 29
Whisky, 201
Wigs, 63
Wine, 186
  red, 73, 201
Witch hazel, 44, 110, 175, 218

Wright, Jonathan, 105

Xylitol, 137

Yarrow, 216
Yellow teeth. *See* Teeth.
Yoga, 21, 32, 62, 90, 99, 128, 131,
    149, 150, 155, 199, 232,
    242–243, 288
Yogasthma, 243
Yogurt, 126, 209
Ysnore, 254

Zeasorb-AF, 111
Zinc, 45, 46, 49, 51, 57, 68, 118,
    158–159, 194, 195, 214, 216,
    217, 221, 226, 227, 281
Zinc oxide, 108
Zinc pyrithione (ZPT), 51
Zincon, 51
Zithromax (azithromycin), 133
Zomig (zolmitriptan), 84
Zovirax (acyclovir), 95, 108
Zyban (bupropion), 212

About the Authors

David Y. Wong, M.D., is board certified in family practice medicine and co-founder and director of the Health Integration Center in Torrance and Santa Monica, California—an innovative educational and holistic health center founded in 1978 that utilizes a variety of healing disciplines, including nutrition, acupuncture, stress reduction, natural hormones, herbal medicine, and energy healing. His goal is to help people achieve optimal heath and balance through the integration of body, mind, and spirit. Dr. Wong has also served as medical director and consultant to the Foxhollow Wellness Clinic in Crestwood, Kentucky. Dr. Wong conducts workshops and lectures frequently to health professionals as well as the general public, and he has been interviewed on radio and television about a variety of health topics.

Deborah Mitchell is a medical writer and journalist whose articles have appeared in professional journals as well as national consumer magazines. She has authored or coauthored more than two dozen books about various health topics, including *The Home Health Adviser, The Dictionary of Natural Healing and What Your Doctor May Not Tell You About Autoimmune Disease,* coauthored with Stephen B. Edelson, M.D. She lives with her husband and a cat, Antonio Carlos Jobim, in Princeton, New Jersey.